"A game-changer for practitioners! *Theraplay®: Innovations and Integration* expanded my clinical imagination. Inspires and motivates to further center Theraplay in my work with children and families."
—*Shannon Murphy Cerise, MSW, LCSW, SMC Counseling Services, PLLC, Dallas, Texas, USA*

"A great addition to existing Theraplay titles from JKP. Exploring not only the history of Theraplay, this book charts its integration with other therapeutic models, with many examples of vibrant innovative practice."
—*Barbara Godden, Director, CairnsMoir Connections*

"This book conveys the flexibility of the Theraplay model both in its application to diverse populations and the ease with which it can be integrated with other approaches. This is a book to take down from the shelf and dip into. New insights will be found each time it is revisited."
—*Kim S. Golding, CBE, DDP trainer, and author*

Theraplay®
Innovations and Integration

Also in this series

Parenting with Theraplay®
Understanding Attachment and How to Nurture a Closer Relationship with Your Child
Vivien Norris and Helen Rodwell
Forewords by Phyllis Booth and Dafna Lender
Illustrated by Miranda Smith
ISBN 978 1 78592 209 1
eISBN 978 1 78450 489 2

Theraplay®
The Practitioner's Guide
Vivien Norris and Dafna Lender
Foreword by Phyllis Booth
ISBN 978 1 78592 210 7
eISBN 978 1 78450 488 5

Theraplay®
Theory, Applications and Implementation
Edited by Sandra Lindaman and Rana Hong
Foreword by Phyllis Booth
ISBN 978 1 78775 070 8
eISBN 978 1 78775 071 5

Theraplay®

Innovations and
Integration

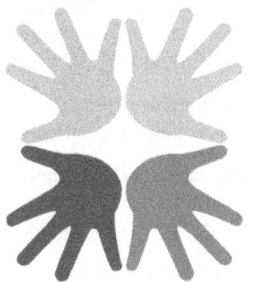

Edited by
Rana Hong and A. Rand Coleman

Foreword by Phyllis Booth

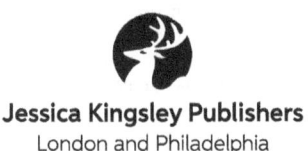

Jessica Kingsley Publishers
London and Philadelphia

First published in Great Britain in 2023 by Jessica Kingsley Publishers
An imprint of John Murray Press

1

Copyright ©
Foreword: Phyllis Booth 2023
Chapter 1: Rana Hong 2023
Chapter 2: A. Rand Coleman 2023
Chapter 3: Andrea Bushala and Nicole Charney 2023
Chapter 4: Sam Bunnyfield and Gloria M. Cockerill 2023
Chapter 5: Lorie Walton 2023
Chapter 6: Dafna Lender 2023
Chapter 7: Helen Rodwell 2023
Chapter 8: Hyunjung Shin and Felicia Carroll 2023
Chapter 9: Fiona Peacock 2023
Chapter 10: Cindy Mitchell Perkins 2023
Chapter 11: Mary J. Ring and Christie Mason 2023
Chapter 12: Jay Vaughan 2023
Chapter 13: Mandy Jones-Fischer and Marshall N. Lyles 2023
Chapter 14: Angela Siu and King-Chi Yau 2023
Chapter 15: Danielle H. Maxonight 2023
Chapter 16: Daniel J. Cane 2023
Chapter 17: Joanna Fortune 2023
Chapter 18: Philip F. Daniels 2023
Chapter 19: David L. Myrow 2023

Figure on page 188 is reproduced with kind permission from Bruce D. Perry.
ROSE model on page 203 is reproduced with kind permission from Raja Selvam.
Figure on page 271 is reproduced with kind permission from The Theraplay Institute.

Disclaimer: The client vignettes that feature in this book are largely composite or
fictional; any real-life vignettes feature with the expressed consent of clients.

A CIP catalogue record for this title is available from the British Library and the Library of Congress

ISBN 978 1 78775 591 8
eISBN 978 1 78775 592 5

Printed and bound in the United States by Integrated Books International

Jessica Kingsley Publishers' policy is to use papers that are natural, renewable and recyclable
products and made from wood grown in sustainable forests. The logging and manufacturing
processes are expected to conform to the environmental regulations of the country of origin.

Jessica Kingsley Publishers
Carmelite House
50 Victoria Embankment
London EC4Y 0DZ

www.jkp.com

John Murray Press
Part of Hodder & Stoughton Limited
An Hachette UK Company

Contents

Part II: Specific Populations, Ages, and Settings

Foreword

Theraplay began as a creative response to a serious challenge, namely to meet the needs of the many children in the Chicago Head Start program who had been identified as needing help. We used basic patterns of playful interaction and nurturing care to form a relationship with each child that felt safe and connected and that changed their internal working model of themselves and the world. Within a few weeks, we were able to see great changes in the behaviors of these troubled children. Angry, acting-out children became calm and were able to interact peacefully with others; fearful, withdrawn children became more outgoing and able to take pleasure in playing with others.

In the more than 50 years since we began our work, Theraplay has benefited from ongoing research into the nature and benefits of attachment. The greater understanding of the neurobiology involved in forming an attachment relationship and in creating secure relationships has also helped us fine-tune our approach. Because it addresses the basic need to build relationships that provide a sense of safety, co-regulation, and connection, Theraplay has appealed to practitioners around the world, and has been easily adapted to fit the needs and values of different cultures.

The first edition of the basic Theraplay book, written by Ann Jernberg, appeared in 1979. The second edition was published in 1999 and the third in 2010. Each edition included descriptions of how Theraplay is being used in various settings. The third edition presented our understanding of the underlying neurobiology of the process of forming an attachment.

As the interest in Theraplay grew, a number of books focusing on particular audiences were published: for example, *Parenting with Theraplay* by Vivien Norris and Helen Rodwell (2017) and *Theraplay: The Practitioner's Guide* by Vivien Norris and Dafna Lender (2020). In 2020, *Theraplay: Theory, Applications and Implementation*, edited by Sandra Lindaman and Rana Hong, was published. This describes how the basic Theraplay model is being used to meet the needs of special groups with special needs.

Over the years, Theraplay practitioners have found it useful to incorporate other modalities into their work with families and groups. The present book provides examples of how Theraplay practitioners around the world have combined Theraplay with other therapeutic modalities to address specific issues that Theraplay alone does not address. They describe how the two modalities support and enhance each other. Case illustrations in each chapter provide a lively view of how the combined treatments are carried out.

Chapter 1 provides an overview of Theraplay integration with other therapeutic models, including fundamental considerations of Theraplay integrative models. It reviews recent Theraplay research and explains key aspects in model integration.

Chapter 2 presents an integration of Theraplay concepts with the neurobiology of trauma and therapeutic change. Key concepts include the systems for emotional processing and how they can be integrated with systems for positive reinforcement and desensitization. Theraplay provides a systems method for changing the neurobiological system.

Chapter 3 describes how Theraplay can be carried out online. The COVID-19 pandemic, with its need for maintaining distance, presented a serious challenge to Theraplay practitioners. How could we continue helping families when our approach depends so heavily on face-to-face interaction and immediate response? The authors of this chapter describe how they adapted their work to online, distance intervention. They provide a detailed description of what is needed for online intervention: how to administer a Marschak Intervention Method (MIM), how to provide feedback to parents and caregivers, and how to prepare them for carrying on the session with the online guidance of the Theraplay practitioner.

Chapter 4 explores the integration of Adlerian Play Therapy (AdPT) and Theraplay based on the congruence of their respective underlying philosophical beliefs, namely attachment theory and individual psychology. It demonstrates how using aspects of both modalities can provide a comprehensive and client-focused treatment approach, resulting in positive and lasting change for clients and their families.

Chapter 5 describes how to effectively incorporate two therapeutic treatment modalities (Theraplay and Cognitive Behavioral Play Therapy, CBPT), which theoretically reside at opposite ends of the psychotherapy spectrum, into a treatment plan that offers support to a child who faces the challenge of severe emotional dysregulation. It also demonstrates the value of incorporating the caregivers into this healing journey.

Chapter 6 describes how Theraplay with Dyadic Developmental Psychotherapy

(DDP) can be combined. When the family has experienced intergenerational trauma, it is important to work on the parent's own attachment history so that they can become aware of how their childhood experiences are affecting their parenting. Theraplay can bring the joy, connection, trust, and safety that is so important for a secure attachment; DDP techniques help parents and caregivers realize how their own attachment history affects their parenting, and also helps them be more accepting and empathic with their child's behaviors and underlying motives.

Chapter 7 describes how Theraplay and Eye Movement Desensitization and Reprocessing (EMDR) can be used as an integrated intervention. Theraplay can be used as the main approach for strengthening a child's relationship with their parents and caregivers and for providing reparative relational experiences, while EMDR is used to address past trauma directly.

Chapter 8 presents a hybrid approach of Theraplay and Gestalt Therapy for children and adolescents. Focused on similarities and differences between Theraplay and Gestalt Therapy, it illustrates how this integration creates a scaffolding of the safe and secure base and self-awareness in the therapeutic process.

Chapter 9 looks at how keeping group analytic theory in mind can deepen the understanding of how to adapt Theraplay groups for various therapeutic situations and contexts, especially with groups where there are multiple and complex needs.

Chapter 10 provides examples of how rhythm, tone, and music are used to regulate children and their families in Theraplay sessions. Voice, tone, bodies, drums, and the Safe and Sound Protocol are used to calm, engage, and enhance relationships for traumatized children and adults. When they are calm, they are then able to access coping strategies.

Chapter 11 presents an introduction to the Neurosequential Model of Therapeutics (NMT), a developmentally informed treatment planning tool designed for use with children who have experienced trauma. It describes how using the NMT can guide the selection and sequencing of Theraplay interventions. Key NMT principles are correlated with the dimensions of Theraplay. It includes examples of Theraplay activities that correspond to the NMT domains of intervention.

Chapter 12 outlines a specialist UK Adoption and Fostering Agency's Neuro-Physiological Psychotherapy (NPP) model for working with traumatized children and young people from the care system. The focus is on how the body-based approach of the NPP model supports and deepens Theraplay interventions.

Chapter 13 presents a model for combining Theraplay and Sandtray Therapy, using Theraplay activities at the beginning and end, with Sandtray in the middle for processing from an expressive part of the brain. The sense of safety that comes from containment in both models is highlighted.

Chapter 14 describes the integration of music in Theraplay for working with children who have social impairment. Different elements of music are used in each of the four dimensions of Theraplay and throughout a Theraplay session.

Chapter 15 explores the social-emotional needs of gifted and twice-exceptional children and families. A case illustration is presented to demonstrate several ways in which Theraplay can be creatively adapted to meet the unique needs of these neurodivergent children.

Chapter 16 describes the principles of Group Theraplay in a school setting with young people with neurological injuries. The chapter emphasizes the importance of attunement to each young person's special needs. The focus is on attunement and on adapting for the physical limitations and the developmental level of each student and the different cognitive abilities resulting from their injuries.

Chapter 17 describes a program using a modified Group Theraplay training format with a broad range of staff who work within homeless services in Ireland. The author describes how this program was funded, supported, and facilitated as well as the modifications involved and lessons learned as a template for others to apply within their countries or work settings.

Chapter 18 describes how play and, more specifically, Theraplay, can be incorporated into Activities of Daily Living (ADLs) for individuals with neurocognitive disorders and their informal caregivers.

Chapter 19 builds on research showing that fathers tend to engage in more large muscle, physical play with their children than mothers, and that the benefits for children are extensive, including better self-regulation and enhanced self-confidence. The chapter shows how large muscle activities can be woven into Theraplay sessions.

Phyllis Booth

Acknowledgments

This unique and innovative book provides, for the first time, state-of-the-art practice knowledge in integrating Theraplay with other therapeutic models. It is the outcome of Theraplay experts' years of clinical practice with clients and considerable collaboration with our incredible mentors and colleagues. Our gratitude goes to children and families who trust and allow us to share their stories and those we learn from daily. We could not have completed this book without their help and support.

Special thanks to Phyllis Booth, who assiduously reviewed all of the chapters and provided constructive feedback and incredible support to improve each chapter—words cannot express our gratitude and appreciation for all your support.

We gratefully acknowledge Bruce Perry's special editing in Chapter 11 (NMT and Theraplay)—we thank you for providing recent knowledge about NMT, and your generous permission to grant the use of NMT's brain image.

We also acknowledge our spouses, family, and friends, who provided the support, time, and encouragement to make this book a reality.

We acknowledge the truly responsive and collaborative efforts from Jessica Kingsley Publishers, particularly Stephen Jones, Publishing Director. Numerous barriers at our end made any deadline seem impossible—we thank you for your support in seeing this book to fruition.

Lastly, we are indebted to the contributing authors—experts in Theraplay and leading clinicians and trainers in the field of child psychotherapy—we are pleased to be in your company and to present your marvelous Theraplay-based integrative work.

Drs. Rana Hong and A. Rand Coleman

The Authors

Editors

Rana Hong, PhD, LCSW, RPT-S, is a Clinical Research Assistant Professor in the School of Social Work at Loyola University Chicago. She is a methodologically grounded Clinical Researcher, Educator, and Clinician who has a depth of knowledge and experience in children, adolescents, and families with issues of attachment, trauma, emotion/behavioral disturbance, and neurodevelopmental disorders. While focusing on research in the areas of neurobiology, thematic analysis, metric development, and program (or intervention) evaluation, Dr. Hong holds clinical expertise with distinguished certifications. She is a Certified Theraplay® Practitioner, Supervisor, and Trainer, Certified Parent–Child Interaction Therapy® (PCIT) Therapist/ Within Agency Trainer, Certified Eye Movement Desensitization and Reprocessing® (EMDR) Therapist and Consultant, and DIRFloortime® Expert Training Leader. As the past president of the board at The Theraplay Institute, Dr. Hong is dedicated to supporting Theraplay research and practice.

A. Rand Coleman, PhD, is a graduate of Hahnemann University Hospital, where he obtained a degree in Clinical Psychology, specializing in Neuropsychology. A Licensed Psychologist and Certified Theraplay® Trainer and Supervisor, his clinical experience includes child neuropsychology, family intervention for children on the autism spectrum, supports for youth and adults with intellectual disabilities, and therapeutic approaches for youth with reactive attachment disorder, trauma, and severe behavior problems. After working for many years in residential care programs that serve youth or adults with serious developmental disabilities, Dr. Coleman now works in a group practice in Malvern, PA, conducting evaluations and providing both individual and family therapy.

Contributing authors

Sam Bunnyfield, LCSW, LIMHP, RPT-S, is a Certified Theraplay® Practitioner, Trainer and Supervisor with extensive experience working with children and families who have experienced acute and chronic trauma. Sam served as President of the Illinois chapter of the Association for Play Therapy (APT) and as a Core Field Consultant for the University of Chicago's Crown Family School of Social Work, Policy, and Practice. Sam is also a specialist in Adlerian Play Therapy (AdPT), Dyadic Developmental Psychotherapy (DDP), EMDR, and Internal Family Systems (IFS) interventions.

Andrea Bushala, MSW, LCSW, is a Certified Theraplay® Practitioner, Trainer and Supervisor at The Theraplay Institute. She is also Co-Founder of Healing Space Therapy in Chicago, IL, a practice dedicated to supporting children from birth to age 10 and their families. Andrea has completed a two-year postgraduate fellowship at the University of Massachusetts in Infant–Parent Mental Health.

Daniel J. Cane, EdD, NCSP, is a Licensed Psychologist, nationally Certified School Psychologist, and Certified Theraplay® Practitioner practicing in Pennsylvania. His research has focused on the application of neuropsychology in everyday environments. He has authored several professional publications, and served as an adjunct instructor for undergraduate and graduate programs in biopsychology and social-emotional learning in schools.

Felicia Carroll, MEd, MA, LMFT, RPT-S, is Founder/Co-Director of the West Coast Institute for Gestalt Therapy with Children and Adolescents, LLC, in private practice in Solvang, California. Felicia is a renowned international Gestalt trainer who teaches clinicians in Europe, Latin America, and throughout Asia in addition to offering training programs in the USA. She has had several chapters and articles about Gestalt Therapy with children published. Her most recent (2019) article, "Gestalt Play Therapy," was included in a special edition of the *Play Therapy*™ Magazine for the APT.

Nicole Charney is a Clinical Psychologist from Chile, and is a Certified Theraplay® Practitioner, Trainer and Supervisor, and Founder of Theraplay Chile. Nicole has been leading Theraplay training in Chile and taking Theraplay into Latin American countries. She has been a speaker at conferences, congresses, and seminars. Nicole has been involved in a variety of public health programs involving mental health issues in populations at risk in her native country, Chile.

Gloria M. Cockerill, LCSW, RPT-S, is a Certified Theraplay® Practitioner, Trainer and Supervisor. She served as the Training Director for The Theraplay Institute and worked as Field Consultant at the University of Chicago's Crown Family School of Social Work, Policy, and Practice, and as an Adjunct Faculty member at the University of Illinois at Chicago's Jane Addams College of Social Work. Currently, she provides clinical services at Kid Matters Counseling in Hinsdale, Illinois, serving as Vice-President of the Illinois APT.

Philip F. Daniels, PhD, LMHC, NCC, BC-TMH, specializes in marriage and family therapy and gerocounseling. He is a Clinical Assistant Professor and founder of a private practice. His research and dissertation stem from his personal lived experience as a caregiver of grandparents who had neurocognitive disorders. This led him to discovering the benefits of Theraplay and the need to utilize play with older adults. He is Level 1 certified in Theraplay®.

Joanna Fortune, DPsych, MICP, MIFPP, CTTTS, Reg Pract APPI, Ap Sup ICP/PTI, is an Accredited Psychotherapist, Supervisor and Trainer. She is a published author of four books, a podcast host, radio broadcaster, and newspaper columnist. She specializes in the field of play and using play to strengthen and enhance relationships, including as part of trauma recovery. She is a fully Certified Theraplay® Practitioner, Supervisor and Trainer, and has more than 22 years' clinical experience.

Mandy Jones-Fischer, LCSW, RPT, JD, is a Certified Theraplay® Practitioner, Trainer and Supervisor. She is also Executive Director at The Theraplay Institute. Mandy has worked almost exclusively with adoptive and foster families since she began her career. She has developed a specialty in helping children with Fetal Alcohol Spectrum Disorder (FASD). While Mandy doesn't regularly practice law, she continues to use her legal knowledge and advocacy skills to help families gain Individualized Education Plans (IEPs) and other essential resources.

Dafna Lender, MSW, LCSW, is an international trainer and supervisor for practitioners who work with children and families. She is a Certified Practitioner, Trainer and Supervisor/Consultant in both Theraplay® and DDP, and co-author of *Theraplay: The Practitioner's Guide* (The Theraplay Institute, 2020). She teaches and supervises clinicians in 15 countries in three languages: English, Hebrew, and French.

Marshall N. Lyles, LPC-S, LMFT-S, RPT-S, EMDRIA Approved Consultant, has over 20 years of practice in family and play therapy. Most of Marshall's clinical practice has focused on attachment trauma and its effect on family relationships. Marshall has contributed multiple written works to journals, professional magazines, and edited books as well as having co-authored *Advanced Sandtray Therapy: Digging Deeper into Clinical Practice* (Routledge, 2021). Marshall owns an expressive arts training center in Austin called The Workshop.

Christie Mason, PhD, LCSW, RPT-S, NMT Level II, is a Clinical Associate Professor in the School of Social Work at Loyola University Chicago. She has more than 20 years' experience of working with children and families, and has expertise in working with traumatized children adopted internationally or via the child welfare system. Christie teaches courses on practice with children, Art-Based Experiential Approaches to social work, and the Neurosequential Model of Therapeutics (NMT). She also maintains a small private practice.

Danielle H. Maxonight, MSW, LCSW, is an Asheville, North Carolina-based Psychotherapist working with school-aged neurodivergent children and their caregivers from an attachment-focused, neurodiversity-affirming lens. She established her private practice, Under Wing Therapeutic Services, PLLC, in 2015, after working with children in diverse settings, including family preservation in homes across rural Appalachia.

Cindy Mitchell Perkins, MA, LCPC, is a retired school teacher, administrator, and counselor of 32 years alongside a private practice of 24 years. She is a Certified Theraplay® Practitioner, Trainer and Supervisor, certified in the Safe and Sound Protocol, and is also a Certified Zentangle Teacher. She has presented at numerous conferences on a variety of therapeutic and educational topics since 1986. She is currently working on a book about her journey after the loss of her daughter, teaching therapeutic interventions, and running groups for the Safe and Sound Protocol.

David L. Myrow, PhD, is a Clinical Psychologist practicing in West Seneca, New York. He is an Affiliate Trainer of The Theraplay Institute in Chicago, where he trained with Ann Jernberg and Phyllis Booth. David is currently a Clinical Assistant Professor in the Department of Psychiatry at the State University of New York at Buffalo. He is a past President of the Psychological Association of Western New York. His scholarly work has been published in a variety of professional journals and books. With his wife, Susan Bundy-Myrow, he received the Ann Jernberg Award from The Theraplay Institute in 2011. The New York APT honored him with its Lifetime Achievement Award in 2022.

Fiona Peacock, PhD, is a BACP Senior Accredited Counsellor and Certified Theraplay® Practitioner, Trainer and Supervisor. She is Co-Lead of the Child and Adolescent Counselling programme at the Faculty of Education, University of Cambridge (UK), and Co-Director of Theraplay UK. She is co-author of *Fostering Good Relationships* (Kamac Books, 2016) and contributing author to *Therapy with Children and Young People* (SAGE Publishing, 2014), *Theraplay: Theory, Applications and Implementation* (Jessica Kingsley Publishers, 2020), and *Relational and Developmental Trauma and Schools* (Oxford University Press, 2021).

Mary J. Ring, MAMFC, MARE, LPC-S, LMFT-S, RPT-S, serves as Family Team Coordinator at the Julianna Poor Memorial Counseling Center in Houston, Texas. She is a Certified Theraplay® Practitioner, Trainer and Supervisor, certified in EMDR, and trained in DDP and Trust-Based Relational Intervention (TBRI). The Neurosequential Network™ acknowledges Mary Ring has completed NMT Training Certification through Phase 2 Level.

Helen Rodwell, DClinPsy, MSc, BSc (Econ), is a Health and Care Professions Council (HCPC) Registered Consultant Clinical Psychologist, Certified Theraplay® Practitioner, Trainer and Supervisor, Certified DDP Practitioner and EMDR Europe Accredited Adult, Child and Adolescent Practitioner. She works in independent practice in Derby in the UK. She is co-author of *Parenting with Theraplay* (Jessica Kingsley Publishers, 2017), *An Introduction to Autism for Adoptive and Foster Families* (Jessica Kingsley Publishers, 2019), and *Supporting the Mental Health of Looked After and Adopted Children* (CoramBAAF, 2018).

Hyunjung Shin, PhD, RPT, is a Certified Theraplay® Practitioner, Trainer and Supervisor. She is also a Certified Therapist and Trainer of Gestalt Therapy for children and adolescents by the West Coast Institute. She is the current President of the Korean Association of Theraplay. Hyunjung is a Professor in the Division of Social Work at Yeonsung University in Korea. She is deeply interested in phenomenology and has had more than 20 research articles and books related to Theraplay, interaction, and mother–child relationships published in Korean.

Angela Siu, PhD, RCP, CPT-S, RPT-S, is a Certified Theraplay® Practitioner, Trainer and Supervisor. She is also a clinical psychologist working with young children and families. She specializes in attachment as well as school and learning issues. She has had book chapters and research studies published on the use of Theraplay for Chinese children and families. She was the Ann M. Jernberg Award Winner for 2018.

Jay Vaughan, MBE, has worked with traumatized children since qualifying as a Dramatherapist in 1989. Jay is also a Certified Somatic Experiencing® and DDP Practitioner, and Certified Theraplay® Practitioner, Supervisor and Trainer. Jay is the CEO of Family Futures CIC. She has dedicated her career to improving the lives of adopted, fostered, and kinship care children and their families.

Lorie Walton, MEd, is a Registered Psychotherapist, Certified Play Therapist Supervisor and Trainer, and Certified Theraplay® Practitioner, Supervisor and Trainer. She is Executive Director of Theraplay Canada and the owner of the Family First Play Therapy Centre Inc. (established in 2000) with two locations in Ontario, Canada.

King-Chi Yau is a Registered Music Therapist (UK, Health and Care Professions Council, HCPC) and Social Worker (Hong Kong, Social Workers Registration Board, SWRB), undertaking a Doctorate in Clinical Psychology at University College London. He is a Module Lead for Safeguarding in Practice at the University of Northampton London. Chi has more than 10 years' experience working with children and their families with attachment and trauma issues. He has had three peer-reviewed empirical papers and a book chapter published.

Special Note

Case illustrations in each chapter are either actual cases with consent or composites from multiple cases by authors who worked with similar children. To protect client confidentiality, any identifying information has been changed. Further, the authors attempt to use inclusive language in their writing, infusing principles of diversity, equity, and inclusion (DEI). For instance, they use the singular "they" when describing a generic person whose gender is irrelevant. In addition, while The Theraplay Institute officially uses "practitioners" for Theraplay providers, in this book, the authors use "practitioners," "therapists," and "clinicians" interchangeably, to make the writing flow more freely. The term "parent and caregiver" is used interchangeably in some situations. If the parent is no longer a caregiver, authors were to make this clear by specific phrasing (e.g., birth parent). The term "caregiver" is generally preferred, as it can indicate a range of relationships (foster parent, adoptive parent, guardian, etc.), but generally carries the connotation of someone who actually delivers regular care to the child.

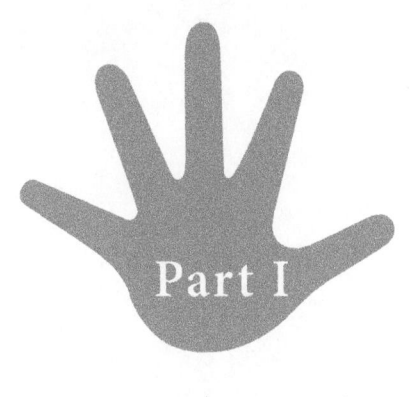

Part I

Introduction

Chapter 1

Overview of Theraplay Integration with Other Therapeutic Models

Rana Hong

Introduction

Theraplay has a 50-year tradition as a clinical intervention that now has practitioners worldwide. Rooted in attachment theory and child development principles, it has become recognized as an effective intervention for children, families, and groups. Advances in modern neuroscience have further allowed for the exploration of its neurobiological underpinnings.

Theraplay practitioners have increasingly experimented with integrative models to address specialized or complex issues among children and families. However, the proliferation of diverse therapies can sometimes distract practitioners, compromising effective integration of models or techniques into Theraplay. Fortunately, many Theraplay experts with specialties in other models have pioneered successful integration of Theraplay with other therapeutic models that are presented in the subsequent chapters with case illustrations.

As the first step to developing appropriate Theraplay integrative models, this chapter aims to help readers understand the fundamental considerations of integrative approaches. It begins by reviewing recent studies on Theraplay and Theraplay-integrated models to outline the converging reasons for Theraplay integration. This segues into descriptions of key aspects in the nucleus of Theraplay-based integrative approaches, and concludes by cautioning against the careless borrowing of other techniques.

Theraplay research

As an example of best practice models with a well-grounded theoretical and practice base, Theraplay has become firmly embedded in the repertoires of many practitioners. Since The Theraplay Institute was founded in 1972, thousands of practitioners worldwide have received high-quality training. Ongoing clinical studies have provided anecdotal examples of the effectiveness of Theraplay (Jernberg 1984, 1988; Mäkelä & Vierikko 2005).

Theraplay research began to flourish in 2009 when the California Evidence-Based Clearinghouse for Child Welfare rated Theraplay as a model of promising evidence for infant and toddler mental health programs. The National Registry of Evidence-Based Programs and Practices by the US Substance Abuse and Mental Health Services Administration further endorsed Theraplay as an evidence-based practice in 2014. As such, Theraplay continues to solidify its effectiveness and research foundation by applying Theraplay to different cultures (Kim & Nahm 2008), settings (Tucker & Smith 2018), disorders (Simeone-Russell 2011), and case studies (Cort & Rowley 2015; Mohamed & Mkabile 2015).

Numerous Theraplay quantitative and qualitative studies establish the efficacy of Theraplay with children's emotional, behavioral, social, and relationship issues (see Table 1.1). Specifically, Theraplay studies using the randomized controlled trial (RCT)—the highest level of evidence (Eruyar & Vostanis 2020; Siu 2009, 2014; Tucker *et al.* 2017; Yazdanipour, Ashori, & Abedi 2021)—and a series of well-designed quasi-experimental studies (Chang, Kim, & Youn 2021; Weir *et al.* 2013; Wettig *et al.* 2011) have consistently increased.

Heterogeneity in clinical research refers to diversity in participants, interventions, and outcomes. As an evidence-based practice—a broader approach to clinical decision making with research evidence—Theraplay has been practiced with a variety of issues (attachment, autism, developmental delays, internalized behavior, externalized, etc.) and in various ways (individual, dyad, family, group, Sunshine Circles®, combining with other models, etc.). The issue of clinical heterogeneity will draw inaccurate conclusions when conducting a meta-analysis or systematic review. A potential solution to reduce heterogeneity in Theraplay is to break them down into various models for specific populations within the parameters of Theraplay. It means the expansion of Theraplay and each Theraplay-based model become empirically supported treatments—specific treatments that have been proven effective in controlled research for particular conditions. The field is already heading in this direction. Many Theraplay-integrated models with specific populations have been developed, practiced, and researched. It is time to learn what they are and how to incorporate them under the umbrella of the Theraplay community.

Table 1.1: Summary of research studies in Theraplay since 2006

Authors	Sample (N)	Study design	Findings	Type of Theraplay
1. Bennett *et al.* (2006)	Children experienced domestic violence (10 children, 15 mothers)	A process of formative evaluation	Improvements in the quality of life for mothers and children	Group Theraplay
2. Bojanowski & Ammen (2011)	Eight children (ages 5–9) with internalizing or externalizing difficulties, three parents	Pre-post design	Statistically significant decrease in internalizing and externalizing behavior	At least eight Theraplay sessions (parent–child)
3. Chang *et al.* (2021)	20 Korean children with autism spectrum disorder (ASD) (ages 2½–9)	Quasi-experimental design	Significant changes in social communication in children with autism	20 individual Theraplay sessions
4. Eruyar & Vostanis (2020)	30 parent–child dyads of Syrian refugees (ages 8–14)	RCTs	Weekly group Theraplay-led statistical significance in reducing attachment-related symptoms with a medium effect (r=0.40) and reduced post-traumatic stress disorder (PTSD) symptoms with a large effect size (r=0.623)	Group Theraplay
5. Francis, Bennion, & Humrich (2017)	40 Children (ages 5–11) Looked After (CLA) who are in local authority care	Mixed-methods (pre-post design and qualitative)	Reduction in overall Strengths and Difficulties Questionnaire (SDQ) in post-intervention but not statistically significant; qualitative findings support noticeable changes in children's relationship, confidence, and engagement with education	Combined (4–16 group Theraplay and 12–18 individual Theraplay) at school setting

cont.

Authors	Sample (N)	Study design	Findings	Type of Theraplay
6. Hiles Howard et al. (2018)	Eight children with mild to moderate autism, eight caregivers	Pre-post design	Improved parent–child interaction and improved behaviors of both parents and children	Two one-hour Theraplay sessions each day for a two-week period
7. Salisbury (2018)	Five children with emotional and behavioral difficulties, five parents	Pre-post design	Improved adult–child relationship, children's mental health, and adult's perceptions about child's behavior	10-minute Theraplay activities for two weeks
8. Salo et al. (2020)	18 Finnish children (ages 4–8) with emotional and/or behavioral problems at outpatient psychiatric clinic, 31 parents	Pre-post design	Weekly Theraplay (M=20.35 sessions) improved the parent–child relationship and reduced child internalizing and externalizing symptoms	Theraplay (parent–child)
9. Siu (2009)	46 children (mean age of 7.84) with internalizing behavior	RCTs	Statistically significant improvements in reducing symptoms of internalizing behavior	Group Theraplay (eight sessions, weekly, 40 minutes)
10. Siu (2014)	38 children with developmental delay (ages 6–13)	RCT with a mixed method	Statistically significant gains for social awareness, social cognition, social communication, and social motivation	School-based group Theraplay (20 sessions, weekly, 30 minutes)
11. Smithee et al. (2021)	Six children (ages 4–7), six mothers with anxiety	Quasi-experimental design	Findings support Theraplay has a potential to be effective in anxiety treatments (no significance)	Theraplay (parent–child), 12 weeks
12. Stubenbor, Cohen, & Trybalski (2010)	53 maltreated preschool children (mean age of 47 months) at therapeutic preschool	Pre- and post-test	Children in Theraplay-guided activities in classroom manifested significant developmental gains	School-based group Theraplay (three days per week), bi-weekly home visits, and monthly family nights

13. Tucker et al. (2017)	206 preschoolers (101 in intervention) from low-income families	RCTs with a mixed method	Statistically significant improvements in social-emotional skills, behavioral regulation, problem solving, and fine-motor control. Qualitative study found improvements in teacher–child relationship and overall classroom behavior	Theraplay group (Sunshine Circle); a full year, weekly, 20–30 minutes
14. Weaver et al. (2021)	21 middle school students	Qualitative (phenomenological approach)	Positive impacts on participants' attachment, emotional regulation, and prosocial behavior	School-based group Theraplay (10 weeks)
15. Wettig et al. (2011)	Study 1 with 22 and Study 2 with 157 children with dual diagnoses of language disorder and shyness/social anxiety in Germany	Longitudinal study (quasi-experimental, pre-post)	Statistically significant improvements in shyness, social anxiety, and expressive and receptive communication	Individual Theraplay (mean 18 sessions, maximum 66 sessions)
16. Yazdanipour et al. (2021)	27 children with hearing loss	RCTs	Positive effects on self-regulation, social competence, empathy, and responsibilities in children intervention group	10 group Theraplay sessions

To our delight, Theraplay's worldwide and broad practice drew the attention of many researchers. An example of model recognition in the research arena is researchers' attempt to conduct a meta-analysis or systematic review to gain aggregated effects of a popular model with enough studies. Money, Wilde, and Dawson (2021) conducted a systematic review of six studies on Theraplay and concluded that the rigorous research base of Theraplay is insufficient. Although their conclusion is not viable because their study presented some fundamental flaws of a skewed bias in the dataset criteria and reporting bias within the review process, they offer some takeaways. Not only did they recognize that Theraplay is a widely practiced model that deserves more research attention, but they also raised the important issue of heterogeneity between Theraplay studies.

Current Theraplay-based integrative models

Theraplay is one of the most suitable models for integration with methods. As a technique, Theraplay activities have been welcomed into other therapeutic models. For example, play therapists have used Theraplay activities as play-based, self-regulation, breathing, and self-esteem building exercises. Eye Movement Desensitization and Reprocessing (EMDR) therapists have used Theraplay activities to assist children in working through the various phases of the treatment protocol. Although Theraplay activities can be useful within an existing treatment protocol, the potential power of Theraplay is minimized compared to a well-designed Theraplay treatment.

Current conceptualizations of the nature of therapeutic change tend to be more complex and multifaceted than ever, so Theraplay practitioners are developing various integrative models. Researchers began to test various Theraplay-based integrative models that best addressed clients' manifesting problems. They found efficacy in combining Theraplay with other models such as Circles of Security (COS) (Sepehrtaj *et al.* 2020), Dialectical Behavioral Therapy (DBT) (Woods-Jaeger *et al.* 2018), Dyadic Developmental Psychotherapy (DDP) (Friend 2012; Robinson *et al.* 2009; Weir 2008), Family Systems therapies (Weir *et al.* 2013, 2021), Filial Play Therapy (May, Mowthorpe, & Griffiths 2014), Neuro-Physiological Psychotherapy (NPP) (Vaughan, McGullough, & Burnell 2016), the Neurosequential Model of Therapeutics (NMT) (Purrington *et al.* 2022), and music (Siu 2021) to address parents' and children's issues. These findings suggest the potential for further development in Theraplay-based integrative models. Table 1.2 shows the list of Theraplay integrative models.

Table 1.2: Studies on Theraplay integrative models

Authors	Sample (N)	Methods	Findings	Other modalities
1. Friend (2012)	Nine-year-old boy with intergenerational trauma (1)	Case study	Significantly improved attachment relationship with caregiver	Family Attachment Narrative Therapy; DPP
2. May et al. (2014)	12-year-old adopted boy (1)	Case study	Moderately decreased anxiety and depression	Filial Play Therapy; directive intervention
3. Purrington et al. (2022)	Adopted children and families (53 dyads)	Pre-post design	Statistically significant reduction in trauma symptoms and behavior symptoms in adopted children	NMT, Theraplay, parenting: A 10-week intervention with one-hour parenting training concurrent with sensory integration Theraplay group for children and one-hour Theraplay-informed family therapy)
4. Robinson et al. (2009)	14-year-old foster boy (1)	Case study	Progressed with affect regulation and self-concept and by meeting adolescent attachment needs	DDP
5. Sepehrtaj et al. (2021)	Siblings of deceased children (4 dyads)	Pre-post design	Prolonged grief symptoms and PTSD symptoms decreased	Theraplay (parent–child), COS arenting, Theraplay, and play therapy: 15 weeks, 45 minutes

cont.

Authors	Sample (N)	Methods	Findings	Other modalities
6. Siu (2021)	Children with special needs (15, 67% with ASD)	Mixed methods (pre-post design and qualitative studies)	Shows statistically significant changes in children's responsiveness to others (effect size >0.80)	Music-integrated Theraplay group
7. Vaughan et al. (2016)	Children with trauma (0)	Conceptual article	Suggestions of Theraplay integration in working with the midbrain	NPP, DDP
8. Weir (2008)	Eight-year-old adopted with Reactive Attachment Disorder (RAD) (1)	Case study	Improved attachment relationship with caregiver	Family Theraplay combined with Structural Family Therapy and DDP
9. Weir et al. (2013)	Parents with substance abuse issues (23; 30 adopted children)	Pre- and post-test quasi-experimental design	Statistically significant improvements in family communication, adults' interpersonal relationship, and children's behavioral functioning	Whole family Theraplay: Theraplay and Family Systems Therapy
10. Weir et al. (2021)	Parents with substance abuse and children with attachment issues (97 children and 78 mothers)	Pre- and post-test quasi-experimental design	Mothers' significant decrease in symptoms of distress and improved mental health; children's improved interpersonal relationships, reduced distress, and improved mental health functioning	Whole family Theraplay: Theraplay and Family Systems Therapy
11. Woods-Jaeger et al. (2018)	86 low-income minority ethnic children (6 therapists; 20 teachers)	A pilot study with a mixed method	100% of therapists and 55% of teachers reported benefits (children's expressiveness, increased interaction with peers, and initiation of activities) of classroom Theraplay	Classroom Theraplay and Dialectical Behavior Therapy (DBT) Skills Training for parents

There are three considerations to develop an effective integrative approach: (1) determining routes of integration; (2) setting up the phases of integration; and (3) determining the parameters of integration.

Routes of integration

Determining a route of integration is foremost in developing appropriate Theraplay integrative models. Although the routes of integration are not mutually exclusive, choosing a route will essentially answer the question of "how to integrate." Commonly, there are four directions to integration (Norcross 2005): theoretical integration, technical eclecticism, assimilative integration, and common factors integration.

- *Theoretical integration* refers to synthesizing elements from two or more theories, potentially creating a new conceptual framework greater than the sum of its parts. Integrating psychoanalytic with behavioral theories is an example of theoretical integration. Another prime example is EMDR Therapy for children by Ana Gomez (2013). In her book chapter with Emily Jernberg, "EMDR Therapy and Adjunct Approaches with Children," they discuss using EMDR Therapy and Theraplay. They conducted 12 Theraplay sessions in the preparation phase before moving on to bilateral stimulations in EMDR. They reported that Theraplay sessions helped the child attain greater levels of stabilization and helped the parents develop attunement and attachment security.

- *Technical eclecticism* refers to a technical blend of models—borrowing techniques (or skills) from divergent models in the approach to a particular case. Borrowing techniques from other models leads to greater flexibility in navigating the treatment process. For instance, if a child experiences anxiety, a practitioner might borrow techniques from different therapies. They may use Theraplay with parents to create a sense of safety and to regulate the midbrain with attachment work. They may develop a toolbox for managing anxious behavior, including shaping techniques, deep breathing techniques, and muscle relaxation techniques from Cognitive Behavioral Theraplay (CBT), DBT, or activities from Gestalt approaches to help clients gain self-awareness. Technical eclecticism, a so-called "mix-up" intervention, combines the best parts of several therapies to facilitate maximum treatment effectiveness.

- *Assimilative integration* involves grounding yourself in a single therapy, but assimilating approaches from other systems. For example, Theraplay practitioners may use a cognitive interweave technique to reinforce the child's internal strengths when playing balloon tennis by saying, "Wow, that's how you can win over it. I am not surprised that you became so brave all of a sudden. It was a powerful hit." Practitioners with strong theoretical and practical roots in Theraplay can selectively extend their repertoire to include techniques or perspectives from other approaches. Drawn from affect attunement, Siu (2021) attempted to facilitate attuned experience in children with social impairment by adding a significant amount of musical rhythms into Theraplay. This music-based Theraplay program follows the traditional sequence of Theraplay sessions, but utilizes musical instruments so children experience "musical arousal" as part of Theraplay-based activities. For instance, it starts with a greeting (with a welcome song), check-up (by choosing and naming instruments), activities (with percussion instruments and/or keyboards using high- and low-arousal activities), feeding (with soothing music), and closing (with a goodbye song). The 11-week music-based Theraplay group resulted in a significant impact of the program on children's responsiveness to others ($d>0.80$).

- *Common factors integration* evolves from the belief that the common core ingredients of different therapies create more effective treatments. This was not well received by individuals preferring particular approaches, but scholars have recently recognized its value in psychotherapy. For instance, the Division 29 Task Force of the American Psychological Association concluded that therapeutic alliance, empathy, collaboration between therapist and client, and a sense of cohesion between therapist and client are common factors for positive treatment outcomes (Ackerman *et al.* 2001). In the Theraplay realm, Theraplay's healing elements, such as attachment, attunement, play, empathy, non-verbal congruence, and up-and-down regulation, can be considered to determine other therapies' commonalities. Integrating Theraplay and DDP is an example of common factors integration. Both models are rooted in attachment theory, work with a similar population (e.g., foster and adopted children and families), involve parents in sessions, focus on building parent–child attachment, and emphasize similar techniques such as reciprocal attuned interactions, play, and empathy. The Integrative Attachment Therapy Program at Chaddock, a nationally accredited residential agency in Quincy, Illinois, is a specific example of common factors integration of Theraplay with DDP. Theraplay was combined with DDP to maximize the development of relationships. The staff at Chaddock found that Theraplay was effective in building a secure relationship with children and adolescents, and there was great efficacy in its use in combination with DDP in treatment (Robinson *et al.* 2009).

Phases in integrative treatments

Once a practitioner decides on a route of integration, the next consideration is when and where to arrange borrowed techniques in the Theraplay process. Ways of setting up the phases in integrative approaches vary. For instance, May *et al.* (2014) used three stages to address the anxiety and depression of an adopted boy. Stage 1 was the Marschak Interaction Method (MIM) and feedback. Stage 2 combined parent preparation sessions with filial therapy. Stage 3 was for adapted Theraplay (starting with Theraplay activities and finishing with non-directive play therapy).

In traditional psychotherapy integration, the transtheoretical model by Prochaska and DiClemente (1992) is used to set up the stages of integrative models. It involves progress through six stages of change: (1) precontemplation, where an individual is unable to recognize issues; (2) contemplation, where an individual recognizes issues but is not yet prepared to change them; (3) preparation, where behavioral changes of an individual are ready to occur; (4) action, where an individual makes changes; (5) maintenance, where an individual is aware of benefits of changes; and (6) termination. Using stage-matched interventions led to positive improvements in treatment progress (Prochaska & Velicer 1997). Preferred models for each stage differ depending on which stage a client is in when referred to therapy. Research suggests some strategies for each stage. For instance, clients in precontemplation stage may benefit from using strategies from experiential approaches to expand awareness, improve defenses, and gain insight. Cognitive and existential approaches are useful for the contemplation stage, and behavioral and structural strategies are effective for clients who are ready for the action stage (Norcross & Goldfried 2003).

Perry's Neurosequential Model of Therapeutics (NMT) (2009) is another framework for guiding the phases of interventions by choosing which brain areas to target when implementing the strategies. For instance, Purrington *et al.* (2022) developed a neuro-collaborative therapeutic package for adopted children and families using NMT guidelines within a Theraplay-based integrative program. Families participated for two hours a week over the course of the 10-week therapeutic intervention. They then did one-hour parenting training for parents, while children participated in group Theraplay with other children. Then, they provided one-hour Theraplay-based family therapy. They found statistically significant reductions in the Trauma Symptom Checklist scale (d=0.31), behavioral issues in the Child Behavior Checklist (d=0.26), and self-monitor/emotional/behavioral regulation in the Behavior Rating Inventory of Executive Function (d=0.38) among adopted children at post-intervention.

Parameters of integration

The third consideration when developing Theraplay integrative models is to determine the parameters of integration, including the format (individual, dyad, family, group), range (partial or full integration), and prioritized principles (hierarchy of theoretical underpinnings to deal with particular behaviors). For example, let's say that practitioners decide to integrate behavioral therapy into Theraplay to support a child with conduct disorder and insecure attachment relationships. Practitioners must first decide whether the format will be dyad, individual, or combined based on the results of the assessments. If they choose to include parents, practitioners also need to decide if parents will be involved in all sessions, partially in each session, in the beginning, or only in the later phase. Helpful questions are: "What are the roots of the child's aggression? Does insecure attachment play a role in the child's aggressive behavior?" The format of Theraplay-based integrative approaches must be carefully considered based on the client's profiles and the root causes of issues. Further, practitioners should predetermine their choice of theoretical principles when dealing with aggressive behavior in session because behavioral therapy techniques are often incongruent with Theraplay in handling aggressive behavior. Deciding how to manage aggressive behavior can prevent serious mishaps in treatments. The helpful question is: "Which theory better explains this child's aggression?" In addition, practitioners must decide the order in which to use borrowed techniques. Helpful questions to consider are: "Which approach needs to be applied first to handle the child's aggression? Do I need to synthesize both theories concurrently?"

To illustrate, some may choose behavioral principles of differential attention by ignoring negative behavior, believing that attention will increase negative behavior. In contrast, others prefer to utilize the Theraplay principle of responding to the underlying meaning of the behavior by being more attentive to the child. How to respond to a child's issues depends on the client's profile and relationship with their parents—remember, one approach prevails over the other. Another critical factor is to be consistent when utilizing a strategy. Inconsistent use of two techniques with the same behavior will lead to chaotic and ineffective results.

Conclusion

When we consider the uniqueness of children in clinical settings, we quickly agree that no one approach is clinically adequate to deal with the complexity of issues. Advances in neuroscience support clinicians' commonsense assumption that children benefit the most from multimodal approaches that can connect different parts of the brain in treatments. Science also guides practitioners on how and what to integrate to meet the needs of children. Theraplay appears to be at the juncture of extending its power to become more integrative with other models. Blending Theraplay approaches with other therapeutic models or incorporating elements from different models offers practitioners flexibility in treatment techniques applicable to clients' pressing issues, developmental levels, and even characteristics. Although integrative clinical models generally stem from clinical experience and training, there are divergent ways of integrating models in Theraplay, as reviewed in this chapter. Careful considerations for integration routes, phases of integration, and parameters in integration are necessary when integrating models. Although it is difficult to specify precisely when to combine another model with a Theraplay-based approach, I hope this chapter helps practitioners understand potential variables that are essential in developing integrative models or carefully choosing a proper existing integrative model. A premature mix-up with models without a clear understanding of their aggregated positive or negative effects may increase the complexity of the client's issues. Further, practitioners should not attempt to integrate models without adequate training in each modality. Haphazard integrations with insufficient training and limited experience will impose confusion or contraindication to reaching clinical goals. Thus, I underscore that developing an effective integrative model requires substantial training and clinical experience, plus careful attention to synthesizing the various concepts.

References

Ackerman, S. J., Benjamin, L. S., Beutler, L. E., Gelso, C. J., Goldfried, M. R., Hill, C., Lambert, M. J., Norcross, J. C., Orlinsky, D. E., & Rainer, J. (2001). Empirically supported therapy relationships: Conclusions and recommendations of the Division 29 Task Force. *Psychotherapy: Theory, Research, Practice, Training* 38(4), 495–497. https://doi.org/10.1037/0033-3204.38.4.495

Bennett, L. R., Shiner, S. K., & Ryans, S. (2006). Using Theraplay in shelter settings: With mothers and children who have experienced violence in the home. *Journal of Psychological*

Nursing & Mental Health Services 44(10), 38–48. https://doi.org/10.3928/02793695-20061001-06

Bojanowski, J. J., & Ammen, S. (2011). Discriminating between pre- versus post-Theraplay treatment Marschak Interaction Methods using the Marschak Interaction Method Rating System. *International Journal of Play Therapy 20*(1), 1–11. https://doi.org/10.1037/a0022668

Chang, Y., Kim, B., & Youn, M. (2021). Changes in children with autism spectrum disorder after Theraplay application. *Journal of the Korean Academy of Child and Adolescent Psychiatry 32*(3), 112–117. https://doi.org/10.5765/jkacap.210001

Cort, L., & Rowley, E. (2015). A case study evaluation of a group Theraplay intervention to support mothers and their preschool children following domestic abuse. *DECP Debate 156.*

Eruyar, S., & Vostanis, P. (2020). Feasibility of group Theraplay with refugee children in Turkey. *Counseling and Psychotherapy Research 20*(4), 626–637. https://doi:10.1002/capr.12354

Francis, Y. J., Bennion, K., & Humrich, S. (2017). Evaluating the outcomes of a school based Theraplay® project for looked after children. *Educational Psychology in Practice 33*(3), 308–322. https://doi.org/10.1080/02667363.2017.1324405

Friend, J. (2012). Mitigating intergenerational trauma within the parent-child attachment. *Australian & New Zealand Journal of Family Therapy 33*(2), 114–127. https://doi.org/10.1017/aft.2012.14

Gomez, A. M. (Ed.) (2013) *EMDR Therapy and Adjunct Approaches with Children: Complex Trauma, Attachment, and Dissociation.* Springer Publishing Company.

Gomez, A. M., & Jernberg, E. (2013). Using EMDR Therapy and Theraplay. In A. Gomez (Ed.), *EMDR Therapy and Adjunct Approaches with Children: Complex Trauma, Attachment, and Dissociation* (pp.273–279). Springer Publishing Company.

Hiles Howard, A. R., Copeland, R., Lindaman, S., & Cross, D. R. (2018). Theraplay impact on parents and children with autism spectrum disorder: Improvements in affect, joint attention, and social cooperation. *International Journal of Play Therapy 27*(1), 56–68. doi: 10.1037/pla0000056

Jernberg, A. (1984). Theraplay: Child therapy for attachment fostering. *Psychotherapy 23*(1), 39–47. https://doi.org/10.1037/h0087526

Jernberg, A. (1988). Theraplay for the elderly tyrant. *Clinical Gerontologist 8*(1), 76–79.

Kim, Y.-K., & Nahm, S. (2008). Cultural considerations in adapting and implementing play therapy. *International Journal of Play Therapy 17*(1), 66–77. https://doi.org/10.1037/1555-6824.17.1.66

Mäkelä, J., & Vierikko, I. (2005). *From Heart to Heart: Interactive Therapy for Children in Care. Report on the Theraplay® Project in SOS Children's Villages in Finland 2001–2004.* The SOS Children's Villages Association, Finland.

May, D., Mowthorpe, L., & Griffiths, E. (2014). Teetering on the edge of care: The role of intensive attachment-based play therapies. *Adoption & Fostering 38*(2), 131–148. https://doi.org/10.1177/0308575914532063

Mohamed, A. R., & Mkabile, S. (2015). An attachment-focused parent–child intervention for biting behavior in a child with intellectual disability: A clinical case study. *Journal of Intellectual Disabilities 19*(3), 251–265. https://doi.org/10.1177/1744629515572711

Money, R., Wilde, S., & Dawson, D. (2020). Review: The effectiveness of Theraplay for children under 12—A systematic literature review. *Child and Adolescent Mental Health 26*(3), 238–251. https://doi.org/10.1111/camh.12416

Norcross, J. C. (2005). A Primer on Psychotherapy Integration. In J. T. Norcross & M. R. Goldfried (Eds), *Handbook of Psychotherapy Integration* (pp.241–260). Oxford University Press.

Norcross, J. C., & Goldfried, M. R. (2003). *Handbook of Psychotherapy Integration.* Oxford University Press.

Prochaska, J. O., & DiClemente, C. C. (1992). The Transtheoretical Approach. In J. C. Norcross & M. R. Goldfried (Eds), *Handbook of Psychotherapy Integration* (pp.300–334). Basic Books.

Prochaska, J. O., & Velicer, W. F. (1997). The transtheoretical model of health behavior change. *American Journal of Health Promotion 12*(1), 38–48. https://doi.org/10.4278/0890-1171-12.1.38

Purrington, J., Glover-Humphreys, E., Edwards, H., & Hudson, M. (2022). The impact of a brief neuro-collaborative play-based intervention on presentations of developmental trauma and attachment difficulties in adopted children: A service evaluation. *International Journal of Play Therapy 31*(4), 237–247. https://doi.org/10.1037/pla0000182

Robinson, M., Lindaman, S. L., Clemmons, M., Doyle Buckwalter, K., & Ryan, M. (2009). "I deserve a family": The evolution of an adolescent's behavior and beliefs about himself and others when treated with Theraplay in residential care. *Child and Adolescent Social Work Journal 26*, 291–306. doi:10.1007/s10560-009-0177-x.

Salisbury, S. (2018). Using attachment enhancing activities based on the principles of Theraplay® to improve adult–child relationships and reduce a child's "overall stress" as measured by the Strengths and Difficulties Questionnaire (SDQ). *Emotional and Behavioral Difficulties 23*(4), 424–440. https://doi.org/10.1080/13632752.2018.1497000

Salo, S., Flykt, M., Mäkelä, J., Lassenius-Panula, L., Korja, R., Lindaman, S., & Punamäki, R.-L. (2020). The impact of Theraplay® therapy on parent–child interaction and child psychiatric symptoms: A pilot study. *International Journal of Play 9*(3), 331–352. https://doi.org/10.1080/21594937.2020.1806500

Sepehrtaj, A., Younesi, S. J., Mousavi, P. S., Jeihooni, A. K., & Jafar, P. (2021). Effectiveness of Theraplay in internalizing and externalizing problems in bereaved siblings of children with cancer. *Iranian Journal of Psychiatry and Behavioral Sciences 15*(2), 1–11. https://doi:10.5812/ijpbs.103992

Simeone-Russell, R. (2011). A practical approach to implementing Theraplay for children with autism spectrum disorder. *International Journal of Play Therapy 20*(4), 224–235. https://doi.org/10.1037/a0024823

Siu, A. F. Y. (2009). Theraplay in the Chinese world: An intervention program for Hong Kong children with internalizing problems. *International Journal of Play Therapy 18*(1), 1–12. https://doi.org/10.1037/a0013979

Siu, A. F. Y. (2014). Effectiveness of Group Theraplay® on enhancing social skills among children with developmental disabilities. *International Journal of Play Therapy 23*(4), 187–203. https://doi.org/10.1037/a0038158

Siu, A. F. Y. (2021). Does age make a difference when incorporating music as a rhythmic-mediated component in a Theraplay-based program to facilitate attunement of preschool children with social impairment? *International Journal of Play Therapy 30*(2), 136–145. https://doi.org/10.1037/pla0000131

Smithee, L. C., Krizova, K., Guest, J. D., & Case Pease, J. (2021). Theraplay as a family treatment for mother anxiety and child anxiety. *International Journal of Play Therapy 30*(3), 206–218. https://doi.org/10.1037/pla0000153

Stubenbort, K., Cohen, M. M., & Trybalski, V. (2010). The effectiveness of an attachment-focused treatment model in a therapeutic preschool for abused children. *Clinical Social Work Journal 38*, 51–60. https://doi.org/10.1007/s10615-007-0107-3

Tucker, C., Schieffer, K., Wills, T. J., Hull, C., & Murphy, Q. (2017). Enhancing social-emotional skills in at-risk preschool students through Theraplay based groups: The Sunshine Circle

Model. *International Journal of Play Therapy 26*(4), 185–195. https://doi.org/10.1037/pla0000054

Vaughan, J., McGullough, E., & Burnell, A. (2016). Neuro-Physiological Psychotherapy (NPP): The development and application of an integrative, wrap-around service and treatment programme for maltreated children placed in adoptive and foster care placements. *Clinical Child Psychology and Psychiatry 21*(4). https://doi.org/10.1177/1359104516635222

Weaver, J. L., Medyk, N. V., Swank, J. M., Daniels, P. F., & Smith-Adcock, S. (2021). A phenomenological study of Theraplay groups within a middle school. *International Journal of Play Therapy 30*(2), 124–135. https://doi.org/10.1037/pla0000139

Weir, K. N. (2008). Using integrative play therapy with adoptive families to treat Reactive Attachment Disorder: A case example. *Journal of Family Psychotherapy 18*(4), 1–16. https://doi.org/10.1300/J085v18n04_01

Weir, K. N., Lee, S., Canosa, P., Rodrigues, N., McWilliams, M., & Parker, L. (2013). Whole Family Theraplay: Integrating family systems theory and Theraplay to treat adoptive families. *Adoption Quarterly 16*, 175–200. https://doi.org/10.1080/10926755.2013.844216

Weir, K. N., Pereyra, S., Crane, J., Greaves, M., Childs, T. S., & Weir, A. B. (2021). The effectiveness of Theraplay® as a counseling practice with mothers and their children in a substance abuse rehabilitation residential facility. *The Family Journal 29*(1), 115–123. https://doi.org/10.1177/1066480720980988

Wettig, H. G., Coleman, A. R., & Geider, F. J. (2011). Evaluating the effectiveness of Theraplay in treating shy, socially withdrawn children. *International Journal of Play Therapy 20*, 26–37. https://doi.org/10.1037/a0022666

Woods-Jaeger, B. A., Sexton, C. C., Gardner, B., Siedlik, E., Slagel, L., Tezza, V., & O'Malley, D. (2018). Development, feasibility, and refinement of a toxic stress prevention research program. *Journal of Child and Family Studies 27*, 3531–3543. https://doi.org/10.1007/s10826-018-1178-1

Yazdanipour, M., Ashori, M., & Abedi, A. (2021). Impact of group Theraplay on the social-emotional assets and resilience in children with hearing loss. *International Journal of Play Therapy 31*(2), 107–118. https://doi.org/10.1037/pla0000175

Yvonne, J. F., Bennion, K., & Humrich, S. (2017). Evaluating the outcomes of a school based Theraplay® for looked after children, *Educational Psychology in Practice 33*(3), 308–322. https://doi.org/10.1080/02667363.2017.1324405

Chapter 2

Neurobiology of Theraplay

LINKING NEUROPHYSIOLOGY TO DEVELOPMENTAL AND THERAPEUTIC OUTCOMES

A. Rand Coleman

 CASE ILLUSTRATION: BENNY'S STORY

Mom Margaret was holding seven-week-old Benny. Wrapped with a blanket and cradled in her arms, she was hoping to play with him, but Benny fussed a bit. "Oh, are you hungry, Benny?" asked Mom in a singsong voice. "Here, Benny, let me get you something to eat." Snuggling Benny close in the crook of her arm, she fed him breast milk while gazing down, warmly, into his eyes. Benny suckled away, occasionally gazing back up at his mother, but seeming intent on consuming the warm milk. When done, he turned away and Margaret immediately noticed, saying, "Oh, are you all done, Benny? That's much better, I think." She propped him on her shoulder, rocking and patting him on the back until he burped, and then she said, "Now we can play, Benny." Facing him toward her and looking into his eyes, Mom sang him a song and told him a story.

At 18 months, Benny is lively and cheerful, exploring the home and yard but always checking back with Mom. When he falls and gets hurt, he cries, runs to his mother, and gets a kiss, a snuggle, and a Band-Aid. He is ready to run and play again, confident; he is supported by his mother.

 CASE ILLUSTRATION: ANNA'S STORY

Anna was screaming again. Mom had picked up three-year-old Anna to cradle her in her arms and rock her, but foster daughter Anna responded by screaming and yelling, "No, it hurts, it hurts." Mom held on and sat down on the sofa with Anna, rocking, rocking, speaking in soothing tones, trying to catch Anna's eye with warm-hearted eye contact, but Anna twisted her head from side to side, avoiding all eye contact, saying, "I will kill you, I will bite you!" Mom tried to calm her with a firm hug and gentle singing, but Anna escalated, kicking, hitting, trying to pull Mom's hair, and turning to bite. She calmed momentarily to spit, then screamed and twisted again. Mom continued rocking, singing, and holding tight with deep pressure. After 30 minutes, exhausted, Anna settled, relaxed into her foster mother's arms, and listened to a song, *You Are My Sunshine*. Seeing that Anna was calm and emotionally self-controlled, Mom set Anna down. Anna walked to her toy box and took out some dolls and pretend food, and played as if nothing had happened.

"Why does Anna scream when I try to comfort her or pick her up?" Mom asked the therapist. "She acts like I am killing her." Later in therapy, when asked to draw a picture of herself, Anna drew a large picture of a girl, putting red dots all over it. "What are those red dots?" she was asked. "Those are where my mom burned me," she said. The number of red dots exactly matched the location and number of cigarette burn marks the pediatrician had documented during intake. During an intensive course of therapy and home practice, the family participated in rocking, feeding each other, telling Anna stories while snuggling in close, and playing early childhood sensory motor games. Near the end of therapy, the foster father and therapist tested Anna's response to nurture. They rocked together in a chair. Dad asked Anna, "How does this feel to rock together?" "Oh, that feels good," she said.

Introduction

These two case illustrations reflect very different outcomes for parent–child interactions, and yet all the same brain systems are at work. In both scenarios, the neural systems of the child were functioning just as nature intended. However, neural systems interact with the environment and with neural systems of other humans; change is triggered and molded by experience. These two children had markedly different parenting experiences that shaped their brains and their behavior. Tracing their relationship development is instructive in understanding the physiology of social engagement, as well as providing a social-physiological model of change in Theraplay.

At birth, Benny and Anna emerged from liquid encapsulation in a stable, warm temperature to an environment of air, hands, and shifting temperatures. The surrounding environment touches Benny and Anna across every square millimeter. They breathe the environment, and it pervades their every cell. They taste and consume their environment, and it becomes their every molecule. The eye is an extension of neural matter, so what they see triggers change. The ear and nasal filaments are directly linked to the brain, so what they hear and smell immediately starts a stimulus–response conditioning process. Their bodies are living and breathing extensions of the environment. This chapter aims to help readers understand the integration of Theraplay concepts with the neurobiology of trauma and therapeutic change. It explains key concepts involving the systems for emotional processing, integrated with positive reinforcement and desensitization systems.

Reflections on environment and neural pathways

Humans are specifically designed for high sensitivity to human contact. Other people are the most powerful agents of change, learning, and regulation for any human. Each infant is an integrated body-neural system that becomes part of the body-neural systems surrounding it. Baby Benny experienced his mother through multiple simultaneous pathways, mapped out in Figure 2.1. Held close to his mother's body, warmth was relayed through unmyelinated C fibers, while Merkel nerve endings relayed the sustained pressure and feel of this mother's arms and hands. Specialized nerve endings relayed the sudden changes of being patted or rubbed on the back or sensed changes in temperature. These cutaneous sensations were relayed through dorsal root ganglions up the spinal cord and to the thalamus, with side relays to the reticular activating system in the medulla, pons, and midbrain, a system that regulates alertness with norepinephrine (NE) projections to the entire brain (Barr & Kiernan 1988). Rocking triggers cilia of the semi-circular canals to register changes in body position and space; the signals are simultaneously sent to the midbrain, thalamus, cerebellum, and lower spinal cord. Singsong vocal tones of his mother triggered cilia of the cochlea, traveling the same auditory vestibular nerve (cranial nerve VIII), to link with midbrain nuclei that register the location of sound with visual nuclei to help orient the eyes toward the sound and with thalamic nuclei that relay the soothing tones to the temporal lobes. Benny turns his eyes toward his mother's face, and in his state of alert but relaxed, warm comfort, he tastes sweet, warm milk and sees kind eyes looking into his own, studying his face.

Benny's warmth, touch, and suckling trigger huge releases of oxytocin, dopamine, serotonin, and opiates in his mother's brain and body. As these neurochemicals arrive on receptors in her ventral tegmental area (VTA), nucleus accumbens (NA), hypothalamus, frontal lobes, and amygdala, she experiences pleasure, relaxation, contentment, and safety. Pain is dulled, and tactile sensitivity to pressure and warmth is activated. The entire body responds. Milk flows for Benny; the mother plays with Benny's hands and feet, they talk and burble at each other, and they look into each other's eyes, exchanging expressions. Benny experiences similar releases of neurochemicals. Day after day, they are both awash in a neuroendocrine bath that is mutually satisfying and positively reinforcing. They have become a single entity, two body-neural systems tied to each other at every level, even at the molecular level of cellular nourishment.

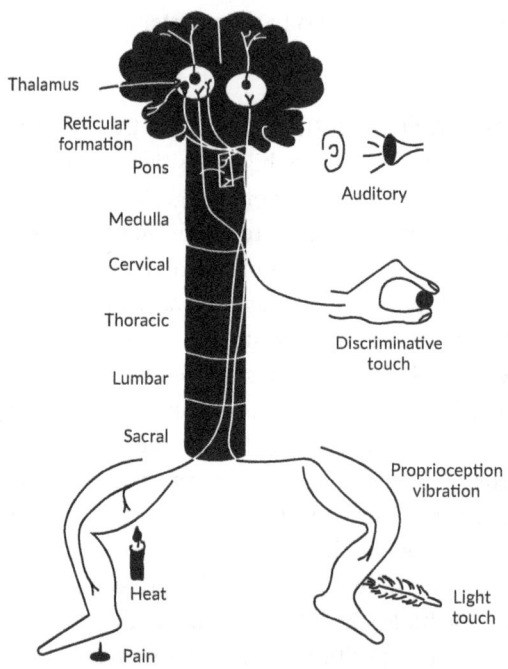

Figure 2.1. Sensory pathways from the body to the brain
ILLUSTRATION BY SHAWNTRELL R. COLEMAN

Anna had a very different experience. Although warmth and food were provided, sometimes the cuddles and holding were accompanied by severe pain. Sometimes the craving for food, comfort, or touch took a long time to be relieved. Cries of fear were met with the infliction of more pain or of rejection. Repeatedly, the humans representing comfort, food, and safety were removed to be swapped out for new ones. The new person might provide safety or might create more pain; sometimes both. Being pulled onto a comforting lap and then repeatedly inflicted with excruciating pain while held in place produced a toxic mix of fear and rage. Anna, too, was experiencing a body-neural interface with another human, altering her neural development at the deepest limbic levels.

Benny is unlikely to need therapy in the near future, while Anna started attachment and trauma therapies at age three. Understanding the body-neural systems involved in sensation, fear conditioning, pleasure response, attachment, social interaction, and emotional regulation helps us appreciate the consequences of different social environments. These systems provide a framework for understanding how and why therapy works, particularly an attachment-based, sensory motor, play-type of therapy, such as Theraplay.

Sensory information of all types (except smell) is relayed to the thalamus. This information is then relayed through fast and slow pathways to the amygdala (LeDoux & Phelps 2008). The fast pathway is direct from the thalamus to the lateral nucleus of the amygdala. A longer pathway travels from the thalamus to the higher cortical regions for processing, after which these regions communicate with the lateral amygdala (see Figure 2.2). By receiving all sensory information at once, the amygdala can correlate pain or pleasure with other inputs, such as sounds, sights, smells, tastes, and different types of touch (temperature, light pressure, deep pressure, balance, vibration). The lateral nucleus receives the inputs, the basal and accessory nuclei integrate the information together, and the central nucleus coordinates a response. Conditioning experiments have demonstrated how a neutral auditory tone can quickly become associated with an electric shock and can then become quickly associated with a movement to stop the shock (e.g., touching a button). Learning involving the amygdala is extremely fast.

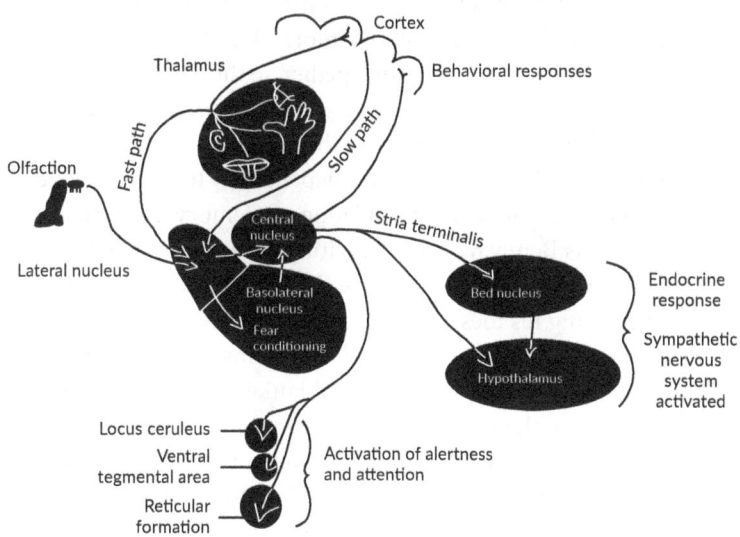

Figure 2.2. Sensory pathways of the amygdala
ILLUSTRATION BY SHAWNTRELL R. COLEMAN

Information is simultaneously relayed from the thalamus to the higher cortical sensory regions. Sensory modalities have individual thalamic nuclei that relay sensation to specialized cortical centers (Barr & Kiernan 1988). For instance, the lateral geniculate nucleus relays visual information only to the occipital lobe, while the medial geniculate nucleus relays sound to the superior temporal gyrus. Surrounding neural tissue uses past experience to make meaning of the data, with sounds interpreted as language, music, or objects, and visual input coded for location and function. Tactile information of all types is received by the somatic sensory region of the parietal lobe, then routed forward to the frontal motor control regions and backward to the parietal regions that make meaning out of it, linking sensations to objects, names, sounds, and past experiences (Petrof, Viaene, & Sherman 2015; Vijayakumar *et al.* 2019). These higher cortical regions allow for conscious awareness of our sensory experience. Conscious awareness is amplified through communication with the frontal lobe, which integrates all information for problem solving, decision making, and predicting the future. The frontal lobes send amplifying or inhibiting signals to the amygdala, completing a comparatively slow circuit of information in the amygdala. This slower circuit is a mechanism for higher-level decision making to suppress initial instinctive impulses in favor of rational choices (Gyurak & Etkin 2014).

Benny sees his mother's face while experiencing sensations of rocking, pressure, and warmth, perhaps hearing his mother sing to him. Occipital, parietal, and temporal lobes integrate this information, causing neuronal-dendritic growth, and they send all this information back to the amygdala. The amygdala also ties the information together, so the next time Benny hears his mother singing, it is associated with a generalized memory of safety and warmth. The hippocampus, situated with the amygdala deep in the temporal lobes, is connected to the amygdala and independently to other brain regions. This region is necessary for the consolidation of memory traces (Lezak *et al.* 2012, pp.83–86). As Benny has fun or exciting experiences with his mother, such as learning words, pointing to new things together, experiencing his mother manipulating his toes for a little piggies game, many environmental features become associated in his mind through amygdala and hippocampal consolidation. Later, seeing his special blanket, smelling his mother's shampoo, or hearing the creak of the wooden rocking chair also become triggers for a myriad of social and emotional memories. Some memories will be explicit, such as the silly name they decided on for a stuffed animal, while others will be implicit (unconscious), such as a smell triggering a sensation of love and security.

Anna may have experienced similar associations to Benny, but her environment contained huge doses of fear conditioning, causing many sensations to trigger associations with pain. Fear conditioning recruits the hippocampus to consolidate memories of the circumstances of the painful or feared experience, but numerous brain regions are involved. The cerebellum is activated (Cheng *et al.* 2008), probably as part of the movement–response system. Cortex areas of the sensory motor region, frontal operculum, middle frontal gyrus, and inferior parietal lobe all become active, representing the distributed memory processing of the cortex (Knight *et al.* 2004). These cortical areas represent key regions, respectively, for sensory awareness, speech output, motor planning, and sensory integration. Thus, a network of sensory–motor–speech actions is linked and integrated within Anna's body-neural circuitry. This has survival value for her because it facilitates high awareness and sensitivity to cues of danger, including adult facial expressions, tone of voice, approaching footsteps, people's smells, and, sadly, the feel of containing warm and human touch.

The amygdala coordinates the fear condition sending signals to the cortex, brainstem, and body. Much of the conditioning is unconscious, meaning that fear is activated without the child being able to describe exactly why. Even people with severe amnesia can experience fear conditioning responses yet have no conscious memory of learning the fear (Phelps & Labar 2006), which helps explain why a child could learn fear at an early age and be unable to verbalize it. A fear response can be measured with electrical skin conductance monitoring, a body-neural response that activates within milliseconds of a stimulus being presented, even at an unconscious level. Anna's reactions were specifically measured in this way, comparing her skin conductance response to a brother who had experienced neglect but less physical abuse and a sister who had experienced no abuse. When being cradled or held for even a brief moment, Anna's skin conductance response strongly activated, while her siblings' reactions showed a calming response.

The emotional circuit runs from the amygdala and hippocampus in a circular manner through the cingulate gyrus, an area of the cortex that runs lengthwise in the interior-medial brain (Barr & Kiernan 1988). Synapsing in the anterior cingulate cortex (ACC), signals are then relayed throughout the frontal lobes to aid in decision making, managing impulses, creating conscious associations between actions and consequences, and marshaling cognitive resources for problem solving. Connected regions in this prefrontal cortex send signals back to the amygdala to allow for a certain amount of conscious control over emotional circuits and amygdala responses (see Figure 2.3 for the entire circuit). Benny started using this part of his brain early to plan ways to keep his mother's attention, getting her to play or talk with him by showing her special toys or pointing out interesting sights on town walks. Anna became highly sensitive to even slight changes in adult facial expressions or body language, planning ways to avoid caregiver contact or control. In the face of an insecure situation or emotional trigger, she would cycle through responses, such as ignoring, acting especially cute, asking a distracting question, or screaming and running away. As stress increased, problem solving quickly declined, and choices became more automatic and reactive. Figure 2.3 shows the circuit from the amygdala to medial frontal regions associated with executive function and conscious control of behavior. Limbic signals from the amygdala provide emotional information for decision making, and the frontal lobes send direct signals back to the amygdala to regulate (inhibit or enhance) its response. When emotional signals from the amygdala become acutely strong, the frontal capacity for flexible decision making is overwhelmed, resulting in less flexible problem solving and reduced emotional regulation (Akirav & Maroun 2007).

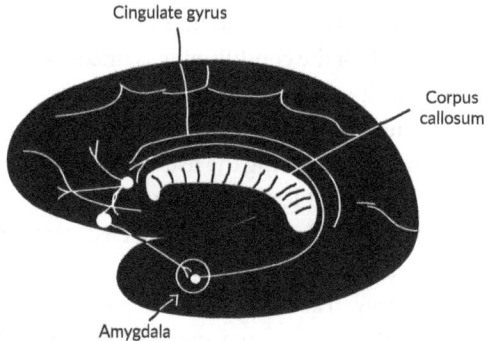

Figure 2.3. Amygdala to frontal lobe network
ILLUSTRATION BY SHAWNTRELL R. COLEMAN

Anna's trauma reactions to her foster mother trying to hold, hug, or comfort her now make neurological sense. Instructed to pick up some toys, her perception is that this may be hard for her or involve stopping an enjoyable play activity, so she stomps her foot and says, "No!" As her foster mother walks toward her, she experiences a neuroception of a looming adult presence, which in the past has been associated with danger. A burst of NE is injected from the locus coeruleus in the brainstem throughout the cortex, raising her brain activation and vigilance level. The stress of this prompts her to throw a toy and run, which prompts the foster mother to scoop Anna up in her arms to prevent a chase. Being scooped up and held tightly sends tactile and proprioceptive signals to the amygdala that danger has arrived and pain will be imminent. Even though this foster mother is loving, the fear response is automatic and overwhelming. The sympathetic nervous system is activated with fast, excitatory, neural connections to the heart, lungs, skeletal muscles, and adrenal glands. The overload of NE in the brain shuts off complex language and complex problem solving in favor of screaming, kicking, hitting, biting, pulling hair, and squirming to escape. Words used are primarily epithets and succinct rejections of "I hate you" or "Help, you hurt!" Fearing her daughter will harm herself, the foster mother holds on, cradling her daughter, taking the hits, and trying to soothe her in natural ways. She rocks her, walks around, pats her on the back, and tries to sing. Anna's body-neural system will have none of this, protesting louder and longer until she stops from exhaustion.

Compounding the parental confusion, Anna tries to get attention and affection from strangers. This seems paradoxical to Anna's foster parents, as they are Anna's primary source of safety, while strangers may represent risks. They notice other children Anna's age peeking out from behind a parent's leg when meeting a new person. The other children have a cautious reserve and use their parents as a base of operations to examine new people and situations, observing parental body language and cues before proceeding. In contrast, Anna walks away from her foster mother in the grocery store to ask strangers for treats. Children have an inherent dependency on adults to obtain things they want, but in situations of attachment trauma caregivers are the ones associated with risk, pain, and rejection, so it feels more comfortable to use strangers to meet personal needs for connection, touch, and affirmation.

Finding the way back home

Adaptability, change, and growth are hallmarks of the human body-neural system. Faith in adaptability and plasticity provided hope that Anna could ultimately experience security and calm and healthy relationships. Ingredients necessary to help Anna are common to all attachment trauma-informed therapies and are integral components of Theraplay. Therapeutic change for Anna can be understood through the neurobiology of play, attachment, and relearning. These biological imperatives occur in the context of developmental stages (i.e., infant through adult) and in the context of learning theory. Therapy as a whole represents a specialized learning situation, and, as such, certain conditions are necessary for change. Each condition is developmentally modulated and is associated with a set of neurobiological conditions, which are as follows:

1. social-environmental security and a safe therapeutic guide

2. emotional and social engagement

3. a reason to change

4. learning and reward conditioning; and

5. new behaviors used with persistence.

Condition one: Establishing social-environmental safety and a safe therapeutic guide

Lacking social safety, Anna was unable to change her conditioned fear response to caregiver nurture and touch. She had undergone intensive fear conditioning in which the normal social cues for connection and support (e.g., being held, looked at, touched, contained) were strongly associated with severe pain. When her foster mother tried to pick her up, it triggered the survival actions of fight or flight. On a normal daily basis, she was continually alert for any signal that harm was impending, which resulted in her maintaining a detached, angry, or resistant approach to adult caregiver relationships. On the other hand, given her developmental age, she was almost totally dependent on adult support. This created a tenuous approach-avoidance relationship to her behaviors, resulting in her accepting some adult rules and guidance but working hard to always maintain an emotional détente. Indeed, she preferred interacting with strangers in many cases, whom she could manipulate with charm, getting accolades and hugs without any semblance of emotional intimacy or requirement to follow their directives.

High structure was used within the therapy office and home to establish some basic sense of safety for Anna. Office sessions were highly routine and predictable, always in the same room and following a basic ritual of activities. Anna's foster parents were coached to use a predictable schedule at home with predictable enforcement of just a few clear rules for safety. The time-limited nature of each session helped create a sense of boundaries in which new activities could be experienced, but with a circumscribed ending point.

Predictability and clear structure are regulating for most human beings and indeed, for all mammals. When a specific stimulus or a general situation is repeatedly experienced in the absence of any painful or aversive experience, the neurological condition of habituation is produced. Something that was emotionally arousing becomes routine, ordinary, and normalized; as this occurs, signals from the amygdala are reduced. Habituation is associated with signals from the ACC and medial prefrontal cortex that reduce amygdala arousal (Gyurak & Etkin 2014). Thus, predictable therapeutic routines and home structure over repeated sessions help to establish safety through the regulatory system of habituation.

The therapist's personal qualities and behaviors help further establish a climate of social safety. Attunement to the emotional responses of the child is a pre-eminent quality in therapy. Attunement is expressed as awareness that the child is emotionally stressed, in physical pain, or is cognitively struggling (Hughes 2007). Empathy for the struggle is expressed (e.g., "Oh, this is hard for you," "You are worried about this"), and action is taken to modulate through changing the task (e.g., making it easier) or increasing the support (e.g., providing extra emotional, cognitive, or physical help). A triad of attunement–empathy–support creates the conditions for emotional regulation. The child experiences the actions of an adult as responsive to their needs and able to downregulate stress. A feeling of safety is promoted, and the underlying communication to the child is that their best interests are valued.

Under chronically stressful and traumatic situations, such as experienced by Anna, the hypothalamic–pituitary–adrenal (HPA) system is continually activated, causing high levels of cortisol in the bloodstream and affecting the body-neural receptors for the stress hormone, which then affects the regulatory feedback system for stress. Supportive attachment relationships reduce stress-based arousal (Cozolino 2006, pp.223–224). Children such as Anna with insecure attachment may find relationships a frequent source of stress, unable to receive the physiological benefits of intimacy and closeness. However, in the context of a third-party therapist providing high attunement to the responses of the child and creating a reliably safe physical and social environment, the high alert system may be dampened enough for new relationship experiences to be tolerated. In this context, the social engagement system may be activated toward emotional health.

Condition two: Emotional and social engagement

Introduced to the Theraplay process, Anna's foster parents engaged in new interactions with her. Touch was included during play periods but in less stress-triggering contexts, such as hand clapping games, little piggies, or writing on each other's back. Nurture was introduced in small, brief moments, such as feeding Anna a caramel or licking chocolate off a spoon after making chocolate brownies together. Excitement and laughter were promoted through having spontaneous music and dance time, or walking across the room pretending to be different types of animals. Sometimes, Anna was invited to sit on her foster mother's lap as she was fed spoonfuls of ice cream; if relaxed, this could be followed by being cradled and rocked while her foster mother sang a special song. *You Are My Sunshine* became their theme song. Eye contact remained hard for Anna, so the foster parents inserted brief moments of warm eye contact throughout the day, such as when asking Anna to pass the salt at dinner or during a playful game.

In the safety and structure of therapist-guided sessions, Anna was able to enjoy being held by her foster parents while they told her stories. Many of the "made-up stories" had parallels to her own life, putting words to feelings they thought she might have. She used these metaphors as a jumping-off point to make sense of things that had happened to her.

Some changes happened rapidly, such as the decrease in tantrums from daily to once per week that occurred over three weeks of intensive work on trauma reactions to touch and being held. Other behaviors were slower to change, such as self-control in the face of frustration or annoyance. After becoming comfortable with touch, nurturing feeding, and hugs, it took over two years to fully receive and give sustained and warm eye contact.

Participation in a learning process requires emotional investment. Unless the process and people are perceived as appealing, limited involvement can be expected. Games or activities are presented that are expected to be appealing to the child, based on developmental level. While adults may find conversation or personality tests appealing and interesting, children are more likely to find social play meaningful. This is the stage at which a personal working relationship with the therapist is established. Through playful interaction and moments of surprise and laughter, the child can experience the therapist's qualities as empathic, accepting, and fun to be around.

Virtually all mammal infants engage in play, and human children are no exception to this biological imperative. Throughout the infant-to-adult developmental process, there exists neurologically determined drives for social interaction, motor development, language development, abstract thinking, and a variety of other skills. Play is merely the exercise of these skills for their pure enjoyment. Given proper conditions, a typically developing child will learn all these skills and find enjoyment in doing them. Social play begins at birth with parental touching, cooing, manipulation of body and limbs, facial expressions, and talking. Body-neural systems reward these experiences with a mix of dopamine, endogenous opiates, and oxytocin, and the body and brain respond with growth and skill acquisition (Cozolino 2006; Vanderschuren et al. 2016).

A critical question for the therapeutic support of children such as Anna, who have sustained attachment and trauma injuries, is how social and play therapy redirects the neurological and emotional systems back toward health. While clinical experience and research have demonstrated the efficacy of attachment-based family and play therapy (Wettig, Franke, & Fjordbak 2006), social and behavioral neurosciences rapidly elucidate the mechanisms of action involved. Two interacting systems are at the heart of change—the reward conditioning system and the social engagement system.

Anna had learned to associate emotional intimacy, touch, and social connectedness with pain, essentially creating a phobia-like panic response to being held, to emotional closeness expressed through touch, eye contact, and tone of voice, and to any conformity to the rules and directives of an attachment figure. While this fear conditioning was powerful, the therapists and foster parents trusted that reward conditioning in the service of social and emotional growth was equally, if not more, powerful.

Like most children, Anna was highly motivated by play and social interaction. Like most humans, she desired and needed touch, but there had to be a way for it to be safely experienced by her body-neural system. In the context of a structured, safe environment, with a third party (therapist) providing social signals and conditions for safety, Anna was able to relax enough to engage in playful and intimate activities with her foster parents, such as being held, rocked, and told stories. In the home environment, the foster parents reduced the intensity of connection through intimate snuggling or eye contact, and increased the intensity of social play, a type of play that involves face-to-face interactions, touch in the context of hand-clapping games, three-legged race challenges, physical safety spotting for somersaults and flips, and physical holding for exciting games of "motorboat" spinning and flying. Food was delivered in the context of hidden treats found by hot and cold games, taste-checking the chocolate brownies, or snuggling with her foster mother for ice cream time in which highly preferred ice cream was spoon-fed directly to her.

These games and activities strongly activated Anna's social engagement system, a body-neural system that operates through the interaction of the brainstem, limbic system, cortex association areas, and autonomic nervous system (Porges 2007). Social interaction involving eye contact, verbal sounds ranging from cooing through actual speech, and matching facial expressions is a neurobiological imperative similar to the developmental imperative to learn language or motor skills. While abrupt and loud sounds or pain may activate the sympathetic nervous system for fight or flight reactions, social signals through a lilting tone of voice, matching affect, coordinated motor play, and eye movements all trigger a reduced stress response through the myelinated portion of the vagus nerve, which causes regulation of the heart, lungs, and facial muscles. Phylogenetically older portions of the parasympathetic nervous system (PNS) are associated with deep calm, resting, digestion, and sleep. In certain life-threatening situations, the motor system shuts down for protection. The newer and specialized portion of the PNS involving vagal regulation of the heart, respiration, and facial expression allows for excitement and socially rewarding, engaging experiences. When social safety is perceived, the body-neural system is specifically primed to listen to vocal tones, share feelings through alternating emotional expressions, and gaze at another person's face. Social play and conversation are activated, the HPA axis is dampened, cortisol output is decreased, and the heart rhythm is regulated

(Porges 2009). Thus, a fear response was suppressed for Anna in favor of enjoyable social play.

Enjoyable social play can set the conditions for the reversal of fear conditioning but is insufficient by itself. Reconditioning through exposure to new nurturing experiences with an attachment figure is necessary. This works the same for all conditioned fears. For instance, if someone wishes to overcome a fear of boa constrictors—as did a colleague of mine who worked in a zoo and needed to demonstrate snake handling for educational programs—it is not enough to just do relaxation exercises; you must actually practice working with the feared animal. Indeed, it was not enough to play with small garter snakes. Although it could be an intermediary step, practicing play with the full-sized boa was necessary. And yes, he did it. I believe this analogy is apt for traumatized youth, for whom intimate social relationships seem to be life-threatening. The advantage for therapists and parents is that human children have an innate need to play with other humans, and a unique biological imperative and responsiveness to vocal tone and facial expressions. For Anna, the social play response was leveraged for reward conditioning that led to experiences of attachment intimacy.

Condition three: A reason to change and learning and reward conditioning

A well-established set of behaviors is difficult to change, and for good reason. Functionally, behaviors have survival value; physiologically, behaviors are neurologically wired to occur. It would be a tremendous hassle if you needed to relearn driving skills each time you got into a car. Learning involves establishing neuronal connections, growing dendritic branches, and potentiating chemical reactions. Automaticity increases the efficiency and usefulness of the learned behavior. For instance, an automatic mathematical calculation may enhance survival in math exams or business transactions, while automatic braking and swerving may increase survival on the road. It is quite foolish to try to undo your learning unless it is quite obviously maladaptive. In this context, there are four conditions for change:

- Current behaviors and experiences are maladaptive and cause suffering.

- New behaviors and experiences are cause for avoiding suffering and obtaining happiness.

- New behaviors and experiences are more effective at getting needs met than old ones.

- The new behaviors are doable at the person's level of development, or experiences can be neurologically accepted.

Pleasure or reward conditioning also involves the amygdala but includes additional regions, among them the VTA located in the midbrain, and has direct, reciprocal connections to the NA, the dopamine reward center. The VTA reciprocally connects with the amygdala, hippocampus, olfactory bulb, and large areas of the prefrontal cortex. In partnership with the VTA, the amygdala appears to assign a reward value to incoming stimuli, alerting the animal or person that a possible reward is coming (LeDoux & Phelps 2008). Hence, walking into your home and smelling a favorite food cooking alerts you that a pleasurable meal is imminent. The VTA's dopaminergic projections then create a cascade of effects: (a) pleasurable feeling state per effect on the NA; (b) visual and verbal memories associated with the smell; (c) motor actions toward the smell; and (d) thoughts related to the significance of the meal being cooked (i.e., who cooked it and why?). Furthermore, the VTA is especially sensitive to novelty and surprise rewards, powerfully conditioning the brain to remember, and associated positively with new, exciting, and fun rewards.

As Anna played with her foster parents, she experienced exciting new games, was surprised by special treats, and associated preferred activities of singing, clapping, popping bubbles, and doing gymnastic tricks with safe touch, parental eye contact, and following caregiver directions. Surges of dopamine output were triggered from the VTA by food, social surprise, and laughter. The associated pleasure response in the NA rewarded her for these connection experiences with her foster parents involving ice cream, chocolate brownies, and caramels. The amygdala creates new associations of the foster parents with safety, social fun, and positive sensations (taste, smell, touch, vestibular change). Repeated experiences over time competed with prior fear conditioning. Being held and rocked underwent rapid reconditioning change so that after three weeks of intensive outpatient attachment therapy, Anna described the experience of being hugged, rocked, and fed as pleasurable and comfortable. In contrast, accepting warm eye contact and following parental directives took a longer period of time to become comfortable for her.

Social play establishes highly specialized body-neural conditions physiologically. Both fear and emotionally engaging play with an attachment figure cause high alert. While fear causes high alert to be associated with sympathetic and HPA activation for danger, and narrows the window of possible actions to basic fight or flight, social-emotional play causes high alert that is associated with an expectation of reward, and it widens the repertoire of social responses. Attachment research with baby rats has demonstrated high amounts of NE release in the context of social interaction, smell, and touch from their mothers (Sullivan 2012). This NE is associated with vigilance, an alert state, and excitement. Humans have the same system, and it responds in a similar manner. Nursing, nurturing grooming, sensory play, and maternal smell are associated with the release of NE and the development of attachment. Oxytocin is also released and triggers pleasurable sensations associated with cuddling and closeness. Of particular significance, the release of these neurochemicals in the context of an attachment directly inhibits fear conditioning of the amygdala. Even after sensitive periods of attachment development have ceased for rats, the presence of the mother can modulate fear responses, promoting exploration and curiosity.

As Anna developed in subsequent years, she increasingly used her foster mother as a secure base, evidenced in being more discriminating about her interaction with strangers, showing increased emotional connection with her family, and progressively more reliance on her foster mother for advice and guidance. From a physiological standpoint, this reflects positive change and growth in neural systems. The VTA and amygdala both have direct connections to the ACC, an area in the mesial frontal lobe just above the corpus callosum. The ACC is critical for certain types of executive functions, particularly inhibiting impulses, performance monitoring, motivation, and regulation of emotions (Gyurak & Etkin 2014). It is intimately connected with surrounding frontal regions (ventral medial prefrontal cortex (vmPFC), dorsal medial prefrontal cortex (dmPFC), orbital frontal cortex (OFC)). These regions project directly back to the amygdala, completing a regulatory feedback loop. Functional MRI research has demonstrated how neglect can result in the disruption of this feedback system (Chugani *et al.* 2001). However, in Anna's case, her capacity for emotional regulation progressively improved over a period of years. Improved emotion regulation is associated with strengthening the feedback loop to the amygdala in the context of approaching the social environment in a more relaxed manner. In the relaxed and regulated presence of a caregiver, the prefrontal cortex (vmPFC/OFC) can assess the importance of a stimulus in the current context, sending a message to the amygdala and motor systems to deactivate survival systems. For example, in the presence of a scary animal (insect or lizard) or a new social situation (public performance), Anna was able to use cues from her foster mother or father to stay calm and approach the situation with curiosity, interest, or confidence.

Condition four: New behaviors used with persistence

Change is impossible without new possibilities. Alternatives must be presented, and these must be with the developmental skills and capability of the person changing. If a boy with autism who is non-verbal uses physical aggression to motivate his parents to get him food and toys, the alternative must be presented and be within his capacity. Learning to speak may be out of the question, but learning a picture communication system might be possible. It must be concretely demonstrated with him in real time using real food and toys. Once the child has experienced exchanging a picture for an item without the stress of a tantrum, the choice is clear. However, training in many pictures, across many communicators, and many foods and toys will be necessary for the new behavior system to be used reliably. Trauma desensitization is very similar to phobia desensitization. Fear of water is counteracted by training the body to first relax in the presence of water, and then to enjoy the experience of water. At this point, the fear conditioning is undone, and a new conditioned response is established.

Changing attachment behavior and trauma reactions are very similar to the examples of Anna and Benny. Anna needed to experience the enjoyable emotional benefits of safety, connection, and touch, in the context of new relationship interactions. For Anna, attachment avoidance was very obvious, with clear and direct fear conditioning. Conditions of safety in which small amounts of connection through touch, feeding, and eye contact could be experienced was the first step to being relaxed in the presence of intimacy and touch. Ongoing practice over an extended period was necessary for the enjoyable context of play and laughter paired with intimacy, touch, and new feelings. In time, the fear conditioning was undone, and a new relationship experience was established. Once a person can experience a sense of holistic love in the absence of fear, it is highly rewarding and self-perpetuating. This becomes the impetus for further change.

For families such as Anna's, persistence and grit are necessary as much for the parents as for the child. Learning new parenting methods requires the parents to undo their own childhood conditioning, to let go of strategies that might have short-term rewards but negative long-term consequences (e.g., yelling), and repeatedly practicing alternatives that feel new or uncomfortable. Faith is required to believe that exercising new skills, behaviors, and attitudes will produce more favorable results. Unfortunately, positive results may be delayed or inconsistent on initial attempts to change. Fear conditioning is very rapid for survival purposes, and extinguishing the conditioning takes multiple trials of a new stimulus–response connection. For this reason, persistence in newly learned skills is essential.

References

Akirav, I., & Maroun, M. (2007). The role of the medial prefrontal cortex–amygdala circuit in stress effect on the extinction of fear. *Neural Plasticity*, 1–11. doi:10.1155/2007/30873

Barr, M. L., & Kiernan, J. A. (1988). *The Human Nervous System: Anatomical Viewpoint* (5th edn). J. B. Lippincott & Co.

Cheng, D. T., Disterhoft, J. F., Power, J. M., Ellis, D. A., & Desmond, J. E. (2008). Neural substrates underlying human delay and trace eyeblink conditioning. *Proceedings of the National Academy of Sciences 105*, 8108–8113. https://doi.org/10.1073/pnas.0800374105

Chugani, H. T., Behen, M. E., Muzik, O., Juhász, C., Nagy, F., & Chugani, D. C. (2001). Local brain functional activity following early deprivation: A study of postinstitutionalized Romanian orphans. *NeuroImage 14*, 1290–1301. doi:10.1006/nimg.2001.0917

Cozolino, L. (2006). *The Neuroscience of Human Relationships: Attachment and the Developing Social Brain*. W.W. Norton & Co.

Gyurak, A., & Etkin, A. (2014). A Neurobiological Model of Implicit and Explicit Emotion Regulation. In J. J. Gross (Ed.), *Handbook of Emotion Regulation* (pp.76–90). Guilford Press.

Hughes, D. A. (2007). *Attachment-Focused Family Therapy*. W.W. Norton & Co.

Knight, D. C., Cheng, D. T., Smith, C. N., Stein, E. A., & Helmstetter, F. J. (2004). Neural substrates mediating human delay and trace fear conditioning. *The Journal of Neuroscience 24*(1), 218–228. https://doi.org/10.1523/JNEUROSCI.0433-03.2004

LeDoux, J. E., & Phelps, E. A. (2008). Emotional Networks in the Brain. In M. Lewis, J. M. Haviland-Jones, & L. F. Barrett (Eds), *Handbook of Emotions* (pp.159–179). Guilford Press.

Lezak, M. D., Howieson, D. B., Bigler, E. D., & Tranel, D. (2012). *Neuropsychological Assessment* (5th edn). Oxford University Press.

Petrof, I., Viaene, A. N., & Sherman, S. M. (2015). Properties of the primary somatosensory cortex projection to the primary motor cortex in the mouse. *Journal of Neurophysiology 113*(7), 2400–2407. doi:10.1152/jn.00949.2014

Phelps, E. A., & Labar, K. S. (2006). Functional Neuroimaging of Emotion and Social Cognition. In R. Cabeza & A. Kinstone (Eds), *Handbook of Functional Neuroimaging of Cognition* (Chapter 13). The MIT Press.

Porges, S. W. (2007). A polyvagal perspective. *Biological Psychology 74*(2), 116–143. https://doi.org/10.1016/j.biopsycho.2006.06.009

Porges, S. W. (2009). The polyvagal theory: New insights into adaptive reactions of the autonomic nervous system. *Cleveland Clinical Journal of Medicine 76*(Suppl. 2), S86–S90. doi:10.3949/ccjm.76.s2.17

Sullivan, R. (2012). Neurobiology of attachment to nurturing and abusive caregivers. *Hastings Law Journal 63*(6), 1553–1570. https://hastingslawjournal.org/wp-content/uploads/2014/03/Sullivan-63.6.pdf

Vanderschuren, L. J. M. J., Achterberg, E. J. M., & Trezza, V. (2016). The neurobiology of social play and its rewarding value in rats. *Neuroscience and Biobehavioral Review 70*, 86–105. doi: 10.1016/j.neubiorev.2016.07.025

Vijayakumar, S., Sallet, J., Verhagen, L., Folloni, D., Medendorp, W. P., & Mars, R. B. (2019). Mapping multiple principles of parietal-frontal cortical organization using functional connectivity. *Brain Structure and Function 224*, 681–697. doi:10.1007/s00429-018-1791-1

Wettig, H. H. G., Franke, U., & Fjordbak, B. S. (2006). Evaluating the effectiveness of Theraplay®. In C. E. Schaefer & H. G. Kaduson (Eds), *Contemporary Play Therapy: Theory, Research, and Practice* (pp.103–135). Guilford Press.

Chapter 3

Tele-Theraplay

A TELEHEALTH MODEL OF THERAPLAY

Andrea Bushala and Nicole Charney

Introduction

Throughout the evolution of psychotherapy and across theoretical models, the common denominator has always been the therapeutic relationship as a critical change factor. It is in this space of listening, connection, and trust where those who seek treatment can safely access their own history, consider their needs, and allow expression of powerful emotions, counting on the practitioner to guide them, assist with reflection, and contain the experience. The same features are true of the Theraplay model, but special features are present when working with children and families within a heavily experiential model.

A Theraplay session utilizes attachment-based play to create a relational experience through activities carried out in pairs, triads, or small groups. The child, practitioner, and parents generate different levels of intensity and rhythms within the session. Theraplay provides an experience wherein facial expressions, tone of voice, energy of movement, and body language are a fundamental part of emotional engagement, nurture, attunement, and connection. Theraplay sessions engage every participant in a multisensory experience involving active and slower moments and using multiple regions of the room. Due to this complexity, it can be difficult to imagine the model being used in a telehealth format.

Until the coronavirus pandemic, online Theraplay sessions were not considered a viable option for Theraplay intervention. The pandemic forced children and families to stay at home while causing a surge in mental health difficulties for children. Mental health worsened due to separation from friends, teachers, and extended family, due to loss through death, fear of illness and death, and adjustment to online learning. The pandemic caused questioning of social predictability and security. Touch among friends and family was reduced. Anxiety and depression problems in children increased worldwide. The COVID-19 pandemic created a humanitarian crisis across the globe that affected both physical and mental health, resulting in an estimated 3 million additional deaths globally through 2021 (WHO 2020, 2021). The need for family and child therapy services grew at a time when access to face-to-face services was necessarily reduced. Tele-Theraplay was developed as a response to this humanitarian crisis. Pandemic conditions put pressure on Theraplay practitioners to make the therapy system more flexible, more available, and more adaptable to help families.

One of the benefits of the pandemic pressure for online care was the acceleration of telehealth services globally (Wong *et al.* 2021). The global therapeutic community quickly adapted to using telehealth, and ingenuity in providing service this way was accelerated. The creation of a telehealth-based system of Theraplay has opened the door for many benefits, including: (1) geographically remote areas can be reached; (2) geographic regions with few practitioners can be reached; (3) cross-cultural and cross-language consultation for immigrants or non-English-speaking individuals is easier; (4) specialist care can be brought to places that lack specialists; and (5) intervention can proceed for patients with autoimmune disorders who are at risk with face-to-face contact (e.g., children with compromised immune systems). In this telehealth context, Theraplay provides a variety of positive experiences for children and their parents, adapting to this new context and using all the advantages of video communication. Theraplay focuses on the here and now through experiences of the body and the senses. While Tele-Theraplay restricts practitioner–client interventions to two senses—vision and hearing (personal communication with S. W. Porges with D. Lender, 2020)—other senses are activated between the participants on the other side of the screen from the practitioner (e.g., the child and parent). The practitioner has the challenge of activating all the senses through verbal instruction and demonstration.

Tele-Theraplay gives an experience of social integration for children. Children experience having someone on a weekly basis who is neither a teacher nor a family member. The practitioner becomes someone who cares, notices them, and connects with them in a safe, positive, and predictable way. The practitioner's presence in the life of children living through the pandemic gives certainty in uncertain moments, and the possibility of trusting and feeling safe in a virtual space different from home. In other words, it sends the message, "There are people other than my parents who can see me and make me feel good." This is a protective and preventive experience.

This chapter reviews the adaptation process to Tele-Theraplay, accompanied by clinical cases that illustrate Tele-Theraplay practice. We explain the challenges and solutions in adapting a face-to-face context to Tele-Theraplay, followed by suggestions on strategies, concrete activities, and the process for carrying out Tele-Theraplay from start to finish. Case illustrations for Tele-Theraplay further explain the step-by-step approaches.

Foreseen challenges of delivering Tele-Theraplay

We identified seven eminent challenges to delivering Tele-Theraplay:

- *Limiting nonverbal interaction:* Theraplay has historically been an interactive, face-to-face therapeutic intervention. Using Theraplay rituals, parents and children experience each other through the senses, and change their relationship through new positive experiences that involve touch, eye contact, surprise, laughter, regulation, and excitement. It can be a challenge to conduct this type of interaction and experiential therapy over the internet.

- *Lack of Theraplay props:* Theraplay often utilizes physical materials such as bubbles or lotion to increase opportunities for interaction between parent and child. Unfortunately, there is no opportunity for the practitioner to transmit these materials through the internet.

- *Inability of therapist to use touch:* Touch is typically an integral part of the therapeutic experience. The practitioner uses touch to connect, structure, engage, and comfort. There is no opportunity for touch to be used by the practitioner when they occupy a different space from the client's.

- *Reduced ability for the therapist to use eye gaze:* The use of eye contact for connection is essential. A steady gaze communicates social attention, and communicates to the client that they are being experienced by the practitioner. Technological limitations exist to the quality of eye contact through a camera and screen transmission.

- *Moment-to-moment revision and repair of social exchanges are part of the therapy.* Social nuances break in attention or connection, and non-verbal communication can be harder to navigate in a virtual environment.

- *Physical unavailability:* Practitioners demonstrate and orchestrate the therapy session at the moment. They typically manage the room by engaging everyone in physical activities in the space. When the practitioner is not physically in the shared space, their presence is minimized, and the parents do not necessarily have the physical support they need to manage their child.

- *Limitations in modeling for parents:* Parents are often learning by observation through the modeling of the practitioner with the child in real time in the session. In telehealth, the practitioner is limited to modeling through voice alone as there is no opportunity to step in and support the parent, or use physical touch to structure and enhance the experience.

Theraplay adaptations for a telehealth model

After many trials, we came up with eight solutions to mitigate challenges in delivering Tele-Theraplay.

Solution one: Increase parent training and parent involvement

In order for the work to be successful, practitioners know that the parent's presence is key to compensating for a clinical practitioner not being in the room. Some parents are able to take on a more central role in the therapeutic process quite quickly. Practitioners meet more frequently with parents alone at the beginning of the therapeutic relationship. Practitioners and parents then work together to brainstorm about the child's possible reaction to activities, so they can be proactive in the face of resistance. Practitioners are more intentional in explaining the activities in detail and the goals behind them. Many practitioners realize that without being able to be in the room with the family, parents' skills improve more quickly than with in-person sessions. Parents are observed to be more structured, more proactive, and more hands-on with their children. Practitioners are observed to be more attuned to the parents, reading non-verbal cues and changes in affect and energy to stay ahead of challenging behaviors due to their diminished ability to regulate through physical support.

 CASE ILLUSTRATION

The parent demonstration was planned to include both parents alone, but the toddler sibling would not go down for a nap, so the practitioner recommended having the child in the session. The practitioner guided the family through a variety of activities that would be as appealing to a toddler as to a six-year-old. This allowed both parents to participate rather than have one parent relegated to childcare while the other parent attended the session. The practitioner walked the parents through a series of structure and engagement activities, including beanie baby drop, sticker match, bubble pop, and lotion/slippery slip. The practitioner processed what the experience was like for the parents and answered a few minutes of questions from each. The parents were able to see their younger child react with delight to the activities, especially the slippery slip and bubble pop, so they could visualize how their other son would enjoy the time with them. They also questioned how therapy could address the angry outbursts that occurred in times of stress. However, they predicted it would go well because of the fun activities and how their child "always does well when he gets all our attention." The practitioner processed the parents' expectations of their work together, explained the concept of being in the present, and how joyful ways of connecting with their child addressed more significant unmet needs. The practitioner also asked the parents to brainstorm other challenging behavioral issues that might come up in session so they could be ready for a wide range of behaviors from the child.

Solution two: Use only supplies that are on hand, or no supplies at all
Thinking through the supplies needed often leads to developing the activity plan with telehealth. Rather than developing a plan and grabbing supplies off a shelf, supplies become the driver of the activities. Some families lack access to supplies, some have limited supplies, and others are fully supplied. For families lacking supplies on hand, it is important to remember that social play requires only two people engaging in some form of physical or vocal interaction. Activities of hand clapping, peek-a-boo, songs, and sound imitation become more important, as do games that require no materials, such as "Mother may I," "Red light/green light," or "Simon says."

CASE ILLUSTRATION

During the COVID-19 lockdown, Steven's parents were rarely shopping and were not bringing their mail into the house more than once a week, so even mailing supplies to them was challenging. Due to these precautions, the session plans included only things the family already had on hand, including aluminum foil, cotton balls, lotion, and newspaper. Most of the activities involved only each other. The standard activity list included:

- Lotion spots (lotion)
- Slippery slip (lotion)
- Lotioned thumb war (lotion)

- Hand stack (no supplies)

- Eye blink game (no supplies)

- Jumping off the couch to a parent on cue (no supplies)

- La la magnets (no supplies)

- Copy my silly face (no supplies)

- Peanut butter and jelly (no supplies)

- Silly walk (no supplies)

- Mirroring game (no supplies)

- "Simon says" (no supplies)

- "Miss Mary Mack" (no supplies)

- Five-part handshake (no supplies)

- Change three things (no supplies)

- Foil prints (foil)

- Newspaper punch (newspaper)

- Newspaper war (newspaper)

- Newspaper basketball (newspaper or tissue paper)

- Cotton ball blow (cotton ball)

- Cotton ball touch (cotton ball)

- Cotton ball pick up with toes (cotton balls).

Solution three: Rely on guiding the parent's touch

Touch is a cornerstone of early childhood experience and essential to healthy development (Courtney, Nolan, & Gil 2017). The challenge with telehealth is being able to teach the parent about and practice touch from another space. The Marschak Interaction Method (MIM) will give the practitioner a strong sense of the parent's ability to use touch and the child's reaction to touch. Based on that understanding, the practitioner will need to assess how much practice time they require to support the parent in being comfortable with and responsive in the use of touch with their child. If there is no co-parent, the parent could bring a friend to the parent demonstration session, so they have the opportunity to practice and truly feel what it is like to touch and be touched. Have the parent experiment with pressure and pacing of touch as well, since every person has their own experience of touch and what feels good for them.

CASE ILLUSTRATION

In the MIM, it was noted that the father was tentative about touch. He read the "Lotion card" and laughed loudly, saying, "This is weird." The child put his arm out for lotion but repeated Dad's comment while looking away from Dad. Dad quickly lotioned the child's arm, then returned the lotion to the MIM kit and moved on without having the child lotion him. The practitioner processed this with Dad, who shared that he didn't think a seven-year-old should be lotioned by his parents. Dad was able to see that his child was open to the experience and was willing to experiment with some playful touch with Mom before starting with the child. The practitioner decided to wait before asking Dad to provide a purely nurturing touch until after the first parent meeting. The practitioner had Dad practice putting lotion spots on the freckles of Mom's hand and then to try to hold on while Mom pulled away. Both Mom and Dad enjoyed the slippery slip game, and Dad immediately said, "Steven's going to love this." The practitioner had Dad practice with some firm grips of Mom's arms and some easier grips, and had Mom talk about what felt best for her body. Then the parents reversed their roles, and Mom went through all the same activities with Dad. By the end of the demonstration session, Dad was able to deliver lotion spots, slippery slips, and the weather report backrub in ways that felt good to Mom. Both parents tried a few activities with their other child and laughed at his delight as they slipped off his arm and rolled back onto the carpet.

Solution four: Providing connection through eye gaze

Eye contact communicates connection, attunement, and trust between people. Eye contact with a calm and loving adult communicates to the child that they are seen and understood. In telehealth, it can be a challenge for the practitioner to establish eye contact long enough to connect with the parent and child, but also know when to transition for the parent to take over and lead the child. The practitioner also needs to practice and rehearse the activities enough with the parent so that the parent is not turned to watch the screen rather than looking at the child's face during the activities. As with touch, practicing and processing with the parents in preparation for family sessions is key to managing eye contact in telehealth.

CASE ILLUSTRATION

During the MIM, Dad's eye contact with Steven was present but inconsistent. Dad could see from the video clips that when he held his child's gaze, Steven appeared to attend to tasks longer and understand more of what was being asked of him. The practitioner role-played a series of games that involved eye contact through the screen, including the eye blink game and "Copy my silly face." After Dad was able to understand the activity, the practitioner had Dad lead with the practitioner and then with Mom. Again, the parents and practitioner tried to guess what the child's reaction would be and brainstormed ways to get around any potential resistance.

Solution five: Rupture and repair

As with in-person sessions, there will be moments that go off plan. Parents may be overwhelmed and unfocused, children may be resistant, and sometimes the internet connection may freeze or fail completely. At each point where there is disconnect or discord, there is an opportunity for repair and reconnection. Even if there is a loss of connection because the internet cuts out, a connection can be deepened through logging on again and reconnecting with a smile and a face that communicates the desire to be back together.

 CASE ILLUSTRATION

The practitioner explained that the protocol for using technology would be to minimize outside distractions that might rupture the connection. The parents selected their basement as the best place for sessions where there would be minimal disruptions from other family members. They were coached to turn off email notifications during sessions, close the basement doors, and keep their phones on and near them should the internet connection go out. When the internet connection was disrupted during a storm, the practitioner could call Dad in less than a few minutes and complete the session via FaceTime.

Solution six: Managing, demonstrating, and orchestrating

Being in separate spaces means the practitioner must engage in more forethought and "what if" thinking before the sessions begin. Each activity should be practiced with the parent beforehand. Parent experiences need to be processed. Talking through the range of possible responses a child may have to any given activity and the parent's reflection on those responses is also critical to the session's success. Only then can the parent and practitioner move on to work with the child. The practitioner will set up the activities and then give verbal support to the parent throughout the activity. The practitioner can also participate as needed. For example, the parent can make a foil statue of a child's body part while the practitioner hides their eyes. The practitioner can guess the body part when the parent and child have completed the foil statue. The practitioner needs to keep track of the energy flow, levels of resistance, and the timing of the session, and lead the parent through with subtle verbal cues (e.g., "Okay, Dad, we have time to do one more game before the feeding" or "Grandma, it looks as if Tommy is a bit tired this afternoon, so we will go right to the feeding activity now").

CASE ILLUSTRATION

To begin with, the practitioner kept the sessions short, going no longer than 30 minutes with the child. At the beginning of each session, the parent would enter the room and log on to the session. The practitioner would allow 10 minutes to check in on the parent's affective state and work to co-regulate the parent before starting the session, if needed. The parent had been briefed the night before about the activities, and supplies were sent if the parents lacked the items at home. Steven had a very positive experience right from the start. He was eager to interact with his father, and because he was complying and enjoying the interaction, Dad's beliefs about his relationship with his son shifted rapidly. Both Dad and Steven began to look forward to the sessions, and Dad started incorporating activities into their daily lives before the practitioner suggested it. After the first parent meeting at the end of the first month, Dad's work schedule shifted so he was no longer available during the session time. The practitioner abruptly shifted to work with Mom, and the tone of the work changed. Sessions with Mom were strained from the start. Her need for compliance in session was much more pronounced than in the MIM. Mom's work stress escalated, and the lack of childcare support after nearly a year had her living in a constant state of worry and exhaustion. Mom explained that she needed her seven-year-old to listen, and found it challenging to be reflective on his experience during the pandemic. It was also challenging for Mom to come to session and have a therapeutic experience different from the experience Dad had shared. It was decided to take a break from Theraplay for a month while Mom started work with her own practitioner. In the meantime, Steven continued 30-minute sessions that combined child-centered work and bibliotherapy.

At month three, Mom returned to the sessions more in tune with her own experiences. A protocol was developed that worked better for meeting her needs so she could meet her child's needs. Every other week was a scheduled parent meeting. The practitioner and Mom met at night after both children were asleep, and each had a cup of tea. The session began with Mom sharing her best parenting moment, and they then viewed video clips from the previous session where things had gone well. With each clip, the practitioner asked Mom to look for anything that felt good to her or Steven. The first parent sessions were awkward, and Mom struggled to identify and share her strengths. Over the next several months, Mom could increasingly identify all that she was doing well. She felt good about her parenting and the practitioner began to notice less resistance in session.

Solution seven: Modeling from afar

Modeling that is used to take place in the session now needs to occur before the session. As parents no longer have the luxury of watching the practitioner execute activities and modifications in session, Tele-Theraplay requires that the modeling takes place beforehand. During the session, the practitioner has only the use of voice, hand motion, and facial expression at their disposal to help create a sense of support and safety. Fortunately, Theraplay practitioners are highly trained in being very emotionally expressive and creative, two skills that help create a playful and connected session whether in person or telehealth mode.

 CASE ILLUSTRATION

During the newspaper punch activity, Mom was unable to get the newspaper taut enough for Steven to punch through. The practitioner held a piece of newspaper in her hands, demonstrating alongside Mom. The practitioner coached by saying, "See how my arms are straight and pulling the paper tight, right along the middle crease of the paper?" and moved her body sideways so Mom could see how to straighten her arms and hold them to the side. While Mom worked on getting her technique down, the practitioner praised Mom and the child each time he punched through the paper. "Wow, look at the muscles on our boy, Mom... Now, Mom, set the paper to one side because we will be using it again for the next activity... Instead of counting 1-2-3, Mom, this time, use your boy's favorite color as the cue to punch." The practitioner stayed present, helping support the engagement between parent and child for six rounds of punching. When the practitioner noticed Steven trying to kick the paper, she helped Mom transition to the newspaper basketball throw activity, again providing the structure needed to create physical and psychological safety for the parent and child.

Solution eight: Use the space beyond the screen

As practitioners, we expect that the child's attention will wander from the screen and that they will struggle to stay still and comply. It is essential to communicate to parents that struggles with attention are expected and developmentally normal. Furthermore, using space outside the screen is acceptable for short periods. Without this reassurance, parents will feel stressed by expecting the children to stay within screen boundaries and always comply. We must provide moments of movement, expansion, and challenge, and accept that participants may move off-screen during these activities. Because the child is at home, we can also expect the child to occasionally run away from the room or leave to get a toy or a snack or say "hi" to the dog, or numerous other things. While working with parents to minimize distractions, the practitioner needs to integrate this need for movement into the session. For example, activities we have used include having the child run and get something from their house that starts with the letter "a," have the child get a toy and the parent guess what it is, or do a piggyback ride with a parent to obtain a snack and bring it back to the area. A fun activity is to have the parent hide an item or two (e.g., jelly beans) somewhere in the house, and at the moment the child needs movement, direct the child to run and look in the hiding place (e.g., "Go look under the cushion of the big black chair and bring back what you find there").

Positive factors to consider

There are some positive factors to consider in Tele-Theraplay. First, capitalize on increased comfort with technology: it may be a comfort for families when they are in their familiar space. For children and parents anxious about new experiences, being in their own homes may lend a greater sense of felt safety than traveling to a clinic, office, or agency. Practitioners may find families settling into session more quickly and being able to stay engaged for longer periods of time. Therapeutic experiences may be more easily generalized in the home when the relationship originated there. Second, many children and parents are very comfortable with technology and relationships that are technology-dependent. For many of the clients we serve, working with technology is a non-issue. Children, and even some parents, grew up with smartphones, iPads, handheld video games, and talking to other family members via video. Families are often used to technology challenges and can move through glitches in connections or services. This makes working remotely fairly easy to normalize and then get to the business of healing. Third, telehealth can be far easier to schedule than in-person appointments. With remote schooling leaving big chunks of the day open, extracurricular activities on hold, and a parent available in the next room, many more times are available to connect with families. As people return to pre-pandemic life, it is still easier to click on a link and be in session rather than drive across town to an office. Families can often fit in an appointment before school or at lunch. And practitioners who only have a down-the-hall commute have extra time to accommodate families. In addition, virtual work requires less dedicated transition and clean-up time. When the supplies and play are happening in the family's home, the clean-up is on them. Finally, Tele-Theraplay has increased the option for including various members of the family. Sessions that could have been desirable but difficult to coordinate can now happen, thanks to therapy reaching into people's homes through the screen. In our experience, including siblings, parents, grandparents, and even pets has generated experiences of self-regulation in the family itself, moments of encounter, complicity, and a sense of belonging for all family members.

Contraindications when using Tele-Theraplay

The use of technology must be consistent with the treatment goals. The practitioner will need to look at each family and their functioning to decide if telehealth can support meeting goals and moving a family towards improved functioning. The client or parent may not fully understand the potential benefits and limitations of technology for therapy. It is imperative that the practitioner has an honest conversation with parents about the limitations of working this way. Concerns and contraindications are reviewed below. In some situations, the client is developmentally incapable of using technology. For some people, the use of technology is stressful. If the technology adds to the anxiety or distress the family is already facing, then it would be best to maintain in-person services if at all possible.

Practitioners must consider whether the technology meets the needs of the client. For clients who are dysregulated or triggered and who act out aggressively, the practitioner may find it more challenging to co-regulate them. If a child becomes very distressed or dysregulated at home, the parent may lack the skills to bring about a state of calm. Resulting tantrums, aggression, or property destruction can be dangerous and costly, and the situation can diminish confidence in therapy. In these situations, face-to-face sessions are preferable, or a very slow pace of therapy and parent coaching will be required.

All possible efforts are made to protect the client's privacy. In some home settings, such as with a number of siblings, extended family, or roommates, lack of privacy may inhibit the freedom of sharing information. Other family members may disrupt sessions, or members of the household not involved with therapy may see portions of a session and become dismissive, undermining practitioner and parent efforts. Confidentiality issues and privacy guidelines must be reviewed with the client and parents. The practitioner must obtain written consent for telehealth services.

Setting up Tele-Theraplay practice

1. Preparing yourself as the practitioner

Before starting a telehealth Theraplay session, some preparations are necessary, similar to how you would prepare for an in-person session. Create a Theraplay space that includes room for your computer and for you to demonstrate or join the activities in session. Ensure effortless transitions up and down from the floor or your seat. Maximize your internet connection—the use of an ethernet cable may ensure a strong connection. It is best when the audio is in sync with the visuals, and the video is fluid.

Optimize your own ability to focus on the task at hand. Turn off notifications on your computer and phone. Notifications can be very distracting to both you and your client. Have the parent's phone number handy should you or the parent lose connection and need to create a plan at the moment for how to move forward with the session. Have all the session supplies nearby, including pen and paper, a drink, tissues, throat lozenges, and anything else possibly needed close at hand. Leaving the screen space can feel to a client like you have left the therapy room, many of whom are already struggling with intense feelings of isolation and/or abandonment.

2. Preparing the family

Similar to how you prepare yourself for a Theraplay session, help the parent prepare for sessions as well. To increase structure and define the boundaries of the play area, parents should create a Theraplay space. They will need a sufficient area in which to stand and play. Any unsafe items should be removed. A blanket or sheet should be placed on the ground to delineate this play space. Pillows should be used to mark where each person is to sit.

Ask the parent to maximize their internet connection either by increasing their home Wi-Fi speed, sitting near the router, or using an ethernet cable. Ask the parent to turn off pop-up notifications on their computer and put away their cell phone or other technology, so as to avoid distraction. The parent and child should have drinks and anything else they may need to make themselves easily accessible. It's also important to work with the parent to prepare for activities, including sending them the list of supplies and perhaps the full plan ahead of the session.

3. Preparing the telehealth session

Planning telehealth sessions starts with the clinically typical therapy sessions. The intake is the first meeting and should be conducted with both parents if possible. Remember that you are both gathering important biopsychosocial information as well as building rapport for a therapeutic alliance. The MIM can be conducted virtually by either sending the supplies and directions for activities in a sealed box to be opened once the parent and child have logged on, or by asking the parent to gather items they have at home (e.g., two little animal toys, paper and pencils, lotions, a dress-up hat, etc.) and putting the directions up on screen via a PowerPoint slide. The parent feedback session should have parents logged on to review the video remotely as you walk them through edited video clips. Have the parents share their thoughts about their experience as well as their child's. The next session, the parent demonstration, will be critical in determining how soon you can bring the child into the work. After the parent demonstration, the parent should clearly grasp how to deliver a handful of activities on the dimensions that have been focused on. They should feel comfortable taking direction from you, and, most importantly, they need to understand the goal of the activities. Keep in mind that the parent is now your co-practitioner. You will not be able to step in to correct or redirect. That will be up to the parent. If you are questioning the parent's capacities for remaining regulated and connected during session, you will need to engage in more intense parent work.

Whether conducting in-person or virtual sessions, it is important to create rituals. Using the entrance to the therapy area as an activity is an important step in setting the tone for the session. The goal is for the child to understand that the adult is focused on creating an experience filled with a joyful connection that begins from the moment the session starts. If possible, have the parent turn on the computer and then join the child on the blanket or sheet or outside the room, to have them enter the Theraplay space together.

As with in-person work, each session should begin with a check-in activity focusing on the child, giving them positive attention and setting the tone for everyone's work together. Similarly, at the conclusion of the session, the parent and child should exit the room together, signaling to the child that the therapy time together is complete for the day. The very same activity used for the entrance may be used for exiting the room. Be aware of the energy level of the start and ending activities. Notice whether the activity used at the start of the session was up- or downregulating, and whether that will be counterproductive to the flow of the session just completed. You want the child to leave the session in a regulated state, setting a tone for adjustment to the rest of the day, which may include school, playtime, chores, or mealtimes in the same environment. As with in-person sessions, the goal is for the adult to be the leader of every part of the experience, from the beginning to the end of the session.

The role of the practitioner using the four dimensions of structure, engagement, nurture, and challenge
Structure in guiding parents in telehealth

1. Create environmental regulation—this is much more challenging when working in a space that is not your own, especially during COVID-19, with so much more distraction than at other times:

   - Review the best set-up of space.

   - Encourage meeting at a time when the child is more likely to be regulated.

   - Support the parent in having all supplies at hand.

2. Create a predictable and organized experience for the parent and child:

   - The parent needs to understand the mechanics of the activity.

   - The parent needs to understand the goal of the activity.

   - If possible, the parent should have experienced the activity themself.

   - The practitioner should lead only until the parent can take over.

3. Create a positive experience for the parent and child:

   - The practitioner should have an informed sense of how the dynamics may play out—they should have adjustments and alternatives prepared.

   - The practitioner will need to be attuning to the experience of the parent and child and supporting joy and moments of connection.

4. Establish relational regulation:

- The practitioner will use themselves as co-regulator, as if they are in the room. For dyads where the energy is low, the practitioner will transmit their energy through the screen. When the dyad moves towards dysregulation, the practitioner will use their social engagement systems to bring them back to their "window of tolerance," the zone in which both parent and child can handle interaction in an emotionally regulated manner.

- Structure activities that translate well into telehealth are peanut butter and jelly, "Simon says," bubble pop, eye blink game, runner bean, land/sea/air, and mirroring.

Engagement in guiding parents in telehealth

The practitioner models for the parent appropriate use of their own social engagement system (SES), to support the feeling of felt safety. The practitioner models eye contact, prosody of voice, and position of the body needed for each activity. Additionally, the practitioner must promote a calm physiological state (neuroception of safety). The practitioner must make accommodations required for the parent to read the practitioner's physiological state through a screen (sit closer to the screen, speak slower, set the camera so the gaze feels close to natural eye contact), allowing for the parent to borrow the calm from a distance. It's important for the practitioner to manage their physiological state, which can be harder than with in-person work. The practitioner must focus on the child in an intensive and personal way, just as with in-person work. The practitioner should direct parents to do all that they would do in session, from sitting closer to each other to using touch to looking directly into the child's eyes. The parent is the "boots on the ground" support. The goal continues to be to engage the parent and child in attachment-enhancing experiences. The practitioner should be the leader so the parent can be free to be in the moment with the child. Depending on the level of the parent's attunement and responsiveness, the practitioner may need to speak for the child's experience when necessary.

Some engagement activities that translate well into telehealth are blow me over, pop cheeks, foil prints (the parent can make prints and the practitioner can guess the body part over the screen), "Copy my silly face," special handshake, imaginary ball toss, and change three things.

Nurture in guiding parents in telehealth

The role of the practitioner for the parent in nurturing activities is to walk the parent through delivering several gentle, caring, and soothing activities to the child. Be sure to provide the psychoeducation parents need to understand the importance of meeting their child's unfulfilled younger needs. This includes helping the parent identify and meet physical needs such as creating a soft place to sit or providing a drink when the child is thirsty, reflecting back, and accepting feelings that arise. This communicates to the child that they are not alone in their feelings, whether positive or uncomfortable feelings arise in session. Lastly, the practitioner should look for opportunities to express appreciation or concern for both the child *and* parent, creating the holding environment they are expecting the parent to create for their child.

Some nurture activities that translate well into telehealth are weather report, warm up or cool down hands, find lines or special shapes in the palm, imaginary face paint, lotion or powder prints, lotion special spots, and feeding.

Challenge in guiding parents in telehealth

The role of the practitioner as support for the parent in challenge activities is to model for the parent how to support the child's growth within the zone of proximal development. The practitioner's role is to help the parent understand what the child is capable of and help take them just a bit further each time. Also, developing a repertoire of activities that should support partnership and collaboration between the parent and child is necessary; challenge is not about direct competition, especially between parent and child. For children who seek challenge, the practitioner can create activities that set the parent and child as a team against the practitioner. Lastly, the practitioner needs to model how to encourage the child to take mild, age-appropriate risks.

Some challenge activities that translate well into telehealth are bubble tennis or bubble catch, feather blow and catch, balloon bop, cotton ball toe pick up, and straight face challenge.

CASE ILLUSTRATION 1

Steven was a seven-year-old adopted child who has struggled with explosive behavior and defiance for the past two years. Due to the pandemic, classes had moved to an online format and his behavior had escalated to daily tantrums that were becoming increasingly violent and destructive. The family was isolated and had lost all of their social support, including friends, neighbors, babysitters, and athletic extracurriculars. Both parents worked full-time in healthcare-related fields, so work was extremely challenging at the time. The parents were increasingly stressed, and their marriage was feeling the strain. There was also a biological sibling (toddler) in the household whose behavior was fairly typical, but the parents felt as if they could not handle any more non-compliance from either child.

The intake session was scheduled for late in the evening so the parents could speak freely about their family life while their children were asleep. Dad presented as disengaged and tired. Mom was weepy and talked quickly, with little focus. The session ran for 90 minutes, and although the practitioner wanted to gather more biopsychosocial background, she realized that the parents needed to feel heard to relieve some of the pressure they were under. The parents shared that until the pandemic, they felt that they could manage their Steven's behaviors. In kindergarten, his behavior became more challenging. He would have two to four tantrums a day, and each could last for up to 40 minutes. The birth of his sister seemed to have caused a decrease in his ability to handle disappointment and frustrations. When COVID-19 forced schools to shift to an online format and the parents were forced to work at home without childcare, their family life "became unmanageable for all of us." The lack of boundaries between work and home, endless days of the same routine, sleep disruption due to the baby, and loss of childcare support exhausted their emotional resources, and they found themselves angry at each other and Steven almost continuously. The parents could remember a time when they adored their son and the time they spent with him. There were still parts of the day that went well, but they were rare. The parents stated their goal for therapy was to get support for themselves so they could have the skills they needed to raise happy, functional children.

The MIM session was set up for a few days later during the daytime, when the youngest would be sleeping. The practitioner mailed the activities and the few supplies she felt the family would not have on hand (two squeaky animals, 16 small blocks, and a few silly hats), and asked the family to gather the other supplies (two pieces of paper, two pencils, lotion, and a snack). The MIM was recorded via Zoom, and was able to be completed with both parents at the same session.

The parent feedback session was also scheduled for later in the evening, so the parents had uninterrupted time while the children slept. The baby woke up crying, though, and Mom spent most of the hour walking in and out of the session, trying to quiet the baby. The practitioner provided a write-up of the key points so Mom would not feel as if she had missed anything while she was out of the room. The parents and practitioner agreed that the lack of structure and engagement led to Steven feeling unsafe in his parents' care. Their understandable distraction had also created an environment where Steven's behavior had escalated in his effort to get some response from his parents. They did not notice when things went well, but had a very big reaction when he misbehaved. Due to Mom's feelings of being overwhelmed at work and with the toddler's demands, it was agreed to begin work with Dad and Steven the following week. A parent demonstration session was scheduled for a few days later, at a time when Steven was attending online school.

Theraplay sessions began the next week. The practitioner provided psychoeducation around developmental challenges as they related to transitions and sibling dynamics. As the summer arrived, a safety protocol opened up, and Mom hired a sitter three mornings a week to reduce the caregiving workload. Mom and Dad began each day the sitter arrived with a 30-minute walk without the children, and reported that it changed their moods for the better part of the day.

Five months into therapy, the family reported that they felt good enough to move to a session every other week. The parents planned the sessions and led most of the activities. When Steven resisted, he could be engaged easily, and the increased confidence both parents had in creating structure was positively affecting the entire household. The family now sees the practitioner once a month, which they have chosen to continue until school resumes in the fall.

CASE ILLUSTRATION 2

Fernando was four years old, living with his parents and a two-year-old younger sister. They lived by the seaside, two hours from the city, and had no access to therapeutic services in their area. The mother was a psychologist and took advantage of the fact that Theraplay was being offered online during the pandemic. The parents' concern was that Fernando had a very low frustration tolerance and was increasingly demanding parental attention. He enjoyed imaginary play, becoming absorbed into characters. The parents were also concerned that the play choices tended to be feminine, like butterflies or ponies; during early interviews, this was particularly worrying and confusing for the mother.

The intake session: Fernando's story unfolded quite normally during the first years of his life, being a very desired and awaited baby by his parents. However, since his sister was born, everything was radically different. The younger sister had been born with a heart condition that caused three cardiac arrests during her first year of life, the last of which caused neurological damage with motor compromise. This situation generated extreme concern in the parents who had to dedicate themselves to their daughter's care and rehabilitation, leaving Fernando in the care of different caregivers, in addition to having no schooling experience due to the pandemic.

The parents were acutely aware of how Fernando's sister's life had negatively affected his emotional development. They wanted to reconnect with him, identify his needs, and be able to repair the emotional damage. At the time of the intake session, the sister was in rehabilitation and in a more stable state of health.

The therapeutic process: this was carried out online from beginning to end, and both parents participated in the sessions. A space in the house where the sessions were held was defined, and they had a bag with previously agreed materials: aluminum foil, a diary, handkerchiefs, balloons, bubbles, pens, cotton balls, paper, pencils, stuffed animals, etc., and always the blanket and a snack.

At first, the sessions were very complicated. Fernando avoided looking at the camera and often failed to follow the practitioner's instructions. The practitioner's perception was that he wanted to take advantage of that special moment when he had his father and mother just for him; however, he became overly excited, sometimes hyperventilated, and wanted to be in charge. The parents tried to make him focus on the practitioner's instructions, especially the mother, for whom this situation generated the greatest frustration.

Despite some difficulty, in the beginning, Fernando greatly enjoyed the sessions. He waited for them with great excitement, and was always ready with a new toy to show the practitioner. However, very few activities worked smoothly, or they were accomplished only for a brief moment before they became disorganized. Fernando threw himself at his mother, hung up on his father, and generally got hyperexcited. The practitioner sought to generate greater regulation by making those same movements in a lower tone, in slow motion, with a whispering voice, and thus be able to give some regulation to the intensity in which Fernando operates.

Fernando was a restless child who wanted to be in control of the sessions and the games. Most of the time, he arrived disguised as a superhero and stayed in that role. At first, the parents were very stressed that he would not follow directions or pick up other toys, or that he became more defiant or disinterested in what the practitioner was trying to generate on the other side of the camera. The practitioner had more sessions with the parents alone, to help them with their anxiety. It was emphasized that they could leave behavior management to the practitioner. The practitioner noted that some avoidance or disruptiveness did not imply that the session was not working. On the contrary, his behavior could be used as his communication, and the challenge as adults was to be attuned to his emotional reactions, including his frustration. The practitioner wanted Steven to feel the supportive presence of his parents and the practitioner, and unconditional positive regard, and only from there could they expect greater flexibility in Fernando.

If Fernando arrived as a superhero, the practitioner and Fernando's parents all put on capes and began interacting from that place. Many times, Fernando would leave the room when the practitioner would talk to the parents and ask them to avoid looking for him. They talked about superheroes, powers, and what powers they saw in Fernando. Meanwhile, Fernando would be listening, ensuring they were still there for him, absorbing their positive thoughts about him. This promoted the self-regulating of emotions by leaving and entering. When he re-entered, he was incorporated, and the practitioner and his parents were always ready to receive him.

The fact that both parents were in the sessions facilitated the execution of the games. As a practitioner unable to control the materials and the space, one of the parents always fulfilled the role of assistant, generating the experiences between the child and the other parent. The parents were very much coordinated with each other, and together they were very supportive, helping them tolerate the most stressful moments of the sessions much better.

The therapeutic process occurred in the midst of a pandemic within the context of total quarantine. Having almost no socialization outside the family walls since preschool, the Theraplay time was the most exciting event of the week for Fernando. As the sessions progressed, Fernando remained active but much more regulated. He was less impulsive and became more accepting of his parents' physical contact, care, and closeness. The parents also managed in a magical way to enter Fernando's imaginary life and connect with his own needs for activity, creativity, and spontaneity.

Fernando and his family participated in the therapeutic process for about six months. At that time, he increasingly took part in the new challenges of the games, even asking for them and accepting the experience. He played with butterflies and ponies as one imaginary game among many, and his interests diversified. He could relax by moving from more intense activities to more neutral and calm ones. During this time, he also became more regressive with his parents, which created an opportunity for them to meet earlier developmental and emotional needs that Fernando still had pending.

Fernando became more flexible in his interests, and was also learning to properly read the social signals of the environment. The parents were very committed to the process of connecting with their son. They more readily saw his diverse traits and increasingly fell back in love with every aspect of him. They managed both their stress and his stress more effectively, and daily life became more enjoyable for them as a family with lower stress.

The completely online therapeutic process was a success and benefit for this family, and if this option had not existed, it is most likely that a long time would have passed before they sought help. Their location would have remained a barrier to services. The participation of two motivated and competent parents was fundamental to the process. The father was essential in supporting the mother in this process, who was actually much more sensitive and fragile.

For Fernando, Theraplay sessions were his contact with the world. It was his social experience beyond his nuclear family, and it was his own special space on the same day at the same time each week. For Fernando, Tele-Theraplay was his opportunity to connect with someone outside his family and read other types of social signals. The experience that Fernando was internalizing, in a context of so much insecurity and unpredictability, was the experience that there might be another adult in the world beyond his parents, who looked at him with appreciation, would take care of him, attend to his needs, and make him feel that the world could be a safe place.

References

Courtney, J. A., Nolan, R. D., & Gil, E. (2017). *Touch in Child Counseling and Play Therapy: An Ethical and Clinical Guide.* Routledge.

WHO (World Health Organization). (2020). Covid-19 disrupting mental health services in most countries, WHO survey. News, October 5. www.who.int/news/item/05-10-2020-covid-19-disrupting-mental-health-services-in-most-countries-who-survey

WHO. (2021). The impact of COVID-19 on global health goals. Spotlight, May 20. www.who.int/news-room/spotlight/the-impact-of-covid-19-on-global-health-goals

Wong, M. Y. Z., Gunasekeran, D. V., Nusinovici, S., Sabanayagam, C., Yeo, K. K., Cheng, C.Y., & Tham, Y. C. (2021). Telehealth demand trends during the COVID-19 pandemic in the top 50 most affected countries: Infodemiological evaluation. *JMIR Public Health and Surveillance* 7(2), e24445. https://publichealth.jmir.org/2021/2/e24445

Chapter 4

When It Is Too Hard to Play

INTEGRATING ADLERIAN PLAY THERAPY (ADPT) WITH THERAPLAY

Sam Bunnyfield and Gloria M. Cockerill

 ## CASE ILLUSTRATION

Seven-year-old Javier was referred by his caseworker for difficulty in school, acting out, refusing to comply with any requests, and overall difficulty in adjusting to his new foster placement. He had been removed from his parents' care due to abuse and neglect at two years old, along with four siblings. The siblings were currently placed in a foster home together, but this was their sixth home in five years. The foster parents were considering providing permanency for all of the children, but were concerned about Javier's struggle to adjust to their home. His foster parents described him as a "sweet boy" at times, but were worried about the behaviors they observed and struggled to help him manage. During an initial phone call, they shared: "Javier is defiant, easily frustrated, struggling to make friends, avoidant, and resistant to physical affection, and at the same time approaches strangers with ease, having emotional outbursts over the smallest changes, controlling, and having difficulty trying new things at home or school."

Introduction

Often practitioners are presented with new clients, like Javier, who exhibit complex symptomatology, a variety of comorbidities, and rich systems in which they are only a part. It is then up to the practitioner's training and experience to determine which therapeutic approach is most appropriate. Due to the complementary nature of Theraplay and Adlerian Play Therapy (AdPT), a seasoned and trained practitioner grounded in attachment and

Adlerian theories will be able to engage in an integrated approach with fluidity and confidence. However, practically speaking, there are some major distinctions between the two, as evidenced by AdPT's use of a more non-directive and playroom-based Phase 1, and Theraplay's specific focus on the parent–child relationship. This doesn't mean that the practitioner should avoid using these two models for a single client; in fact, just the opposite—it is imperative that when the need arises, the practitioner not only finds a way to meet the relational needs that many children come to treatment with, but also provides a space for processing and gaining conscious insight into their experiences and beliefs of the world. In facing these various challenges, as in the case of Javier, utilizing Theraplay with AdPT allowed for a clear path toward scaffolding the therapeutic work and needed interventions for the child and family system to experience healing.

At their core, sharing key underlying theoretical constructs outlined in attachment theory and individual psychology, Theraplay and AdPT allows practitioners to utilize aspects of both modalities to maximize the impact of the interventions in meeting the needs of complex children and families. While Theraplay is often utilized with children in foster care and adoptive families to foster a primary attachment (Doyle Buckwalter 2018), it has also been implemented successfully with biological families in which the behaviors of a child or caregiver have created stress, negatively impacting the attachment relationship (Lindaman, Booth, & Cockerill 2018). In addition, current research supports Theraplay as an evidence-based practice when working with internalizing behaviors and a promising practice when working with children on the autism spectrum.[1] It is important to note that due to the ability of practitioners to easily adapt the model to meet varying developmental needs and cultural values, practitioners have long provided anecdotal evidence that the model can be utilized with a broad range of issues in which relational dynamics have been stressed. Like Theraplay, AdPT has also been utilized successfully to provide treatment for a broad range of issues. Among these, practitioners have found that AdPT is particularly helpful when working with children and families who present with concerns regarding power and control, traumatic experiences, low self-esteem, and difficulty with social interactions (Kottman & Meany-Walen 2016). In addition to the broad range of clinical issues that AdPT can address, its recognition of the important role culture plays in shaping the individual's lifestyle allows for application across cultures. Where both modalities may be implemented in tandem is when the lack of sense of safety

---

[1] See https://theraplay.org/wp-content/uploads/2020/02/SAMHSA-approval.pdf

and limited attachment relationship hinder the child's ability to engage in the play therapy treatment process—when the playroom overwhelms, and at their core the child finds it too hard to play.

This chapter looks at how to integrate Theraplay with AdPT. Specifically, we (1) present an overview of AdPT constructs that are pertinent to integrating with Theraplay; (2) examine how to integrate AdPT with Theraplay by reviewing assessment and determinant factors; and (3) contextualize AdPT with Theraplay approaches through Javier's case illustration.

Adlerian Play Therapy (AdPT)

AdPT, developed by Terry Kottman in 1987, is based on Alfred Adler's individual psychology theory. Key tenets that underlie Adler's beliefs about individuals include: individuals are driven to be socially connected, their behaviors are purposeful and goal-directed, their perspective of life is subjective, and they are creative in nature (Kottman & Meany-Walen 2016). The underlying constructs of Adlerian theory draw from attachment theory as they each highlight the intrinsic need for the infant to connect with their caregiver, and they similarly note that the early caregiver–infant interactions shape the child's ability to develop relationships and their overall level of functioning (Weber 2003). According to Adler, through early life experiences with our family, we develop a lifestyle that implicitly organizes and shapes future interactions. Much like the development of the internal working model in attachment theory, the lifestyle represents the unconscious blueprint that guides relational interactions and coping style (Kottman 2011).

Key constructs: personality priorities, private logic, Crucial Cs, and goals of misbehavior

Assessing and developing a clear understanding of a client's lifestyle is a critical aspect that aids in the treatment planning for working with a particular client and their family. AdPT relies on several constructs as they strive to develop a clear picture of the lifestyle of the child, caregiver(s), and family, as outlined (Kottman & Meany-Walen 2016):

- *Personality priorities.* These can aid in helping the practitioner conceptualize and understand a client's lifestyle. Kottman and Meany-Walen (2016) describe personality priorities as a critical component of how each individual endeavors to experience a sense of connection and belonging/comfort. They are typically defined in four categories: comfort, pleasing, control, and superiority. While it is generally considered typical for each individual to possess all of these priorities in some capacity, the "priority" can be identified as the main approach an individual relies on for managing experiences and relationships.

- *Private logic.* Adler's underlying belief that people experience life through a subjective lens leads to the development of their private logic. An individual's private logic is how their life experiences have shaped their perceptions of themselves; their reality shapes their belief system about self, others, and the world (Kottman & Meany-Walen 2016). Through these perceived misconceptions in our relationships and life experiences, we develop a belief system (private logic) in which our truth is based on mistaken beliefs that shape our responses and future interactions. One of the aims of AdPT interventions is to shift this private logic to a system that relies more heavily on common sense.

- *Crucial Cs.* Developed by Amy Lew and Betty Lou Bettner, the construct of the Crucial Cs highlights the idea that children who engage in healthy relationships also tend to demonstrate their sense of security in four critical internal beliefs. These include their relationship with others (connect), their ability for self-care (capable), their sense of being seen as important (count), and their ability to engage in appropriate developmental risk (courage) (Kottman & Meany-Walen 2016).

- *Goals of misbehavior.* In accepting these constructs, we can further develop our understanding that a child's misbehavior is motivated by their striving to attain one or more of these needs. The development of intervention strategies will be guided by the practitioner's understanding of the underlying purpose of the child's maladaptive behaviors (which typically present as attention, power/control, revenge, or proving their own inadequacy) in seeking fulfillment of one of their Crucial Cs.

Phases of treatment

AdPT follows a typical progression through four phases: Phase 1: Building the relationship; Phase 2: Investigating the child's lifestyle; Phase 3: Helping the child gain insight; and Phase 4: Re-orienting/re-educating (Kottman & Meany-Walen 2016). In Phase 1, the development of the therapeutic relationship is viewed as a critical component of the success of the overall treatment process. AdPT focuses on the development of an egalitarian relationship in which the child is provided with options, and their decision is ultimately respected. While AdPT begins from a non-directive approach to engage the child in the therapeutic relationship, as treatment progresses into the second and third phases of treatment, the practitioner takes a more hands-on and practitioner-led role, combining non-directive and directive play techniques. Directive activities are selected to aid in conceptualizing the child's lifestyle and increase their understanding of the underlying motives for their behaviors, the Crucial Cs, the make-up of their family, and their thoughts, feelings, and perceptions of self, others, and the world (Kottman 2011). Progress of a shift from the implicit to explicit and unconscious to conscious is the focus of Phase 3. During this phase of treatment, the practitioner begins to help the child consider and decide what behaviors and attitudes serve them well, and which need to be replaced by alternative and more constructive approaches. The child will have opportunities to practice them in the final phase, called re-orientation/re-education. It is important to note that these phases are parallel to the work with the caregivers. The practitioner works through each phase to support the caregivers in developing and strengthening the insights and teaching and practicing parenting skills.

Phases 1 and 2: Building the relationship and investigating lifestyle

The assessment and relationship building in AdPT begins with the practitioner's initial contact with the caregivers. It may be a brief intake call and/or the first appointment. Regardless, the practitioner needs to focus on setting the stage for the importance of caregiver involvement, understanding the presenting problem, and considering underlying motivators of the behaviors caregivers are reporting. Kottman and Meany-Walen (2016) emphasize that while forms can be used to guide the assessment process, it is not customary to ask all the questions. Still, the practitioner should carefully consider what questions may be most valuable for their conceptualization of the work ahead. In addition, they highly recommend incorporating play-based techniques such as sandtray, expressive art, and other creative methods to aid in gathering relevant information. In doing so, the caregivers may also gain a deeper understanding of the play therapy process their child will experience. While the assessment is initiated by an intake with the caregivers, the practitioner continues assessment in their beginning work with the client, further taking into consideration family and relationship dynamics. This continues through the second phase of treatment and culminates with the development of a collaborative treatment plan.

Phases 3 and 4: Gaining insight and re-orientation/re-education

In AdPT, the primary goal of treatment is to utilize the therapeutic relationship with the client system to aid in developing insight into their sense of self and interactions with others (Kottman & Meany-Walen 2016). By developing insight into their behaviors, thoughts, and feelings, the practitioner can support them in shifting their perceptions of self and others, leading to positive interactions with others and long-term positive changes. Goal development focuses on recognizing personal resources, enhancing social interest and collaboration, and decreasing feelings of inferiority and negative views of self and others (Kottman & Meany-Walen 2016). Within these categories, the practitioner, in collaboration with the child, caregivers, and other key stakeholders, develops a plan that highlights specific, targeted goals connected to the identified issues at intake and clinical observations to maximize the child's overall levels of functioning. The treatment culminates in Phase 4 with a focus on creating opportunities to practice and strengthen specific skills, and strengthen insight for the child and their caregivers.

Contraindications

The concept of safety becomes critical in determining contraindications for implementing AdPT in working with children and their families. Kottman stressed that in the beginning, to use AdPT with a client, the underlying assumption must clearly be that the child has the capacity for a relationship (personal communication, March 26, 2021). Their inability to engage in relationships would significantly hinder their ability to benefit from treatment. Another consideration that would hinder progress is the caregiver's limited ability to actively engage in the treatment process, whatever the underlying cause may be, as it is considered an important element of the treatment process. Finally, taking into account the child's developmental stage would also play a role in determining the appropriateness of AdPT for a particular child. Engaging anyone in an intervention in which one of the primary goals is to achieve a degree of insight into their thoughts, feelings, and behaviors assumes a certain degree of cognitive capacity. For children who have endured traumatic experiences at an early age and stage of development, the therapeutic process may be hampered by their inability to engage at a level that requires this higher level of cognitive functioning. Children with these experiences likely require and would benefit most from a treatment approach that matches the experiences they missed at a fundamental level. Subsequently, the focus on therapeutic interventions needs to be initially right brain to right brain in nature.

Theraplay with AdPT

Theraplay and AdPT are distinct play therapy approaches that have been proven to meet the needs of a variety of clients. Based on the theoretical congruence between the models, practitioners can engage in a symbiotic treatment process that includes aspects of both modalities while also working to honor the unique practical applications of these distinct play therapy approaches. Peluso and colleagues (2004) identify that Adlerian constructs of Individual Psychology align with Bowlby's Attachment Theory. They both recognize that the individual's sense of self and the world is developed through their early social interactions with caregivers. In essence, Theraplay's acknowledgment of and the goal toward shifting the internal working model (IWM) mirrors AdPT's assessment of lifestyle and work to support the client in gaining insight into their lifestyle to engage in productive change. This also highlights how both modalities value that early childhood relationships and experiences impact the development of the child's IWM and, thus, lifestyles. The similarities between the two models do not end there. In fact, as we consider both approaches, it is evident that there is an overlap between the Theraplay dimensions (structure, engagement, nurture, challenge) and Adlerian theory's Crucial Cs and goals of misbehavior (Michigan State University 2016).

The dimension of structure in Theraplay refers to the caregiver's leadership role in ensuring a sense of safety through organized and regulating experiences. These experiences lead to the child experiencing a sense of feeling the Crucial C of "capable," allowing them to explore their world, learn about themselves, and develop an ability to self-regulate. The underlying goal of misbehavior is seen as a child striving for power and control. When these underlying needs are met in their interactions with their caregivers, a feeling of belonging is achieved.

Similarly, the dimension of engagement refers to the attuned responses to all affective states, utilized by the caregiver to entice the child into moments of joyful connection as well as acknowledging and supporting in negative states. In these experiences, the child is seen and heard and feels "connected" (Crucial C). Children seeking this sense of attuned responsive connection may resort to negative attention-seeking patterns to have these needs met.

Nurture as a dimension of caretaking focuses on the day-to-day interactions that provide a child with the comfort, reassurance, and downregulation as needed, resulting in the Crucial C of feeling as though they "count." Nurture provides a child with a sense of their value and significance within the context of self and other. When these needs have not been adequately met, children can engage in revenge-like patterns of behavior in an effort to secure their value and strengthen their sense of self.

Finally, the challenge dimension highlights the role of the caregiver to provide developmentally appropriate risks while supporting the child's ability to manage the tension created by the risk, leading to the sense of mastery or the Crucial C of "courage." When these underlying needs are met, the child can face new opportunities with confidence and capacity, diminishing the negative behaviors associated with giving up or avoiding new or difficult tasks. This alignment in fundamental views of client needs and behaviors allows practitioners integrating Theraplay and AdPT to assess, plan, and cultivate a treatment process that meets the distinct needs of more complex cases.

An integrated assessment

By engaging in thorough assessment, Theraplay practitioners trained in AdPT can help determine which route to take for meeting client needs and achieving treatment goals. It is not typical for Adlerian Play therapists to engage in the administration of the Marschak Interaction Method (MIM). However, in personal communication with Terry Kottman (March 26, 2021), it could be a valuable assessment tool as the dimensions align with the Crucial Cs. It may provide useful information about the child's lifestyle and the caregiver's responses to their behaviors. We have found this to be true, as it also allows for the practitioner to observe the family dynamics through a Theraplay lens and, as outlined above, from an AdPT perspective. The practitioner can then determine whether the treatment needs to prioritize fostering a relationship between the caregiver and child, or whether individual play therapy would be more appropriate.

Determining factors in integrating Theraplay and AdPT

There are a number of factors that must be considered when deciding the best course of treatment for blending Theraplay and AdPT. While theoretically there is a lot of overlap between them, each modality approaches how to best support the client in vastly different, though complementary, ways. The practitioner should explore the following factors when determining the best way to blend these two modalities:

- cultivating a neuroception of safety
- developing therapeutic relationships
- exploring and addressing goals of behavior
- involvement of caregivers

- role of the practitioner in enacting change.

Cultivating a neuroception of safety

The first factor is how to best achieve a neuroception of safety. It is well known that fostering a sense of safety is paramount for the therapeutic setting. Clients must feel safe enough to be vulnerable in order to explore and shift their patterns of engaging. This is even more important when working with children, and especially children with complex needs or experiences of relational trauma. Attachment theory explains that healthy development requires an attuned and co-regulating caregiver. The practitioner has a unique opportunity to support healthy development in their clients by providing a safe environment through their own attuned and co-regulating responses. This further leads to the client experiencing a felt sense of safety or "neuroception" of safety (Norris & Lender 2020). Stephen Porges (2018) describes this autonomic response to feeling safe/unsafe as the social engagement system (SES), expressed through prosodic vocal tones and soft facial features that communicate an openness to positive interpersonal connection.

Whether a client presents in a state of fear or something within the treatment process activates their fight, flight, freeze, or appease response, it is of the utmost importance that the practitioner works to support the client in bringing their system back online and activating their SES. From the very first meeting to the last session, a Theraplay practitioner does this by activating their own SES and communicating non-verbally to the client that they are safe, but also adapting and shifting the environment, pacing of activities, and their overall engagement to engender this sense of safety in a practitioner-directed and structured way. Kottman and Meany-Walen (2016) similarly emphasize the importance of developing a relationship involving cultivating trust and respect between the play therapist and the child, as well as between the play therapist and the caregivers during the initial phase of AdPT. However, it is an egalitarian relationship developed through a non-directive play therapy approach that communicates safety and a willingness to engage in an intersubjective experience.

 CASE ILLUSTRATION

The practitioner entered the waiting area to meet the child for the first time, and observed him clinging to the case aide in an overly familiar way, and noted the discomfort in the case aide's expression and stiff posture. Javier quickly shifted his attention to the practitioner and greeted her with a tight hug. On entering the playroom, the practitioner oriented Javier to the room and shared, "In this playroom, you can play with the toys in most of the ways that you want to. Sometimes I will choose what we do, and sometimes you will get to pick what we do. Other times, we will figure it out together. Today, you can explore the playroom and pick what we do." Javier wandered the playroom for a few moments and then slumped on the small couch in silence. The practitioner, focused on developing a positive, egalitarian, therapeutic alliance with the child, focused on tracking his behaviors, reflecting his feelings, attempting to explore why he was coming for play therapy, and explaining the play therapy process. Javier's eyes continually scanned the room, but he verbalized little. As the session was coming to a close and the practitioner shared with him that the session would be ending in 10 minutes, Javier began to cry and moved to hide under a table in the room. The next several sessions seemed to be a repeat of the first, with Javier spending time disengaged, physically hiding, and clearly experiencing significant distress.

Relationship development

For Javier, it was becoming clear to the practitioner that establishing the relationship was a significant challenge and was serving as an obstacle to progress. In considering the integration of the two models, the practitioner must consider which approach is most appropriate for how to cultivate the relationship. AdPT devotes an entire phase of treatment to building rapport and an egalitarian relationship through providing respect, consistency, and acceptance (Kottman & Meany-Walen 2016). Theraplay, similarly, values the relationships that are built between practitioner and child, child and caregiver, and caregiver and practitioner as the cornerstones for shifting the IWM. Norris and Lender (2020) explain the concept of intersubjectivity that focuses on the reciprocal attuned mirroring experiences that occur between caregiver and child and that are foundational to the development of healthy relationships. Through intersubjective experiences, which require safety within the relationship, the child is able to experience new possibilities for their interactions and alternatives to their previous assumptions about themselves, the world, and others. It is through healthy and typical caregiver–infant interactions that babies first learn intersubjectivity. Theraplay recognizes that the child may have missed out on this opportunity to connect through primary intersubjectivity with their caregiver. Primary intersubjectivity emerges when the caregiver has the capacity to understand what is in the mind of the child, whereas secondary intersubjectivity develops when the caregiver and child share an interest in objects or play materials (Trevarthen & Aitken 2001). Providing those connecting experiences will need to be an important piece of the treatment. While AdPT values the relationship, and believes intersubjective experiences are an important aspect of treatment, there is an assumption that the child is capable of such relationships on entering the playroom, thus engaging the child in a more secondary intersubjective experience. While the practitioner was offering consistency and acceptance, and attempting to provide the child with an egalitarian relationship through AdPT, Javier had not yet experienced a relationship grounded in these types of interactions. His lack of a positive IWM to support the practitioner's efforts to provide such a relationship appeared to conflict with his private logic, limiting progress from the start. This may be one determining factor that points to the practitioner starting with Theraplay to provide the client with these early developmental connecting experiences before shifting to the AdPT protocol.

CASE ILLUSTRATION

Despite the practitioner's best efforts to create a sense of safety, Javier continued to struggle to use the toys in the playroom or to engage with the practitioner. All efforts to engage Javier in a therapeutic relationship focused on respect, and his ability to make his own choices were met with resistance. The practitioner felt stuck and grew increasingly concerned regarding the impact Javier's experiences in relationships had on his ability to engage. It was clear to the practitioner that something was not working for Javier, and a change was warranted. Through consultation, the practitioner received support with shifting the approach to working with this client system. Based on the initial observations of the practitioner, consultation with the foster mother, caseworker, and a colleague, a shift to providing Theraplay was implemented, and the MIM was administered.

Goals of behavior

The third factor in determining how to best utilize these modalities in tandem recognizes the importance of practitioners being curious about a child's underlying motives, as this is the key to understanding them as individuals and as part of their larger family system. Throughout Theraplay treatment, the development of insight is geared toward the practitioner and caregiver's understanding and empathic response to the child's behaviors. The practitioner is looking at the child's verbal and non-verbal cues to determine the dimensional need underlying the behaviors in the MIM and during caregiver–child sessions. For example, suppose the child is running around the playroom. In that case, the Theraplay practitioner is cued to structure the energy into something organizing and engaging in supporting the regulation of the child. On the other hand, AdPT may or may not be as directive, depending on the phase of treatment. Still, it works to increase awareness of the child's behavior and develop insight across the system, utilizing techniques of metacommunication and tracking. Importance is placed on the client gaining conscious awareness of their behaviors that no longer serve them in prosocial ways. In contrast, Theraplay focuses on in-the-moment experiences that challenge negative perceptions that lead to unhelpful behaviors.

CASE ILLUSTRATION

The MIM was marked by Javier's need to control, and he was resistant throughout to engaging in tasks. His foster parents' efforts to provide nurture were met with avoidance and dysregulation. They had a clear sense of his developmental capacities and scaffolding challenges, and yet he struggled to experience a sense of success, as noted by his negative self-talk. The foster parents acknowledged his negative sense of self and attempted to provide support, but ultimately they appeared frustrated, and Javier's experience was invalidated. The practitioner identified goals in all dimensions with a primary focus on structure, engagement, and nurture, knowing that progress toward managing challenges would develop with a clear sense of felt safety. This aligned with the Crucial Cs identified in the initial caregiver meeting of capable, connect, and count.

Caregivers

The fourth factor to consider is *how and when* to work with and utilize caregivers. Both treatment modalities value the contributions of caregivers and other important adults in the child's life, working to create a therapeutic alliance and provide a parallel process. Caregivers can struggle to provide what they have not adequately received in their own attachment histories. This requires the Theraplay practitioner to offer caregivers experiences across dimensions, as a co-regulating other, to facilitate their ability to provide these experiences to their child. Similarly, Kottman and Meany-Walen (2016) outline the importance of consulting with caregivers and engaging with them through their four-phase approach as individuals and caregivers of the child. The place where the two models diverge is when determining who is in the room. For Theraplay, the caregiver is an active participant in all sessions, and importance is placed on the relationship and dynamics between the caregiver and child (Norris & Lender 2020). Both modalities work to support caregivers in increasing their skills of attunement and co-regulation, and strive to help them with understanding and reframing their child's behavior while increasing their sense of hope through encouragement and recognition of effort. When determining the initial needs of the client system, the practitioner should explore the benefits and necessity of the caregiver and child being in the room together in order to meet those needs.

CASE ILLUSTRATION

Following the initial parent feedback session, Javier's foster parents began to see his behaviors from a different perspective: the oppositional behavior was an effort to maintain control and safety, and his lack of acceptance of physical love and connection was a result of the lack of consistency with which he received loving touch as an infant and toddler. His foster parents were eager to learn and make sense of his behaviors. They worked closely with the practitioner, asking questions and quickly integrating their new understanding of Javier into their interactions with him in Theraplay sessions and at home, providing consistent structure and nurture, and attuning to his underlying needs through engagement to all affect states.

Role of the practitioner for enacting change

The final factor to consider is the role of the practitioner, and determining what level of directiveness the practitioner feels would be beneficial for the client system and how to navigate the child's representation of consciousness in play. Yasenik and Gardner (2004) created the Play Therapy Dimensions Model to provide a framework for play therapists to examine these factors more closely when doing integrative work. Their model looks at the degree of directiveness utilized by the practitioner as well as the child's conscious understanding of their experiences. They explore these degrees through a quadrant approach of directive/non-directive and conscious/unconscious.

Both approaches, AdPT and Theraplay, are found toward the more directive side of the quadrants. Practitioners must be playful, engaging, attuned, and confident leaders. Whether that is during the more observational and exploratory phases of treatment, or during the phases in which practitioners are working to enact change and support shifts in client IWM, practitioners are always paying attention and taking an active role in guiding the client and making adjustments to their verbal and non-verbal cues. The point at which these two modalities diverge is when exploring the level of consciousness of clients within the treatment. Kottman explained that one major goal of AdPT is to support the child and caregivers by making the unconscious conscious (personal communication, March 26, 2021). Theraplay, on the other hand, utilizes preverbal, in-the-moment intersubjective experiences that tap into the unconscious nature of the IWM, while also guiding every aspect of the interaction to foster safety and regulation. A practitioner will need to decide where they align and fall in their integrative approach, while also considering the client's external systemic needs and their developmental capacity.

When supporting clients with accessing their unconscious beliefs and experiences, there needs to be a foundational amount of cognitive and developmental capacity to engage in relationships and more symbolic play. As Bruce Perry's Neurosequential Model of Therapeutics suggests, practitioners must provide treatment that is going to match the level of brain development in which the trauma occurred (Mason, Kelly, & McConchie 2020). Theraplay works on lower levels of brain development (the limbic and diencephalon areas). While AdPT *can* engage clients on these lower levels, the focus on gaining insight and re-education necessitates engaging higher levels of brain development. Javier's experience with Theraplay created a sense of safety and an ability to engage developmentally at a higher level of functioning, utilizing symbolic play and demonstrating his increased capacity for intersubjective experiences.

 ## CASE ILLUSTRATION

After several months of weekly Theraplay sessions, Javier's foster mother was not available to come to a session, so a return to the playroom occurred. Javier entered the playroom, and to the practitioner's surprise, without prompting, he moved to the dolls houses, set both up, and began to move figures and belongings between the two, narrating the story of the figures as he played. Having firmly established a positive relationship and sense of felt safety through Theraplay, the practitioner shifted to Phase 3 AdPT techniques, metacommunicating about the patterns in Javier's play and their connection to his experiences and relationships. In addition, there was a focus on using movement to help him regulate his body as he engaged in abreactive play.

Treatment continued alternating between the two modalities: Theraplay to continue to enhance and support the development of a positive attachment relationship and AdPT to help Javier continue to process and gain insight into his behaviors and the role his early life experiences had played in maintaining his sense of safety and avoidance of "healthy" relationships. His foster family reported positive shifts in his behavior at home and school; he was less resistant, more open to accepting affection, and willing to try karate class.

In his final sessions, Javier constructed a letter to his practitioner thanking her for helping him to see that he no longer needed to be afraid, that he was safe with his new family, and they loved him and he loved them in return. Through the treatment process, not only had Theraplay provided Javier with the early missed relational opportunities, but AdPT also allowed for him to shift his private logic, making the unconscious conscious in understanding, at a developmentally appropriate level, why he used to have such a hard time.

Conclusion

After considering the determining factors for utilizing Theraplay and AdPT in tandem, we recommend an integrated approach to the assessment, from intake to the administration of the MIM. This information will be critical in the conceptualization of the treatment plan, taking into consideration dimensions, lifestyle, underlying components, and caregiver and client capacities. Theraplay excels at fostering the early experiential attachment needs of the child, and supports a healthier dyadic relationship and positive IWM. In addition, AdPT offers the opportunity to expand the therapeutic potential for growth and a shift in private logic due to the increased focus on insight and skill development. While distinct approaches, their congruence in their underlying belief systems grounded in attachment theory affords practitioners the ability to meet a wider array of client needs and complexity.

When Javier entered treatment, he found it was "too hard to play." His complex early experiences led to attachment insecurities that negatively impacted his ability to engage in AdPT from the start. Considering the tools available in the practitioner's play therapy toolbox and the congruence in the underlying theory, the practitioner was able to meet Javier's complex younger needs while moving him forward to process his experiences when he was ready. The strengths of utilizing Theraplay, in conjunction with AdPT, ensured positive and lasting change for Javier and his family.

Key takeaways

- AdPT and Theraplay align theoretically. Both share practitioner-guided techniques resulting in a symbiotic and integrative treatment approach that can meet the needs of complex cases.

- Theraplay's acknowledgement of and goal toward shifting

the IWM mirrors AdPT's assessment of lifestyle, and works to support the client in gaining insight, leading to productive change.

- An overlap exists between AdPT's Crucial Cs and goals of misbehavior and Theraplay's four dimensions of structure, engagement, nurture, and challenge:
    - Structure, capable, power and control, resulting in the child feeling a sense of belonging.
    - Engagement, connect, attention, resulting in the child feeling seen and heard.
    - Nurture, count, revenge, resulting in the child feeling valued in the context of relationship.
    - Challenge, courage, giving up, resulting in the child feeling confident with a sense of self-efficacy.

- Both modalities value cultivating a neuroception of safety and fostering a therapeutic relationship; determining the capacity of the client in each of these areas at the onset of treatment determines with which modality to begin.

- Goals of behavior and the meaning underneath the child's (and caregiver's) actions are important factors when completing the assessment, developing treatment plans, and moving through the different phases of treatment.

- The importance of the contributions of caregivers and other important adults in the child's life cannot be understated in both of these modalities; working to create a therapeutic alliance and providing a parallel process with caregivers are key to both Theraplay and AdPT.

- As playful, attuned, and confident leaders, practitioners must be comfortable and flexible when moving between the consistently guided interactions of Theraplay toward a balance of directive and non-directive approaches in AdPT.

References

Doyle Buckwalter, K. (2018). Overview of Attachment Theory and Clinical Application. In K. Doyle Buckwalter & D. Reed (Eds), *Attachment Theory in Action: Building Connections Between Children and Parents* (pp.3–16). Rowman & Littlefield.

Kottman, T. (2011). Adlerian Play Therapy. In C. E. Schaefer (Ed.), *Foundations of Play Therapy* (2nd edn) (pp.87–104). John Wiley & Sons.

Kottman, T., & Meany-Walen, K. (2016). *Partners in Play* (3rd edn). The American Counseling Association.

Lindaman, S., Booth, P., & Cockerill, G. M. (2018). Theraplay: Creating Felt Safety, Emotional Connection and Social Joy in Relationship. In K. Doyle Buckwalter (Ed.), *Attachment Theory in Action: Building Connections Between Children and Parents* (pp.93–104). Rowman & Littlefield.

Mason, C., Kelly, B., & McConchie, V. (2020). Including neuroscience in social work education: Introducing graduate students to the Neurosequential Model of Therapeutics. *Journal of Teaching in Social Work 40*(4), 352–371. doi:10.1080/08841233.2020.1788692

Michigan State University. (2016). 4 goals of misbehavior: Crucial C's and goals of misbehavior. *Very Important Parents.* May. https://adler-prod.s3.amazonaws.com/uploads/resource/filename/273/Crucial_C_s_and_Misbehavior.pdf

Norris, V., & Lender, D. (2020). *Theraplay®—The Practitioner's Guide.* Jessica Kingsley Publishers.

Peluso, P. R., Peluso, J. P., White, J. F., & Kern, R. M. (2004). A comparison of attachment theory and individual psychology: A review of the literature. *Journal of Counseling & Development 82*(2), 139–145. https://doi.org/10.1002/j.1556-6678.2004.tb00295.x

Porges, S. W. (2018). Polyvagal Theory: A Primer. In S. W. Porges & D. Dana (Eds), *Clinical Applications of the Polyvagal Theory: The Emergence of Polyvagal-Informed Therapies* (pp.50–69). W.W. Norton. https://integratedlistening.com/wp-content/uploads/2020/10/polyvagal-primer-from-clinicalapplicationofpolyvagaltheory-3.2019.pdf

Trevarthen, C., & Aitken, K. (2001). Infant intersubjectivity: Research, theory, and clinical applications. *Journal of Child Psychology and Psychiatry, and Allied Disciplines 42*, 3–48. https://doi.org/10.1111/1469-7610.00701

Weber, D. A. (2003). A comparison of individual psychology and attachment theory. *Journal of Individual Psychology 59*(3), 246–262. https://psycnet.apa.org/record/2003-08854-002

Yasenik, L., & Gardner, K. (2012). *Play Therapy Dimensions Model: A Decision-Making Guide for Integrative Play Practitioners* (2nd edn). Jessica Kingsley Publishers.

Chapter 5

Theraplay and Cognitive Behavioral Play Therapy (CBPT)

CALMING "THE BIG MAD"

Lorie Walton

Introduction

Combining Theraplay with other modalities effectively supports the complexities of many childhood mental health issues (Beacon House 2017; Tucker & Smith-Adcock 2017). Theraplay's magic is in helping early foundational healing components via a bottom-up approach, and is aligned with the neurosequential models of thought (Tucker & Smith-Adcock 2017). Cognitive Behavioral Play Therapy (CBPT) treatments offer a top-down approach and are at the other end of the spectrum when considering mastering control over triggered responses (Brickel 2019). This chapter will demonstrate how to effectively incorporate these two treatment modalities (Theraplay and CBPT), which theoretically reside at opposite ends of the psychotherapy spectrum, into a treatment plan that offers support to a child who suffers from severe emotional dysregulation challenges. It will also demonstrate the value of incorporating the caregivers into this healing journey.

The foundation of regulating emotions

Early childhood is a period of rapid brain development that paves the way for the growth of self-regulation skills. Self-regulation is defined as controlling one's behavior, emotions, and thoughts by managing disruptive feelings and impulses. Research suggests the level of self-regulation skills children manifest during early childhood can consistently predict a multitude of short- and long-term outcomes, such as school readiness, primary school academic achievement, adult educational attainment, self-worth, and an ability to cope with stress (Montroy *et al.* 2017). It is normal for developing children to experience many emotions as they grow, but it is how they learn to master control over those emotions that will help them cope in healthy ways later in life.

Multiple factors contribute to self-regulation, from biological predisposition to caregiver support to environmental context. It can be extremely difficult for a child to learn how to independently master control over strong overwhelming feelings without a co-regulating caregiver. The infant's brain is profoundly influenced by the attachment bond. Research reveals that a positive or negative primary attachment relationship supports the ability or inability to manage stress, attune to one's inner emotions, be playful in a mutually engaging manner, and be readily forgiving with others (Robinson, Segal, & Jaffe 2022).

Because children's emotional, brain, and body systems are still developing, they require help being soothed as they often cannot soothe themselves without an attentive adult's help. If left alone, their overall emotional development may be negatively impacted in the long term, potentially predisposing them to anxiety and future mental health issues. In addition, disturbances of the brain's rhythm-keeping regions are often causes of depression and other psychiatric disorders (Perry & Szalavitz 2006). Therefore, if young children's primary regulating system functions poorly, this will negatively affect the modulation of hormonal and emotional reactions to stress and other systems, such as sleeping and eating, learning motor functions, and even responding positively to others.

The regulation of emotions is an essential component of facilitating healthy attachment. Attachment research has demonstrated that attuned, engaging interactions between a baby and mother lead to secure attachment, positive internal working models of self and world, and the capacity to regulate emotions and actions (Sroufe 2005). Attachment theorists have described the caregiver–child attachment relationship as a foundation for developing children's capacity for emotion regulation and coping with stress. Brumariu (2015) concludes that securely attached children internalize effective regulation strategies based on their primary attachment relationship, and can successfully employ adaptive emotion regulation strategies when the attachment figure is absent. Bundy-Myrow (2005) references how attachment-based interventions assist children who experience difficulties in self-regulation.

Can Theraplay be paired with CBPT?

Mental health practitioners who work with young children know that helping them learn how to master control over their emotions is no small feat. Unlike adults, children cannot make significant emotional changes without a supportive, attuned caregiver co-regulating them through the process. Often, a child unable to appropriately regulate emotions may experience cycles of dysregulated states of anger with an inability to master control of their emotions, which then becomes a chronic cycle of frustration, disappointment, and shame responses. These intensive episodes can easily lead to further dysregulated states. Frequently, children with dysregulated emotional systems require interventions that help their bodies unconsciously experience soothing and calming from an external source (e.g., an attuned co-regulator) *before* they can consciously begin to master their triggered emotions in a controlled and motivated way. Growing evidence endorses the concept that children require a secure relationship with a supportive adult to help them master control over their emotions before working on regulating triggers from past experiences of trauma (Saarni 2011).

Theraplay has evolved over its inception and has become known as a primary foundational therapeutic intervention for its ability to effectively support children with emotional regulation issues (Bundy-Myrow 2005). It helps children experience emotional regulation by participating in playful, attuned experiences with an attentive, supportive parent or caregiver. It offers structure to the dyad of the child and caregiver by endorsing in-sync, nurturing responses through playful interactions that effectively co-regulate the child. One of Theraplay's many assets is its ability to assist the caregiver in incorporating attuned responses to help the emotionally dysregulated child's body internalize new reactions to stress. Attunement, by definition, is the process of feeling emotional synchronicity with another person. This involves sharing and understanding those feelings (Gray 2007). Empathy develops out of affect attunement and helps a child make sense of their own feelings from this shared unconscious experience. Theraplay endorses the building of synchrony by providing activation, support, and foundational healing and by incorporating attuned, empathic responses during playful engaging moments to assist the dyadic dance.

Baylin (2018) described how specific attachment figure-based methods help to disarm the child's defense system and promote the awakening of the child's social engagement system (SES). The child needs to engage the prefrontal regions of the brain to achieve emotional regulation and to be able to work on a more conscious level of mastering emotions. Polyvagal theory affirms that mammals have a social engagement system that has evolved to employ cues from face-to-face interactions. These interactions efficiently calm our physiological state and shift our fight or flight behaviors to trusting relationships (Porges 2015). Play is considered an important neural exercise for practicing the detection of trust versus danger in relationships (Norris & Lender 2020). The physically active, face-to-face play used in Theraplay combines safety cues with upregulating states of arousal and downregulating states of overstimulation. These playful moments promote co-regulated experiences (often called face-to-heart connections), provide integration to the SES, and prompt safety signals. Over time, the children's inner responses begin to solidify towards security, which then supports the child's eventual ability to self-regulate emotions and stress-like situations on their own without the caregiver's presence.

CBPT is rooted in an evidence-based theory of Cognitive Behavioral Therapy (CBT). CBPT can support the healing journey of a child who experiences uncontrollable emotions by offering them the ability to learn the science of how their body works in conjunction with emotions. Hierarchical in nature and problem-focused, CBT involves teaching skills and coping strategies to help children effectively deal with a wide range of emotional responses (Castagna, Long, & Upton 2020). Skills and strategies are practiced in session and within other environments (such as home and school) to support the generalization of skills into everyday life and to build a sense of efficacy and positive affect. There is an abundance of research that demonstrates the effectiveness of CBPT in helping children manage not only anxiety but also other emotional challenges, such as sadness and anger (Knell 2009; Weiss *et al.* 2018).

You may wonder how attachment theory can contribute to CBPT's treatment goals. CBPT utilizes play and play-based interventions to help children change their thoughts, feelings, and behaviors by restructuring each in developmentally appropriate ways (Drewes & Cavett 2019). CBPT is predominantly a structured, directive, and goal-oriented play-based treatment modality that systematically integrates empirically validated techniques. It includes cognitive and behavioral interventions that help children to gain mastery over their environment while being active participants in change (Drewes & Cavett 2019). Practitioners using CBPT with children do not typically invite the caregivers to participate in the play therapy room, although there are options to do so. Typically, CBPT is done with the child alone, and promotes the child's ability to cathartically utilize the CBPT tools to reframe emotional responses and behaviors.

Recent studies are now demonstrating how the inclusion of a supportive attachment figure can positively support the healing journey of a child in the long term. Cavett (2018) developed a relation-based alternative to traditional CBT and CBPT called Integrative Attachment Informed Cognitive Behavioral

Play Therapy (IAI-CBPT). This therapeutic technique captures the strengths of CBT/CBPT while addressing their noted weaknesses, particularly their neglect of the importance of relationships in treatment. IAI-CBPT is a tiered, prescriptive, attachment-based treatment rooted in and dependent on attachment and therapeutic relationships for its efficacy (Cavett 2018). With its additional grounding in and focus on attachment and the therapeutic relationship, this model brings a more holistic approach to child trauma treatment and the challenging realm of medical trauma. Bosmans' (2016) review of CBT and attachment interventions asserts that restoring trust to insecure caregiver–child attachment relationships can be integrated within CBT and could contribute to its treatment outcomes.

Although at different ends of the treatment paradigm, Theraplay and some CBT-based treatments stress the importance of integrating trauma-informed teaching to caregivers about their child's dysregulated presentations. Theraplay incorporates several opportunities for caregiver practice and learning within the model. By providing caregivers with the opportunity to experience firsthand what Theraplay sessions will entail and have deeper discussions regarding the physiology of attachment, dysregulation, and attunement, caregivers become more trauma-informed. This leads to the building of their confidence and the motivation to instill structure, attunement, and nurture within their parenting routines. Similarly, Trauma-Focused Cognitive Behavioral Therapy (TF-CBT) provides explanations to caregivers about how a child's changes in mood, behavior, or thinking might be attributed to trauma (Cohen & Mannarino 2008). TF-CBT methods strive to give caregivers the resources and skills necessary to help children cope with the psychological ramifications of abuse or other trauma. This method offers both caregivers and children tools to process emotions and thoughts relating to traumatic experiences.

Combining Theraplay with CBPT

A combination of supports such as the implementation of Theraplay with age-appropriate CBPT techniques can make a long-lasting impact of change for a child who struggles with emotional vulnerabilities and dysregulated trauma responses, as well as attachment insecurities. Consideration of which therapeutic modalities to use first and/or which modalities can be effectively used simultaneously should be made to support long-lasting and effective change.

First and foremost, when formulating a treatment plan, it is essential to consider two important aspects of the child's presentation to identify and structure therapeutic support most effectively: (1) Does the child's emotional system appear younger than their chronological age? (2) Does the child have a significant attachment caregiver who can learn how to attune to their internal dysregulated state and provide soothing and nurturing experiences to effectively help their brain and body systems begin to regulate? With structure and an attuned caregiver by their side, a child can make significant gains and learn to master control over emotions through evidence-based interventions.

The following case illustration will demonstrate how the combination of using Theraplay and CBPT helped a little boy master control over "The Big Mad," and helped him to form a secure bond with his primary carer.

CASE ILLUSTRATION

Sammy was a smart but aggressive seven-year-old boy. He had a history of neglect, abuse, and a transient lifestyle until he was placed in foster care with his two younger sisters at the age of four. Sammy had been placed three more times in foster care until he found a home at age six with Rachael (his foster mother). Sammy's sisters were placed in a separate home with a kinship relative. Rachael was an experienced carer who understood childhood trauma and was open to doing all she could to help Sammy feel safe and settled in her home, but she readily admitted it was hard work and exhausting at the best of times. It was reported that Sammy was vulnerable to episodes of intense anger, recurring nightmares, sleep challenges, and controlling behaviors, especially during transition times. Struggles with social issues at school were prevalent and often caused him to be sent home on suspension. In addition, he was repeatedly in trouble for violent behavior, such as fighting with his peers, and for physical aggression toward his teachers.

Child psychotherapy was requested to support Sammy's healing journey and to assist Rachael with therapeutic parenting strategies in the hope that moving Sammy again could be avoided. Treatment planning occurred after several observational assessments were conducted to assess Sammy's relationship with Rachael as well as to assess Sammy's trauma and grief responses. The Marschak Interaction Method (MIM) assessment was implemented to observe the strengths of the relationship between Rachael and Sammy, and assess areas that required support.

Results from the MIM demonstrated Sammy's vulnerabilities. He appeared to be in a constant state of hypervigilance, which presented as oppositional defiant behavior. He constantly moved around, checking the room and doors that led to the hallway. It was positive to see that he often circled back to be physically close to Rachael, which demonstrated his ability to use her as a "secure" base. Sammy showed his need to take control. This was especially prevalent each time a new MIM activity was read aloud by Rachael. For example, Sammy grabbed the cards out of Rachael's hand and insisted he held on to all of them during each task. When Rachael read a card aloud, Sammy would take any of the materials needed (even before he understood what was required) to do that play task. This unsettled behavior appeared to sabotage Sammy's ability to enjoy anything playfully offered by Rachael.

Rachael presented with many strengths. She was observed to be calm and often used a soft voice that Sammy appeared soothed by. Rachael attempted structure by stating simple guidelines for Sammy to follow during each task without question inflections. Matter-of-fact positive comments and statements were consistently observed during her attempts to engage Sammy in the MIM activities. Although Rachael appeared with many strengths, Sammy's hypervigilant presentation and controlling behavior appeared to exhaust her. Sammy was hard to engage, and after many attempts to complete each directive card activity unsuccessfully, Rachael would move on to the next task.

Sammy's biggest vulnerability was observed during the "Leave the room" task. Rachael prepared Sammy by suggesting he sit and play with the blocks. Sammy demonstrated anxiousness and hesitancy on leaving, but when the door closed behind Rachael, Sammy froze, as if in a dissociated state. He sat on the floor before the door and stared into space. He did not move, and his breathing appeared slow. When Rachael re-entered, Sammy jumped up as if startled, and appeared disoriented and defensive.

Individual play therapy sessions were conducted to assess Sammy's emotional development and offer an opportunity for Sammy to provide some perspective on his life story thus far. Directive play therapy tasks and non-directive play opportunities were provided within the play therapy room without Rachael across four hour-long sessions. During the directive play assessment tasks, Sammy shared that he felt scared "a lot" at night and that he had bad dreams about "wolves trying to eat" him. He also stated that he disliked waking up on school mornings to go to school, and that he liked it when Rachael let him sleep in some mornings. He also expressed sadness and felt lonely for his two younger sisters, stating, "I miss my sisters 'cause we're apart." Often, Sammy could not sit for a directive task for long and would state, "I can't do this" or "Can I play now?" If games included feeling states or the people in his life, he would become quite guarded and defensive, and then become angry and state, "It's too hard. Stop," and he would remove himself from the table where the game was being played.

On completion of the assessment phase, it was determined that Sammy would benefit from a combination of therapeutic supports. Children who experience early traumatic events, including disrupted attachments, often present with many symptoms and challenges in their social, emotional, behavioral, and cognitive development. Sammy's presentation was certainly an indication of his emotional vulnerability. His need for control, his presentation of anger, and his symptoms of fear and resistance in discussing his own feelings were indicative of the emotionally dysregulated state he constantly hovered in. Impairment of the brain from early chronic stress can impact virtually every aspect of development. Because both the emotional and cognitive components are vital to relationships, their proper development, functioning, and reciprocal regulation are essential to the healing journey, especially for a young child (Cozolino 2006). Thus, it was recommended that the therapeutic treatment plan include a combination of Theraplay and play-based techniques, including directive CBPT-based activities, including some non-directive play, to support this little boy's healing journey.

The structure of each session included 40 minutes of CBPT time alone in the playroom with the therapist and then a 20-minute rejoining segment with Rachael for Theraplay. Directive CBPT tasks initially included activities that would help Sammy become more comfortable with his feelings. To help Sammy become more consciously comfortable with feeling states, pictures with feeling faces and playing directive feeling games, such as feelings tic-tac-toe[1] and feelings bean bag toss[2] were used. This was a little boy who needed to move his body and was unable to relax and enjoy the play if too much "talking" occurred. However, while Sammy tossed bean bags at the feeling face holes, he was able to verbalize personal incidents connected to those faces. These experiences began as recent events and then evolved over time to include past traumatic memories. The CBPT activities encouraged Sammy to slowly process emotions connected to individual experiences, and supported the mindfulness of his internal responses in a safe

---

1   A directive CBPT game that is similar to the old game of tic tac toe. Instead of using Xs and Os, the grid is left blank and each person draws a feeling face in an open space. Once drawn, the person tells what the feeling is and when they felt that feeling.

2   A directive CBPT game where the participants throw a bean bag into a large grid drawn on the floor that has feeling faces in each grid. Wherever the bean bag lands, the person gets to name the feeling, act out the feeling, and/or say when they experienced that feeling.

space, encouraging a cathartic release of pent-up energy and triggered responses.

As therapeutic rapport began solidifying, Sammy started to comfortably share more specific details of his world with the therapist. He shared openly when he felt mad at school or at home, and would tie memories from the past into these sharing moments. Sammy had recently labeled the term "The Big Mad" when he recalled an incident at school when he had thrown a chair in his classroom. He stated, "I think 'The Big Mad' made me do it!" This was the open window the therapist was waiting for. Sammy loved to chat about science and scientific facts learned from one of his favorite educational television programs. When Sammy labeled "The Big Mad," the therapist knew he was ready to consciously work on methods to help him become in charge of his feelings rather than the feelings being in charge of him. By using CBPT activities, Sammy became motivated to learn how to master his overwhelming emotions. Sammy was a curious and smart little boy. He was easy to engage when the therapist brought in specific mediums to demonstrate concepts, such as a picture book on how bodies work or materials to make a volcano erupt (to demonstrate how emotions can get the best of us and make us blow up out of control). Sammy responded to these directive play-based activities and was eager to learn how to control his feelings so they didn't feel so big and out of control. He was also excited to share these strategies with Rachael when it was time to join her for "Theraplay-ing."

The joining at the end of each session was to implement Theraplay to include Rachael as Sammy's co-regulating caregiver. The theory behind scheduling the sessions in this way was to help Sammy feel nurtured after working emotionally hard during the individual component of the sessions. Experiencing being soothed, nurtured, and delighted at the end of processing difficult memories was the goal of using Theraplay in this way. Sammy would eagerly run into Rachael's waiting arms and receive her welcoming hug. He responded enthusiastically to his favorite magic carpet and blanket games, and welcomed the opportunity to cuddle with Rachael while being fed fishy crackers. During these moments, Sammy would sometimes share openly about "The Big Mad" and would tell Rachael what strategies he had learned to be in charge of it. His favorite technique was what we called "feather blowing" fingers—he would wiggle his fingers across Rachael's hand and blow on them as if they were feathers. This became their magical way of greeting each other and, as later reported, their way of helping Sammy transition from Rachael onto the school bus. The CBPT strategies he learned were providing Sammy and Rachael with a common language to communicate about his feelings as Sammy learned and gained mastery over these emotional experiences. It was affirming to hear Rachael report that she was incorporating Theraplay's nurture and structure into her daily routines with Sammy. She also reported that she explained some of the simple CBPT techniques Sammy was learning to his educational assistant and teacher at school. She reported that school personnel noticed Sammy's affect was more stable and that his learning techniques were beginning to improve his ability to self-regulate without her during school days. Although everyone involved knew Sammy had a long road of healing ahead of him, he was well on his way to mastery over some of his emotions. He was beginning to form a trusting relationship with his carer. This was most likely the first relationship he had ever had that was consistent, attuned, and nurturing, and provided a balance of structure, engagement, nurture, and challenge to create a sense of feeling enjoyed, cared for, and protected.

Conclusion

The combination of implementing CBPT and Theraplay within a therapy session, although completely different in style, works well and can be quite effective at supporting a client's healing journey. By introducing CBPT strategies, the child can consciously learn age-appropriate yet effective ways to master control over emotions and triggered responses, which can then be encouraged and supported by the attuned caregiver. The caregiver welcomes the child via Theraplay and provides immediate co-regulating, attuned, synchronized experiences, which ultimately aid in the child's foundational development and blueprint the child's IWM as secure, safe, and adored. The combination of the two provides a strong, comprehensive model for renewal, growth, mastery, and all things necessary to repair a hurting heart.

Although every child client is unique, the richness of pairing Theraplay with CBPT activities within a treatment plan can make for a comprehensive therapeutic approach that supports the healing from the bottom up as well as from the top down to meet in the middle to support healing, regulation, *and* long-lasting mastery.

References

Baylin, J. (2018). Attachment-Focused Treatment and the Brain: A Neuroscience Perspective. In K. Doyle Buckwalter & D. Reed (Eds), *Attachment Theory in Action: Building Connection Between Child and Parents* (pp.35–50). Rowman & Littlefield.

Beacon House. (2017). The repair of early trauma: A bottom up approach [Video file]. August 7. www.youtube.com/watch?v=FOCTxcaNHeg

Bosmans, G. (2016). Cognitive behaviour therapy for children and adolescents: Can attachment theory contribute to its efficacy? *Clinical Child Family Psychology Review 19*, 310–328. doi: 10.1007/s10567-016-0212-3

Brickel, R. E. (2019). Why a bottom-up approach to trauma therapy is so powerful. June 4. https://brickelandassociates.com/bottom-up-approach-to-trauma

Brumariu, L. E. (2015). Parent–child attachment and emotion regulation. *New Directions for Child and Adolescent Development 148*, 31–45. doi:10.1002/cad.20098

Bundy-Myrow, S. (2005). Theraplay for Children with Self-Regulation Problems. In C. Schaefer, J. McCormick, & A. Ohnogi (Eds), *International Handbook of Play Therapy: Advances in Assessment, Theory, Research, and Practice* (pp.35–64). Jason Aronson.

Castagna, P., Long, A., & Upton, S. (2020). Cognitive Behaviour Therapy for Children with Emotional Regulation Challenges. In C. Maykel & M. Bray (Eds), *Promoting Mind-Body Health in Schools* (pp.317–333). American Psychological Association.

Cavett, A. M. (2018). Integrative Attachment Informed Cognitive Behavioral Play Therapy (IAI-CBPT) for Children with Medical Trauma. In L. C. Rubin (Ed.), *Handbook of Medical Play Therapy and Child Life: Interventions in Clinical and Medical Settings* (pp.131–153). Routledge. https://psycnet.apa.org/record/2017-43459-008

Cohen, J., & Mannarino, A (2008). Trauma-focused cognitive behavioural therapy for children and parents. *Child and Adolescent Mental Health 4*, 158–162. doi:10.1111/j.1475-3588.2008.00502.x

Cozolino, L. (2006). *The Neuroscience of Human Relationships: Attachment and the Developing Social Brain*. W.W. Norton & Co.

Drewes, A., & Cavett, A. (2019). Cognitive behavior play therapy. *Play Therapy 14*(3), 24–26. doi:10.1207/s15374424jccp2701_3

Gray, D. (2007). *Nurturing Adoptions: Creating Resilience after Neglect and Trauma*. Perspective Press.

Knell, S. M. (2009). Cognitive Behavioral Play Therapy: Theory and Applications. In A. A. Drewes (Ed.), *Blending Play Therapy with Cognitive Behavioral Therapy: Evidence-based and Other Effective Treatments and Techniques* (pp.117–133). John Wiley & Sons.

Montroy, J., Bowles, R., Skibbe, L., McClelland, M., & Morrison, J. (2017). The development of self-regulation across early childhood. *Developmental Psychology 52*(11), 1744–1762. doi:10.1037/DEV0000159

Norris, V., & Lender, D. (2020). *Theraplay®—The Practitioner's Guide*. Jessica Kingsley Publishers.

Perry, B. D., & Szalavitz, M. (2006). *The Boy Who Was Raised as a Dog and Other Stories from a Child Psychiatrist's Notebook: What Traumatized Children Can Teach Us About Loss, Love, and Healing*. Basic Books.

Porges, S. W. (2015). *Social Connectedness as a Biological Imperative: Understanding Trauma Through the Lens of the Polyvagal Theory*. [Published presentation at the Kinsley Institute, Indiana University, Bloomington, IN.]

Robinson, L., Segal, J., & Jaffe, J. (2022). How attachment styles affect adult relationships. *HelpGuide*, December 5. www.helpguide.org/articles/relationships-communication/attachment-and-adult-relationships.htm

Saarni, C. (2011). Emotional development in childhood. *Encyclopedia on Early Childhood Development*. www.child-encyclopedia.com/emotions/according-experts/emotional-development-childhood

Sroufe, L. A. (2005). Attachment and development: A prospective, longitudinal study from birth to adulthood. *Attachment & Human Development 7*, 349–367. doi: 10.1080/14616730500365928

Tucker, C., & Smith-Adcock, S. (2017). Theraplay: The Evidence for Trauma-Focused Treatment for Children and Families. In R. L. Steen (Ed.), *Emerging Research in Play Therapy, Child Counseling, and Consultation* (pp.42–59). Information Science Reference/ IGI Global. https://doi.org/10.4018/978-1-5225-2224-9.ch003

Weiss, J., Thomson, K., Burnham Riosa, P., Albaum, C., Chan, V., Maughan, A., Tablon, P., & Black, K. (2018). A randomized waitlist-controlled trial of cognitive behavior therapy to improve emotion regulation in children with autism. *The Journal of Child Psychology and Psychiatry 59*(11), 1180–1191. doi:10.1111/jcpp.12915

Chapter 6

Dyadic Developmental Psychotherapy (DDP) and Theraplay

HEALING OF INTERGENERATIONAL TRAUMA

Dafna Lender

Introduction

One of the most important decisions a therapist makes is how broadly to define the problem that clients bring into treatment. In an individualistic culture such as ours, it's common to focus narrowly on whoever is exhibiting problem behavior without understanding the wider family context shaping the issues of immediate concern. Often, the key to working effectively with a family is expanding the therapeutic perspective to include the history of intergenerational trauma underlying the present-day issues, even if that's not the family's view of the origins of the presenting problem.

It's not easy to introduce this perspective to parents. When parents bring their child for therapy, they don't expect or want to be the focus of work. That's why one of the first things I tell parents is that I work from an attachment perspective and will be working as much with them as with their child, or sometimes more. The real work can begin when they're willing to look into their own childhood history and how it may contribute to the situation. Theraplay can bring the joy, connection, trust, and safety that are so important for attachment. However, Dyadic Developmental Psychotherapy (DDP) (Hughes 2011) is needed to help parents realize how their attachment history affects their parenting and guide them towards being more accepting and empathic with their child's behaviors and underlying motives.

Theraplay and DDP

The best way to illustrate the integration of Theraplay and DDP is through a story. I worked with a father named John and his son Adam. John's entire identity was his family business. He owned a wood-processing plant and a small horse farm and worked all the time, even on weekends. He never meant to become a client, but when he brought his 11-year-old son, Adam, to see me, I insisted he come too since I specialize in Integrative Attachment Family Therapy (IAFT). I'd have asked that the mother join us, but she worked the swing shift as a nurse and wasn't available after school. Adam had anxiety and executive functioning deficits and had been diagnosed with attention deficit disorder and oppositional defiant disorder. He was on three different psychotropic meds, including a sedative for sleeping. When I asked for details, John said, "Adam's in his own world: he doesn't listen. He needs to be told three times just to do simple things, like clearing his cereal bowl from the table. Same with going to school, going to bed—whatever we say, he stalls and doesn't listen."

Unlike in Theraplay treatment, in DDP we talk to the child in the presence of their parents about the reasons that brought them to therapy and what they would like to work on. When I asked Adam what he thought he struggled with, he told me what he thought the problem was: "I can't think straight sometimes. I forget. When my dad tells me to do something, it sounds far away. Then he gets mad and yells at me." I then asked Adam about the anxiety and fears that the psychiatrist was medicating him for. "I can't sleep at night because I'm scared someone is gonna crawl through the window," he said. "My dad tells me that's impossible because we're so high up, but my sister can climb the tree. Also, I'm scared of Kiko, one of our mares, because she gets scared by critters, and twice she kicked me when she saw a mouse."

"How do you deal with these fears?"

"I try to tell my dad that I don't want to muck the stalls. I'll fill the trough and the water buckets and stuff, but I don't want to go in behind her because she gets spooked so easily."

I turned to John and asked, "Is that a fair deal? He'll take care of the chores outside the stall but won't go in?"

"That's fine for now, but it's not a solution. Adam has to learn that he's in charge. Horses are social animals. If you're scared, they're scared. But if you're confident, they're as calm as can be."

It turns out that was John's entire parenting philosophy. Whenever Adam was scared, John told him he had to put his mind over matter and be courageous. This also applied to the bully Adam was contending with on the school bus, and when he had fears about going to sleep alone at night.

Understanding DDP

One main goal of DDP is to let the child (or parent in parental consultations) clearly see that they have a positive impact on you, as the therapist, and how they affect you. It's about discovering a person's strengths (which the practitioner responds to with delight and recognition) and vulnerabilities (which are responded to with empathy and compassion). This means developing a shared meaning of experiences, behavior, and events, past and present, that the child understands, makes sense of, and could tell as their story, should they choose to do so. It is crucial to be able to tell a clear story about your life—your memories, experiences, and emotions—including the good and the tough times, and to share it with someone else. This helps to define who you are and to make sense of your feelings and your responses.

There is an important DDP tool that we always teach parents, for responding to children when they are first working on solving behavioral problems or disagreements. This tool is the PACE attitude. PACE is comprised of the words "playful, accepting, curious, empathic." It allows someone to focus on a person's inner life, not on specific behaviors. In other words, it is to discover what their underlying wishes, motives, feelings, or thoughts are under the behavior. This will allow the person to take in the feelings of empathy and acceptance that we want them to experience without feeling overwhelmed or shame or defensiveness.

Examples of playfulness, acceptance, empathy, and curiosity
Playfulness

- Making silly faces together.
- If the child said, "You're weird," responding by saying, "You're right, my boss pays me a lot to be weird, so thanks!"

Acceptance

- "Thanks for telling me."
- "I understand."
- "That makes sense."
- "I could see how you could feel that way."
- "I'm glad to know what's on your mind."

- "I didn't know you felt that way before."

- "I get it."

Empathy

- "That must be hard."

- "I would be sad too if that happened to me."

- "That sounds confusing."

- "That would be a lonely feeling."

Curiosity

- "How long have you felt this way?"

- "Have you felt this way a lot before?"

- "What else would you want to tell me about this situation?"

I talked to John about responding with the PACE attitude at home, and John always nodded in seeming accordance and said he would try. However, the next week, Adam would report the same things happening. John would ask Adam to go to bed but wouldn't tuck him in; John would tell Adam to muck the stalls, even though we agreed they'd do it together; John yelled at Adam for dawdling before school, even though we talked about his fear of being bullied on the bus.

I had four Theraplay sessions with John and Adam where I tried to model the dimensions of nurture and engagement on a simple level. I did this because Adam was very fearful and needed his dad to help him nurture him during bedtime and before school. I found that John would superficially try to participate in the nurture activities like the weather report or powder print, but he looked stiff and was rough, and Adam also stiffened and couldn't relax. When they played the feather blow game or the special handshake game, John got competitive and teased Adam when he didn't remember the sequence.

In the parent-only session, I asked John why he couldn't implement our strategies when dealing with bedtime problems or struggles with chores. First, he said he was tired and couldn't muster the energy. Then, in exasperation, he said, "Adam is going to have to manage the factory when he's older. If he can't stand up to a horse or a kid on the bus, how is he going to be the boss of 35 workers at the factory?"

Attachment relationships

In our individual session, I asked John questions about his own childhood, such as how his parents showed affection and how they punished him. Were there any family secrets, alcoholism or other addictions, any significant losses or deaths? Did anyone other than his parents take care of him? Did he feel rejected as a child? These questions are adapted from the Adult Attachment Interview, which asks adults to recall attachment-related memories from early childhood. The responses lead to adult-attachment classifications in three main areas that can help inform therapy.

Autonomous or secure adults tend to value attachment relationships. They can coherently describe the impact of attachment-related experiences, such as being sick and needing comfort, or losing an important relationship because of death, moving away, or divorce. *Dismissing adults* tend to devalue the importance of attachment relationships or to idealize their parents without being able to give any examples of their goodness. *Preoccupied adults* are still very much involved with their past attachment experiences and can't explore them productively. They often express anger when discussing current relationships with their parents. Dismissing and preoccupied adults are both considered to be insecure.

When I asked John about his relationship with his father, he told me he revered him. He described his father as a hard-working war hero devoted to his community. Rather than sounding personal, John's description of his father seemed like a reporter's account of a man on a pedestal.

When I asked for specific adjectives to describe his relationship with his father, John said: *kind, strict, and inspiring.* I asked if he had specific memories of those adjectives. For *strict*, he described the work ethic his father had imposed on him and his brothers, requiring them to help at the factory and around the property, as well as maintain excellent grades and play football in high school. For *inspiring*, he said his father had helped rebuild the church with his own hands after part of it had burned down. For *kind*, he recalled that he'd once disobeyed curfew, and when he'd come home, his dad was sitting in the dark with a rifle across his lap. John laughed and said he jumped five feet in the air, but his dad didn't say a word and didn't punish him. "That was his way of showing mercy on me."

Noticing a dismissive pattern of attachment, I pointed out that John's father seemed quite frightening—which prompted John to defend his father adamantly, invoking the wisdom of his ways. He kept repeating that he was much softer than John's grandfather, a volatile, angry man who'd beaten John's father. "He was a tough SOB," he told me. "He came to the US as a poor immigrant at 19 with nothing but his work ethic. My grandfather provided for his family, and he's the reason I was able to go to college."

"Wow," I said, "your grandpa had some really admirable qualities, but I saw you shudder as you spoke about him. What do you think made you shudder just then?"

"He died when I was six, but the stories my dad told—he was *not* someone you wanted to cross!"

I pointed out that dealing harshly with boys seemed to be a repeated pattern in their family.

"Well, you had to back then!" John exclaimed. "You don't understand the generation of men who came here and built their lives from scratch." As he smirked with derision, I noticed how small and naïve it made me feel, and I thought about how Adam must feel when his dad lectures him in that tone.

"John, you seem to think I'm saying your grandfather and father are bad, or that I don't appreciate their struggle. I think it's admirable that you're defending them, but you seem worried about my pointing out that they were scary men at times. I wonder why that's so hard for you to talk about."

"Because you don't understand! They had to do what they did to me in order to get me where I am!"

"What did they do to you?"

"My dad did scare the shit out of me at times. Once, he locked me in the tool shed for a whole evening because I'd gotten in trouble at school for punching another kid's science fair display. We'd both done a project on solar eclipses, except his diorama had electricity wired in and looked really good. I'd worked so hard on mine without any help. So when I saw this kid's project and what his dad had helped him do, I just flipped my lid. The teacher called my parents, and I knew I was in trouble. I ran home and hid under the bed until my dad came home and put me in the tool shed. It was so hot in there I thought I was going to die. He brought me water once in a while but then just closed and bolted the door. When he finally let me out, the only thing he said was, 'You're not going to get anywhere by being jealous.'"

As John talked about his experience, I could see he had flashes of fear, anger, and sadness, and I made a point of demonstrating an intense focus and presence, nodding my head and expressing empathy in my voice. I asked John, "Do you think it's possible to respect your father and understand why he felt he needed to do that to you while also honoring that, as a 10-year-old boy, you were scared by what he did?"

"I don't know," John responded in a faraway voice.

"I want you to consider that you were a boy who had his own thoughts and wishes, his own feelings, who wanted to be accepted and recognized."

Again, John got a faraway look as if contemplating this idea, and then he seemed to come to. He looked at me and said, "What does this have to do with Adam's problems?"

"I think Adam feels he can't have fears or need your help without you scaring him and making him feel bad for those feelings, just like your father did to you and your grandfather did to your father," I responded. "I don't think Adam has anxiety or attention deficit. I think that he senses from you that it's not okay to feel scared or unsure. So when he feels that way, he has to hide those feelings, but they don't go away. They get pushed down and then come out as having irrational fears and an inability to concentrate."

"Well, I was raised that way, and I turned out okay!" John barked.

"At what cost?" I asked.

He paused. "What cost? I'm happy the way I am. I don't have any problems."

"Well, maybe, but do you ever feel lonely or empty? Do you ever isolate yourself from your wife, even though she wants to be with you? Do you yell at Adam for not wanting to fall asleep alone, even though we'd agreed in here that you'd sit with him until he falls asleep?"

John then told me he spends every night in his garage playing video games and gambling online. He hasn't lost any money, he assured me, but his wife is furious at him for staying in there and ignoring her feelings.

"John," I said, "you have to decide whether you're satisfied with the way you're functioning in your family right now. I can't decide that."

John tried one more time to defend himself. "But how is sitting in Adam's room until he falls asleep going to teach him independence and courage?! He's almost 12 and needs me to read him a story and hold his hand on the bus? If he can't get his act together, he'll run the factory to the ground when he's older!"

"I want the same thing for Adam as you do. I want him to have a clear, healthy mind and be able to hold down a good job and function in society. But here's the thing: forcing Adam to do things he's afraid of is impeding his ability to gain the independence you're striving to teach him. By forcing him to muck out Kiko's stall, even though he's been kicked by her twice already, he doesn't respect his experience of fear—just like your father misunderstood and humiliated you for being jealous of your classmate's project. Your dad didn't ask you what made you feel so bad that day when you saw your classmate's project. Instead, he made you feel really ashamed, lonely, and scared. Imagine if he'd asked you what it was like to feel so proud and then so crestfallen when your classmate had such a superior science project?"

John became quiet.

"What do you think it would've been like?"

John choked back tears as he mumbled, "That boy's father was at the science fair helping him rig up the electricity, and they looked so happy together. My dad would never have had the time or even thought to help me."

"That makes so much sense, John. You wanted your dad to be with you, to enjoy you. And seeing your classmate get that was too painful, so you got angry and violent instead. And then you got scared of what your dad would do. You were taught to hide when you had feelings that were 'weak.' But actually, being able to be with someone who loves you when you have those feelings is what makes you feel stronger."

This was the beginning of my therapy with John. It took us about five months of weekly sessions for him to see the impact of his own experiences as a child and how the legacy of violence, loss, and fear had been playing into his parenting attitudes toward Adam. Trauma is transmitted between generations when frightening experiences go unnamed and cause a child to internalize.

Stopping intergenerational trauma
One of the most important things John and I worked on was honoring the fact that John's father had done the best he could *and* acknowledging that as a child John had harbored real and legitimate emotional needs that had gone unmet. The next step was to have empathy for John's young self as he endured isolating and invalidating experiences with his father. In the process, John remembered several other disturbing and frightening incidents when his father had intimidated and humiliated him in his efforts to raise him up to be "a strong man." Since a persistent and corrosive feeling that John and many trauma survivors have is that they deserve the treatment they received, we provided him the opportunity to "reparent" his child self through self-compassion, modeled through my compassionate attitude.

Once John had come to terms with his childhood trauma, we turned our attention to his ability to repair with Adam. John had to take responsibility for invalidating and scaring Adam. In one touching DDP session, John looked his son in the eye and apologized for forcing him to muck out Kiko's stall, even though Kiko had kicked him in the head, and said how sorry he was for making him feel that his fears were not valid. John told his son how hard it was to allow him to express his fear because he was taught that being sad or afraid was wrong; he added that he was learning to approach things differently from how his father had handled them.

The final piece of the therapy between father and son was teaching John about facilitating joyful play, physical proximity, and touch, through the use of Theraplay sessions. As a result of using a sequence of engaging and nurturing activities in weekly sessions, Adam began to feel calmer and less fearful about going to school and going to sleep. John had had no experience of affection, tenderness, and nurturing in his childhood. Therefore, he had no idea how to be present for another person on a physical level. Theraplay helped John learn how to do that.

Our therapy involved showing John how to stay close to his son during bedtime by doing the weather report. We also practiced simply sharing a snack towards the end of the session and doing simple things like sitting shoulder-to-shoulder or stroking Adam's hair. We also read stories to practice the importance of storytelling as a way to calm Adam's anxious brain. When given the freedom to be by Adam's side, it turns out that John enjoyed lying next to Adam and making up adventure stories. As a result, Adam's nighttime problems went away.

Regarding Adam's school fears, now that John had more empathy for his childhood self, we were able to have more compassion for Adam's fears and be more supportive of him. John tried to advocate for a bus monitor to prevent the bullying, but that didn't work. He tried meeting Adam at the bus stop to give the bully an intimidating look, but that only made things worse. Then, one session, when they came in, and I checked in on how the week went, Adam said, "It was great. Dad drove me to school every day." My eyes widened in surprise, and I looked at John.

"Yeah," he shrugged. "I don't want Adam to waste his energy worrying about some twerp on the bus. I figure let him start out his day without that hassle so he can focus on learning." Adam nodded. It was a much better week.

Conclusion

In the end, the power of Theraplay coupled with DDP transformed the family's problems. The family members became motivated to see their struggles in a new light. The key to change in this case was creating a new narrative for John, the father, by using DDP, which then superseded the patriarchal legacy and opened the way for John and Adam to join together to create a new, more fulfilling relationship through Theraplay.

Reference

Hughes, D. (2011). *Attachment-Focused Family Therapy Workbook*. W.W. Norton & Co.

Chapter 7

Eye Movement Desensitization and Reprocessing (EMDR) within a Theraplay Intervention for Children

Helen Rodwell

Introduction

Children can be traumatized by a wide range of experiences, including single events, such as a road traffic accident, or more prolonged experiences, such as abuse and neglect within their child–parent relationship. This latter realm of trauma, often referred to as "developmental trauma" (van der Kolk 2005) or "relational trauma" (Schore 1994), can have profound and wide-ranging effects on a child's development, state of regulation, and sense of self. Theraplay has developed as an effective way for a child to build new relational experiences with their current parent. At its core, Theraplay uses a model of healthy child–parent relationships that contain the four dimensions of structure, engagement, nurture, and challenge. Through the vehicle of interactive physical play activities, the focus is on assisting a traumatized child to experience their parent as being organized and predictable (structure); regulating, attuned, and enjoyable (engagement); soothing, calm, and safe (nurture); and supportive of the need to master new experiences (challenge).

Traumatic experiences shape a child's brain and body and provide a child with an internal working model (IWM) of themselves and others (especially their parents) and the world (Bowlby 1969). Within the world of fostering and adoption, when a child moves to a new home and parent, the child's existing model, or survival strategy, will influence how they relate to their new parent and environment. Their existing model of how to "be parented" may not fit with their new parent; the child may show rejecting, controlling, overly compliant, and confusing behaviors. Theraplay has developed as an effective intervention for assisting parents in understanding their child's existing IWM and behavior while also providing the child with new reparative experiences of being parented, which will, over time, reshape their model.

The impact of traumatic relational experiences on a child's IWM will be uniquely influenced by many factors, including the child's age, resilience, availability of supportive relationships, and their perception of their experiences. This means that there is no therapeutic "one size fits all," so the goal of Theraplay is to tailor the activities to best fit the child's unique experiential and relational needs.

In this chapter, I describe how I use Theraplay with Eye Movement Desensitization and Reprocessing (EMDR) as an integrative intervention. I begin with an overview of EMDR before focusing on how this model can be integrated within Theraplay. I then illustrate this using a composite, fictionalized case study. My intention is to illustrate how Theraplay, my "go to" model of child–parent intervention, can be used as the main approach for strengthening a child's relationship with their parent, and for providing reparative relational experiences while using EMDR to directly address past trauma. My hope is that this chapter will inspire you to explore the potential superpower that EMDR could add to your Theraplay practice.

Throughout this chapter, I use the word "parent" to describe any adult who is in the parenting and caregiver role.

EMDR and Theraplay

EMDR has become well known as a trauma therapy and is recognized in national and international guidelines as an effective evidence-based treatment for post-traumatic stress disorder (PTSD) (e.g., England's 2018 NICE guidelines and WHO 2013). What may be less well known is that EMDR is used for strengthening positive memories so that they become internal resources. EMDR also fits well within a range of therapeutic models. Within a Theraplay intervention, EMDR can be used to resolve disturbing memories of trauma and loss while also being used to strengthen a child's relationship with their parent. EMDR can be used to strengthen a parent's personal resources for parenting, which is incredibly helpful since many parents experience secondary trauma or "blocked care" (Hughes & Baylin 2012) when parenting their traumatized child.

Adaptive Information Processing (AIP) model

EMDR is based on the Adaptive Information Processing (AIP) model (Shapiro 1995), which proposes that our brains have a natural process for recovering and growing after traumatic experiences, that memories are processed and stored in either a helpful (adaptive) or unhelpful (maladaptive) way. Adaptive memory processing happens when positive or negative memories are successfully processed so that they are stored and integrated with similar experiences we have had about ourselves, others, and the world. Memories tend to get linked to other memories that share similar information, such as physical sensations, senses, emotions, and beliefs. This memory linkage is illustrated by the common experience many of us have had of a memory having been brought back to our awareness by a specific smell or song. Memories that have been successfully adaptively processed tend to become neutral in their affect (i.e., they no longer disturb or bother us) or are remembered positively (i.e., memories that give us nice feelings). Adaptive memories give us positive resources, behaviors, self-beliefs, and skills. Memories may be explicit (conscious) or implicit (unconscious). A memory is multisensory (images, sounds, smells, tastes) and has associated emotions, body sensations, thoughts, and beliefs.

According to AIP, memories are maladaptively stored when there are disruptions to the information processing system. These disruptions can occur for many reasons—for example, dissociative responses that happened at the time of the traumatic event. When the information processing system is disrupted, this can lead to the disturbing memory being easily triggered by stimuli long after the original event has passed. To the person, it can feel as though they are right back reliving the original event. Sometimes the triggered past experience can be named, while at other times the triggered feelings and sensations are not consciously tied to an event but "the body remembers" it (van der Kolk 2014). Children who experience trauma at a very early age are more likely to re-experience these implicit body memories. Distressing and confusing feelings, thoughts, and body sensations can be triggered by a plethora of daily, ordinary things. Ordinary parts of a child's current relationship with their parent may trigger a child to show sudden changes in their mood and behavior, like a kind of flashback to early relational trauma memories. Ordinary daily life can lead a traumatized child to fall down into "time holes" (Hobday 2001) and elicit natural fight, flight, freeze, or fawn responses (Walker 2003).

EMDR assists the brain's natural memory processing system so that disturbing memories are adaptively stored. This is done by having the person focus their attention on the disturbing memory, specifically the negative image, cognition (belief), emotion, and body sensation related to it, while also engaging in bilateral stimulation (BLS). BLS means that both sides of the brain are stimulated. This can happen via eye movements—for example, moving the eyes by watching something move horizontally from left to right, comically referred to as "finger waggling" by some children I've worked with. BLS can be delivered via tactile taps (such as using hands to tap both sides of the body or by using electronic vibrating pulsers such as TheraTappers™[1]), or it can involve auditory tones (such as hearing tones that alternate from left to right). It is thought that this dual attention on both the target memory and the BLS enables the brain to resume its normal healing process, so that disturbing memories are stored without the original associated physical and sensory sensations, emotions, and thoughts.

The role of the EMDR therapist

The EMDR therapist's role is to guide the process, use specific techniques to support the person to stay within their "window of tolerance" (Siegel 2012) during processing, and use strategies to assist the information processing system to keep going when it gets stuck or blocked. EMDR therapists have had specialist training and are skilled at knowing when the brain's processing system needs extra stimulation to enable information to be adaptively resolved and for new learning to occur. Brains will always want to create new meaning from experiences and to grow—with this being especially true during childhood. EMDR is effective for assisting children in developing new meaning from early childhood adversity, although it is more complex because of the developmental challenges inherent during childhood. It's essential that specific child EMDR training is undertaken after the basic adult EMDR training, as set out by EMDR Europe and the EMDR International Association.

Phases of EMDR

EMDR is an eight-phase treatment consisting of:

- Phase 1: Client history and planning

- Phase 2: Preparation

- Phase 3: Assessment

- Phase 4: Desensitization

- Phase 5: Installation

---

1   www.dnmsinstitute.com/theratapper

- Phase 6: Body scan

- Phase 7: Closure

- Phase 8: Re-evaluation.

These eight phases contribute to the child's therapeutic goals in specific ways, as outlined below.

Phase 1: Client history and planning

This phase mirrors the Theraplay process of gathering initial intake information about the child's presenting problem and daily life. The EMDR therapist wants to identify what has happened in the child's history because the AIP model hypothesizes that the child's current difficulties are being driven or influenced by earlier memories that have not been adaptively processed. The EMDR therapist wants to identify a potential map of the child's memory experiences with potential targets for memory processing. Information is gathered from the child's current parent(s), school, other key people, and historical documents, although we are mindful that these sources do not accurately tell us how the child actually experienced their life events. We tell parents why and how we understand the child's history using the AIP model. In EMDR, we use a three-pronged protocol of past, present, and future to organize a treatment plan:

- *Past:* We map out the child's past memory network of experiences that potentially inform their presenting issue.

- *Present:* We identify the current people and situations that trigger the child's negative reactions and symptoms.

- *Future:* We identify the child's desired future response and prepare for potential future challenging situations.

We introduce EMDR to parents and talk with them about the idea that poorly processed memories can lead a child to develop distortions in how they view themselves and their world. These distortions usually fall into the broad themes of responsibility, safety/vulnerability, self-defectiveness, and power/control/choices. An EMDR goal is to identify the cognitive distortions that a child has attached to their experiences and assist them in developing a more helpful and healthier cognition. For example, a child moves from believing "I am not lovable" to "I am lovable."

We talk with parents about how EMDR can be used with them, too, in their parenting role, in terms of strengthening memories that support their parenting and/or processing distressing memories that negatively influence their current parenting. It's important that we get informed consent for EMDR, and it's useful to obtain this early in the intervention process so that opportunities to use EMDR can be captured as they arise during Theraplay.

Phase 2: Preparation

This phase focuses on preparing the child and parent for EMDR memory processing. Traditional EMDR preparation includes sharing psychoeducation about trauma and EMDR with the parent and child (in an age-relevant way); stabilization of the child; resource building; and developing the child's strategies for self-regulation. This phase of EMDR is usually longer for traumatized children compared to children without a chronic or relational trauma history.

In traditional EMDR, we prepare a child for trauma processing by first installing a "safe" or "okay" space within them. Children are encouraged to imagine or recall a safe space. When possible, we invite the child to imagine this place, draw it, or create it in a sandtray. We then assist the child with identifying the emotion and location of positive sensations in their body, before providing slow, short sets of BLS to install this as a resource.

Traumatized children often find it hard to imagine what "safe" or "okay" would look and feel like because they have had few or no experiences of this. They do not have robust memory networks that contain information about what "safe" feels like. Considerable time can be spent creatively exploring and finding experiences of feeling "safe" and "okay" using various mediums, such as smell (e.g., a particular smell that a child finds relaxing) or physical movement (e.g., a particular yoga pose that elicits a feeling of strength in a child, hugging a cushion, or being wrapped in a blanket). These experiences can then be installed and strengthened as a resource using BLS.

Traumatized children, especially those who are dissociative, will need lots of stabilization and resourcing. EMDR can be used to assist children to become able to identify and label their emotional state—for example, using scripts such as "When I am feeling butterflies in my tummy, that's a signal from my brain that I'm feeling anxious" and adding BLS. The child can then be taught grounding or self-regulation strategies to help them manage these feelings—for example, "When I'm feeling anxious, that's a sign for me to press my hands down on the seat next to me and count to 10" (Darker-Smith 2020, adapted from Omaha 2004).

We sometimes encourage children to practice mentally eliciting their "safe" or "okay" space using a "cue" word. For example, in traditional EMDR with older children and adults, we practice "cueing with disturbance," which involves having the person imagine a minor annoyance and noticing how they feel, before then asking them to use their "cue" word (which is attached to their "safe" space) to bring up better feelings. This can be useful for allowing older children to practice having some control of their experiences.

During EMDR, it's important that children know that they will have control of the process, particularly when processing distressing memories during Phase 4: Desensitization. For example, we can teach children to use a "stop" signal (such as a hand signal) so that they can indicate the need for a pause during desensitization.

Preparation also involves assisting a child in being able to identify feelings and cognitions in age-relevant ways. This could involve teaching a child emotional literacy skills.

The preparation phase is aimed at the child and their parent to acquire and strengthen personal resources before processing traumatic memories. This goes hand in hand with the EMDR therapist developing a therapeutic relationship with the child and parent.

Parent preparation

It is important that parents are well prepared for their child's EMDR so they know what their role will be during EMDR and how they can support their child. Children need the presence of a safe, stable, and supportive parent for EMDR. Parenting a traumatized child can be hard, and it is common for parents to feel overwhelmed and experience "blocked care" (Hughes & Baylin 2012). Trauma can feel contagious as traumatized children often seem to trigger any unresolved, soft spots within a parent's own history. We can use the EMDR three-pronged protocol of past–present–future to assist parents with their current difficulties with their child. Past events in the parent's history could be triggered by their child's current behavior, so we can use EMDR to process this. For example, the standard EMDR protocol can be used during parent-only sessions to process previous experiences of loss and grief, such as miscarriage and infertility. EMDR with parents can be used to desensitize child behaviors that trigger current feelings of distress in a parent. EMDR can also be used to install a "future template" for how a parent wants to respond to their child in the future.

Phases 3 and 4: Assessment and desensitization

Assessment refers to the process of the child accessing the target memory network and identifying the cognitions, emotions, and body feelings associated with the memory. For example, this could involve a child being asked to remember a specific event (the target memory) while they also notice and identify the thoughts, emotions, and body sensations that come up. Some children are developmentally able to do this, while younger children cannot. During Phase 3, we create a baseline of the target memory by using two measuring scales called the Validity of Positive Cognition (VOC) and Subjective Units of Disturbance (SUDs). We can use cards, cubes, and balls that have negative cognitions (such as "I am bad," "I am going to die"), positive cognitions (such as "I am a good kid," "I am safe"), emotions, and physical body sensations written on them. We help the child to measure the intensity of these cognitions, emotions, and body sensations by using creative methods such as visual scales, numbered blocks, dolls of different sizes, or hands (e.g., "Use your hands to show how much it bothers you right now"). Gomez (2013) provides an excellent resource for creative tools.

Desensitization of disturbing memories

When therapy moves on to processing disturbing memories, traditional EMDR involves asking children to identify the negative cognition or thought, emotions, and body sensations that are associated with the disturbing target memory. Children will vary in their capacity to use language and identify thoughts, emotions, and body sensations, so the EMDR therapist makes developmental adjustments for this.

A traditional EMDR process would invite children to recall a disturbing target memory by asking the child to "think of the worst part of it" and then asking them to identify the cognitions, emotions, and body sensations currently associated with it. The child is then asked to focus on these and to do repeated sets of BLS. We'll invite the child to "notice" what comes up and to "just go with that." Between sets of BLS, we encourage the child to "take a deep breath in and out." This dual process of having the child access the disturbing target memory network and its associated current cognitions, emotions, and body sensations, while receiving BLS, continues until the memory reaches a state of resolution (i.e., when it's no longer disturbing). We use faster and longer sets of BLS during desensitization, rather than the slow, short BLS sets we do when installing a resource. We use the child's SUDs rating (e.g., "How much does the memory bother you now?") to know when this memory has been desensitized.

The value of EMDR with children is that they can have considerable control over what memories they focus on for processing. EMDR also does not require a child to talk about the event during processing, which is helpful for children who experience shame about what happened to them or cannot talk about the event for other reasons. Traumatized children will often avoid focusing on disturbing memories; avoidance may have been a useful survival strategy for them previously. It's therefore essential to take the time needed to use Theraplay to build trust and resources within the child before we take them back to their difficult past.

A storytelling (narrative) approach is useful for children who cannot recall an explicit memory and its associated cognitions, emotions, and physical sensations. With the parent, we write a story that reflects the child's experience so that the action of listening to the story becomes the trauma memory target. We can also use doll figures to recreate the story while the child watches and listens. Preparing the narrative with the parent allows us to be sure that the parent is ready and able to listen to the story with their child. Narratives can be hard to listen to, so it's essential that parents are able to self-regulate during its telling.

A good narrative is short and focused with a beginning, a middle, and an end (Logie *et al.* 2020). It can focus on a specific event or a period of time. The parent or therapist tells the story to the child while the other adult delivers BLS to the child. Traumatized children will often need a range of narratives to address different periods of their life and themes of trauma, loss, and attachment. We can also develop resource narratives that help reconnect the child with times in their life when they felt brave or loved.

When the desensitization phase is first used with children, it's important for them to experience EMDR in a way that is not too much for them so that they gain confidence and trust in how it works. I've found many children to be tentative at first. Still, after experiencing EMDR with low-intensity (i.e., less disturbing) events, they discover that their brain really can process events in a helpful way, especially when they feel supported and are not rushed to face past events that they are not ready for. It's not uncommon for children to then start coming to sessions with their own list of EMDR memory targets. We invite children, especially older children, to identify the experiences (past, present, and future) they want to work on so that these become less muddled and confusing. We often develop a timeline with children.

For some children, the intense focus on the target memory coupled with BLS is all that's needed to process a memory. However, many children will need the addition of an interweave during desensitization. An interweave assists processing by adding in psychoeducation or making changes to the child's imagery, thought, action, or physical movement. For example, if a child becomes stuck during desensitization with the cognition that they were to blame for their abuse (a responsibility cognition), we might ask, "Whose job is it to keep children safe?" and add in BLS. There is a plethora of interweaves available for an EMDR therapist to use.

Phase 5: Installation

This phase is focused on installing a positive belief (cognition) connected to the past disturbing memory. For example, a child who believes "I am not safe" in connection with past abuse is assisted in having the cognition "I am safe now" installed with that experience. This phase involves the child holding both the target memory and the positive belief in mind while BLS is used. The VOC scale is used to gauge how much the child believes the positive belief—for example, "When you think about the memory you've been working on, how true do the words, 'I am safe' feel to you now?" Some children will not have the developmental skills for this kind of rating, so adaptations are made.

Phases 6 and 7: Body scan and closure

The body scan phase is used to make sure that the child's positive belief is congruent with their body's experience. The EMDR therapist checks whether the child has any residual body sensations associated with the target memory that needs more processing.

Some children may fully process a target memory during one session, while others, especially traumatized children, will need more than one session. All EMDR sessions are closed carefully, especially if disturbing material has come up for children. We want to ensure that a child leaves a session in a good, stable state.

Phase 8: Re-evaluation

This phase focuses on the changes that occur following EMDR processing. Many children's play and behavior change quickly after EMDR processing sessions. For example, immediately after processing a target memory, a child may laugh more genuinely or play differently. It's important that we check in with parents after EMDR sessions so that they can share any changes they have seen in their child. As EMDR therapists, when we hear about new or more intense distressing behaviors, we consider these as potential future targets for EMDR processing.

Once a child's past target memory has been processed, we move on to the second step of our three-pronged protocol of past–present–future. We focus on processing the child's present triggers. This involves us identifying the current situations that trigger emotional disturbance or distressing behaviors and then using EMDR to desensitize these. Specifically, in the eight-phase process, we use Phases 3: Assessment through to 8: Re-evaluation. This process could begin, for example, by asking the child to "bring up a memory of [recent event]" and notice the current thoughts, feelings, and sensations. Or we could use a narrative storytelling approach that focuses on the current situation.

The final step of the three-pronged protocol involves a focus on the future. We identify the future situations that could potentially lead to the child experiencing distress, and we use EMDR Phases 3 through to 8 to process these. The aim is to assist the child in developing a future template (or IWM) that is adaptive, healthy, and helpful.

Theraplay with EMDR

EMDR's AIP model and Theraplay both share the premise that the human brain and body work towards health, resolution, and social connection. Both EMDR and Theraplay are supported by theories of attachment, affective neuroscience, and neurobiology. For traumatized children, I've found that it is better for EMDR to be incorporated into Theraplay rather than vice versa. This is because Theraplay's clear protocol, session sequence, and relationship-focused goals provide the essential stabilization experiences needed for EMDR. The power of pure stand-alone Theraplay should not be underestimated.

Theraplay practitioners will be familiar with the Theraplay process that comprises the initial intake information gathering; Marschak Interaction Method (MIM) assessment and analysis; MIM feedback sessions with parent(s); parent demonstration sessions; and dyadic (parent–child) sessions (Booth & Jernberg 2010). I follow the standard Theraplay plan and incorporate EMDR within this.

Phase 1: Integrative intake and integrative assessment

The usual Theraplay process of gathering information about the child and parents is followed to develop an understanding of the dyad's strengths and needs across the structure, engagement, nurture, and challenge dimensions. From an EMDR perspective, we want to begin identifying the potential memory networks, both for adaptive and maladaptive memories. EMDR desensitization of disturbing memories is more successful when it can be linked to adaptive memories.

The MIM observation is used in the usual Theraplay way to identify and think about the child's and parent's strengths and needs across the four dimensions of structure, engagement, nurture, and challenge. From an EMDR perspective, the MIM provides a rich window into how a child's earlier experiences (i.e., memory networks) may be influencing their current strengths and struggles with their parent and during daily life. We can use the MIM observation and our subsequent MIM feedback sessions with parents for EMDR's Phase 1: Client history and planning. For example, if a child shows the capacity to be playful with their parent during the squeaky animals task, this could mean that the child has an adaptive memory network of earlier positive play experiences. These earlier positive memories could become a potential resource for strengthening within the child using EMDR.

In terms of current struggles, if, for example, the child shows distress when being touched during the lotion task, this could be connected to earlier unprocessed memories of abusive or neglectful touch. Such memories become potential EMDR targets for processing later on during dyadic Theraplay sessions when the child is ready.

The process of identifying past, current, and future targets for memory processing tends to be ongoing throughout the intervention. It is typical for initial memory targets to be easily identified—for example, the past traumatic events that adults know of. However, it is common for previously unknown memories to come up for a child during EMDR processing sessions. This happens because memories tend to be connected; for example, memories with common themes or feelings tend to be linked in our memory networks. This means that EMDR is used flexibly in response to what a child experiences and recalls. The regular parent-only sessions during Theraplay are important spaces for the practitioner and parents to continually recheck what EMDR should focus on.

Many traumatized children, who have experienced chaotic, emotionally neglectful, and physically abusive early environments, have developed memory networks that contain little, if any, adaptive and positive information. This means that the reparative healthy child–parent experiences that can be developed through dyadic Theraplay are essential. The MIM assessment often painfully highlights the scarcity of adaptive memories of safe, healthy, and attuned attachment relationships for many traumatized children.

Phase 2: Integrative preparation
MIM feedback
During the MIM feedback parent sessions, we share our hypotheses and ideas about the strengths and needs of parents and their child across the Theraplay dimensions. We encourage parents to reflect and mentalize on their own and their child's experiences during the MIM. We can incorporate EMDR into these feedback sessions by, for example, using it to strengthen a parent's positive memories of being with their child. For example, a parent could be shown a positive MIM clip and be asked to focus on the positive thoughts, feelings, and body sensations they felt at the time. This can then be installed with a short set of slow BLS. Other positive resources for parenting can also be installed with EMDR. For example, we could ask the parent to bring to mind their "best ever parenting day" (Darker-Smith 2020) or recall a moment when they felt deep love and empathy for their child. Using EMDR in this way with parents helps to strengthen their parenting resources and helps prepare them for EMDR with their child. Anecdotally, parents who have experienced EMDR themselves have said that it has helped them to understand EMDR, giving them greater empathy and insight into what EMDR might feel like for their child.

Parent demonstration session
The parent demonstration session occurs in the usual way. From an EMDR perspective, this session provides more opportunities to learn more about

the child's and parent's memory networks. For example, parents often share memories while doing Theraplay activities with us. The parent demonstration session can also be used as a space during which EMDR is used directly with a parent. For example, I have used EMDR during cotton ball or feather guess with a parent (who was experiencing "blocked care") to install this as a resource for them, having felt genuinely attended to.

Resource development

Pure dyadic Theraplay offers a traumatized child the opportunity to experience much-needed safe and healthy interactions with their parent. The Theraplay practitioner leads the session and uses carefully chosen activities to meet the child's needs. A traumatized child may need activities that involve more physical distance, less physical touch, reduced eye contact, and quieter voices. Polyvagal theory (Porges 2011) helps to conceptualize what happens within a child during Theraplay and their daily life. A traumatized child may move easily and quickly into mobilization/fight or flight (sympathetic state) and immobilization/freeze (parasympathetic dorsal vagal state). Theraplay activities are used to move children through this hierarchy of states, from immobilization, to (and through) mobilization, to the ventral vagal state of being safe and open to social connection. Knowing the child's nervous system state is crucial during EMDR because we do not want to overwhelm a child during the processing of disturbing memories. Close viewing of the video-recording of Theraplay sessions can help us to identify what state of arousal a child is in.

Pure dyadic Theraplay sessions provide a child with important experiences of stabilization, which are an essential foundation for EMDR. Strategically chosen Theraplay activities can assist a child in learning regulation. For example, the firm physical regulating pressure inherent during Play-Doh squeeze can be installed as a resource using EMDR.

In traditional EMDR, we usually install a "safe" or "okay" space during the early stages of treatment. When using Theraplay, I incorporate "safe" space work after a series of pure dyadic sessions, when we've reached a stage where a parent is able to successfully do some Theraplay activities with their child, and the child has experienced co-regulation, connection, and relational synchrony during some Theraplay activities.

Relationship building with dyadic Theraplay

Sessions of pure dyadic Theraplay provide much-needed positive adaptive memory networks within a traumatized child. This means that dyadic Theraplay sessions occur in their usual way, with Theraplay activities being chosen to fit the specific needs of the child. As Theraplay progresses, EMDR can be used to strengthen new positive attachment experiences as they occur at the moment, and to install the experience as a resource. For example, when a child and parent are enjoying an activity together, in the here and now, the child can be directed to "notice your body, heart, and mind," and BLS can be added in. This strengthening of new healthy relational experiences is important for EMDR because disturbing, traumatic memories are processed more effectively when they are linked with existing, adaptive memory networks (Shapiro 1995).

We can incorporate BLS into a Theraplay activity so that it becomes a logical part of it. For example, when a child is genuinely enjoying playing balloon tennis with their parent, we can encourage the child to "notice how good it feels to have fun with your dad," and incorporate BLS by having the child slowly bat the balloon with their alternating left and right hand while we say, "It's important to notice moments like this to help us remember them."

We can also install moments of calm during the Theraplay session. For example, during the calmness of sticker match, we could verbalize, "Notice how calm it feels to be with your mum" and then place a few stickers slowly onto the child's left and right shoulders alternately. The EMDR lens invites us to notice and capture positive moments as they occur during Theraplay activities.

Pure Theraplay does not involve much talking. For EMDR, it is helpful to introduce the child to the concepts of mind (thoughts), heart (feeling), and body sensations (Gomez 2013). During a Theraplay mirroring activity, we may ask the child, "Your body looks really relaxed right now. I wonder what your heart and mind are saying?" We accept and acknowledge the child's responses. When the child identifies positive feelings and good-feeling body sensations, we can direct the child to "notice that" and continue mirroring using slow, left-to-right actions.

Using Theraplay activities to install a "safe" or "okay" space

The process of installing a "safe" or "okay" space within a child can be facilitated with Theraplay. Traumatized children often find it hard to imagine what "safe" or "okay" would look and feel like. Theraplay activities can become the vehicles for finding this state within the child. For example, when a child shows calmness and "felt safety" (Purvis, Lyons Sunshine, & Cross 2007) during cotton ball soothe, we can ask the child, "What is your heart and body feeling?" and if the feelings and body sensations are positive, we can add in a short and slow set of BLS to install this good feeling as a resource.

Positive feelings that a child has felt during interactive Theraplay activities with their parent can also be stored inside an imaginary "heart jar" (Gomez 2013) so that they are always carried within the child.

Safe place exercises can be deliberately incorporated within dyadic Theraplay sessions as a goal-directed activity. For example, we could add in "Build a fort" to physically make a safe place for the child to sit in (ideally with their parent), and then use EMDR to strengthen this feeling.

Theraplay activities as vehicles for BLS
We introduce the idea of BLS to children as a way to help the child's whole brain notice a moment with their right and left hemispheres. We tell children that BLS can "turn both sides of our brain on," and we introduce different types of BLS to find a child's preference. One child may prefer to watch a finger puppet being moved horizontally, while another child may prefer taps on their shoulder by their parent, or a self-directed butterfly hug (Artigas et al. 2000).

In typical Theraplay, the activities are chosen as vehicles for achieving therapeutic goals. For example, feather blow can provide a child with the joy of a serve-and-return interaction with their parent. Theraplay activities can also be used for BLS. Slow and short sets of BLS are used to install and strengthen positive resources, while faster and longer sets of BLS are used for processing disturbing memories. Using Theraplay, we might do slow pretend strokes of paint on a child's alternating hands while enhancing a positive memory, or we might do fast bilateral hand clapping while remembering disturbing events.

Using Theraplay activities to establish a "stop" signal with the child
Theraplay activities that incorporate instructions such as "ready, steady, go" can assist children with knowing how and when to stop and pause, and show them that we listen and respond to them. This is a good precursor for helping a child to develop a "stop" signal that they can use during EMDR, which they trust us to respond to. I often give children a concierge bell for them to ding when they want to stop during EMDR processing.

The relational and attuned focus of Theraplay provides an essential platform for us to notice a child's non-verbal signs of where they are in their "window of tolerance." Desensitization of distressing memories can be scary for children, so they need to know that they will not become overwhelmed. It's essential that we know when to pause and help the child to "put the bad stuff away" using some form of imaginary container, and when to continue with desensitization using techniques to help the process move quickly and smoothly. We often use a metaphor such as "It's like you're watching old movies," to remind children that their memories are in the past.

Parent feedback sessions

Throughout the Theraplay intervention, regular parent-only sessions occur with the usual aim of developing the parent's understanding of Theraplay and how they can provide their child with goal-focused experiences. As the intervention begins to incorporate EMDR, more frequent parent sessions will be needed for preparation (e.g., identifying target memories and preparing the parent for their role during EMDR); for checking how a child has responded during the days following EMDR; and for possible direct EMDR processing with a parent themselves.

Phase 3: Desensitization

Once pure Theraplay has become established, and the child has been introduced to EMDR, we can begin to process disturbing memories in a titrated way using EMDR. One pattern is for the child to do an enjoyable Theraplay activity, and then do EMDR desensitization on a disturbing memory, before then doing a reconnecting and calming Theraplay activity.

My preferred mode is to use Theraplay as a structured wraparound for EMDR, meaning that dyadic sessions begin and end with pure Theraplay, using a consistent sequence of activities, with the core EMDR processing of disturbing memories occurring during the middle of the session.

Desensitization of disturbing memories

EMDR is a flexible model, which means we can adapt it to the needs of each individual child. For example, we can use attachment-focused narratives to address a child's attachment wounds. We can use trauma-focused narratives. Or we can use more traditional EMDR, which involves asking a child to recall a particular memory. We have flexibility in terms of which part of a child's trauma timeline we focus on, whether to begin with the older memory first and work forward in time or start somewhere else. Traumatized children can find it hard to focus on disturbing memories, so it can be helpful to begin with a less intense past memory or a positive future event first.

Within Theraplay, an EMDR narrative storytelling approach can fit nicely with the feeding activity. One adaptation for dissociative children is to read the story to different parts (or ego states) of the child—for example, the "baby" or "little me" part (Gomez 2013). The parent can feed the "little me" while adding in BLS. If we are going to use the idea of "parts" then we would introduce this to the child before we use it. This is delicate therapeutic work because a child may reject their younger, hurt parts, and struggle to connect with them.

During desensitization, between sets of BLS, we usually want a child to pause and take a deep breath. We could do this via a short Theraplay activity. For example, we could invite the child to blow a feather from their parent's hand on the out-breath. This can also be a useful way for the child to know that their parent is physically close during the processing of disturbing material.

Using Theraplay activities as an interweave during processing

When desensitizing early attachment trauma, Theraplay can be used as a reparative interweave (Gomez 2013). For example, we could have the parent cradle, rock, and sing a gentle lullaby to a doll that represents their child's "baby" part. During desensitization, we activate an old memory and we can then do an action, which, in essence, goes back in time and meets the unmet need. For example, when a child recalls a time when they were hungry and ignored, we can ask their current parent to do the Theraplay feeding activity while saying the words "This is for the young, hungry part of you" and adding in BLS.

Installation

Theraplay activities are useful for enhancing and amplifying positive cognitions. For example, the positive cognition "I am safe now" can be enhanced by doing a special delivery activity that ends with the parent cradling and holding their child while saying, "I'll protect you."

It is important that the positive cognition is meaningful for the child (Shapiro 2001). Incorporating playful elements will make it developmentally appropriate and appealing to a child (Gomez 2013). Positive cognitions may be sung using a tune known to the child or chanted in a rhythmic way.

While installing the positive cognition, we have to notice the child's non-verbal communication so that the positive cognition is congruent with the child's state. Pure Theraplay's acute focus on noticing a child's state helps us know whether an experience is genuinely integrated within the child's right and left brain hemispheres.

EMDR proceeds through to Phase 6: Body scan to check whether there is any residual disturbance held somatically within the child. Again, we can use imaginal tools such as an "internal camera" to assist children with noticing their body (Gomez 2013).

Phases 6 and 7: Integrative body scan and closure

During the EMDR body scan phase, if a child has not fully processed a disturbing memory, and we are coming to the end of our session time, it's important that we close the session in a way that helps the child feel safe and contained. We can use Theraplay to connect to calm, soothing body states. For example, if a child notices that part of them feels disturbance, we can invite their parents to care for that part by touching it with a soothing cotton ball.

For most traumatized children, it usually takes more than one session of desensitization to process relational trauma memories. We can use metaphors of "strong containers" to create places where children can mentally store unprocessed trauma memories in between therapy sessions. After an EMDR session that has involved desensitization, Theraplay activities can help children to find balance, re-orient back to their present-day self, and feel connected with their parent. It's important to have a segment of Theraplay activities after desensitization. The activities chosen should match what the child needs so that they leave the session feeling "just right."

The closure part of EMDR basically means that we want the child to leave the session in a regulated state. Theraplay activities, with their inherent playful, connecting, and nurturing aspects, are brilliant for ensuring that children leave the session in a good state.

Phase 8: Re-evaluation

The needs of the child and parent are monitored throughout the intervention. Our partnership with parents is key so that we know how they and their child are responding to Theraplay and EMDR. It's common for children to engage in Theraplay activities in a different way straight after processing. For example, I've experienced children looking more relaxed during activities following EMDR processing.

In terms of ending the intervention, for Theraplay we usually work towards a time when a parent has developed confidence in their parenting and use of Theraplay as a model. It's important that the goals of therapy are revisited with parents so that we can decide when enough EMDR work has been done. For EMDR, we typically end once we have completed the three-pronged protocol of past–present–future. This means that we finish the intervention by doing a future template, which processes future events that could elicit disturbance within the child. For example, a child who has difficulty with new activities or situations could create a future template where they are able to successfully seek adult support and co-regulation.

 CASE ILLUSTRATION

BACKGROUND

Olivia, aged seven, lived with her adoptive mother Michelle. Olivia's early life was complicated and traumatic, having been born to a young mother who was herself traumatized by a domestically abusive relationship. At age four, Olivia sustained a broken arm, which led to a child protection investigation, a move into foster care, and then adoption. Olivia initially appeared to settle well with Michelle but then, within weeks, showed aggression, defiance, and sleep disturbance. Michelle described Olivia as being a "whirlwind of distress" and "impossible to get close to." At school, Olivia struggled to settle in class and frequently hurt other children with her over-boisterousness and need to be in control.

THE INTERVENTION PROCESS
History and MIM
Intervention began with the usual intake information gathering. I read Olivia's social care chronology and began to gather a timeline of what she had lived through. I noted down key attachment experiences, traumatic events, and positive events (including, for example, positive experiences from Olivia's contact visitations with her birth mother prior to adoption).

I met with Michelle to gather information from her, and we began to build our therapeutic relationship. Michelle shared that her own childhood had involved periods of separation from her birth parents because of illness. Alongside getting to know Michelle, I gathered information about Michelle's relationship with Olivia, their current home situation, and concerns. I used the Attachment-Focused Questionnaire (shared during Level One Theraplay training; adapted by Dan Hughes from Siegel & Hartzell 2003). From a Theraplay perspective, my focus was on Olivia and Michelle's attachment and parenting relationship. From an EMDR perspective, I wanted to identify their respective adaptive and maladaptive memory networks. My main focus was Olivia, but I was also interested in Michelle's memory network. My hypothesis was that Olivia's memory networks were informing her current behaviors and ways of relating, which would activate Michelle's memory networks.

Olivia and Michelle completed the standard MIM. Analysis and MIM feedback conversations with Michelle led to strengths and needs being identified across the Theraplay dimensions. Together we identified specific Theraplay goals:

- To increase moments of connected joy and playfulness between Olivia and Michelle.

- To increase moments of Olivia being focused on an activity rather than showing fight or flight behaviors (such as running around the room or throwing objects).

- To increase moments of Olivia being able to enjoy nurturing physical touch from Michelle.

With EMDR in mind, we added the additional goals:

- To notice moments when Olivia is genuinely feeling good and connected to Michelle during Theraplay activities so that these could be enhanced and installed as a resource using EMDR.

- To increase a segment of time when Olivia could sit calmly with Michelle and listen to a short story. This would allow us to create a space during Theraplay sessions for an EMDR narrative approach.

MIM feedback sessions

It's beneficial to front-load dyadic Theraplay with more than one parent session so that ample time is spent on developing a therapeutic relationship. I had more than four MIM feedback sessions with Michelle. During these, in addition to watching MIM segments together, I introduced the idea of EMDR and explained its use in installing and strengthening Olivia's resources before using it to process traumatic experiences. I openly discussed how Olivia's trauma experiences could trigger difficult memories and feelings for Michelle, which EMDR could help with. It was important that Michelle knew that any difficult memories that came up for her were a common response when parenting a traumatized child. I intended to ensure that Michelle felt supported so that we could address any signs of "blocked care" together. I shared YouTube videos that explained EMDR to children and adults (created by the EMDR Association UK).

During an MIM feedback session, Michelle and I watched an MIM activity that had felt good to her at the time. We enhanced this with EMDR so that Michelle had a resource called "I can connect with Olivia." We also used EMDR to install a future template that comprised Michelle imagining herself comforting Olivia.

A sequence of Theraplay activities was chosen for the first dyadic session, which was practiced with Michelle during our parent demonstration session. These activities consisted of:

- Entrance: How many big steps to get from the waiting area to Olivia's sitting cushion in the therapy room

- Check-in, by noticing Olivia and counting her fingers and freckles (engagement)

- Create a special handshake (engagement)

- Bean bag drop (structure)

- Balancing a bean bag on the head while being supported to stand up (challenge)

- Balloon tennis (challenge)

- Balloon balance (challenge)

- "Red light/green light" (structure)

- Floating on a raft (nurture)

- Special delivery (nurture)

- Feeding (nurture)

- Hand stack (structure)

- Exit by using the same entrance activity.

During the parent demonstration session, some of Michelle's own attachment needs and memories were elicited. With Michelle's agreement, I began to keep a note of potential EMDR memory targets for Michelle—for example, particular behaviors from Olivia that triggered distress within Michelle. During the parent demonstration, I spoke with Michelle about how we could use Theraplay activities for BLS.

Dyadic Theraplay sessions

The initial set of dyadic sessions was typical pure Theraplay because I wanted to ensure the integrity of Theraplay and provide Olivia with the experience of predictability and relational attunement. I was aware that the relational safety that Olivia could develop with Michelle would provide the most optimal preparation for EMDR.

An EMDR-related adaptation used in early sessions was the inclusion of a bean bag animal for bean bag drop. Olivia quickly became attached to this animal by naming it. This meant it could become an EMDR resource later on, although I was mindful that Olivia might become focused on the bean bag animal as a symbolic play object rather than something for reciprocal social interaction (Norris & Lender 2020). During feeding, I read a short, rhythmic children's picture book to Olivia. Her attention span was short, which meant a quick reading pace to get to the story's end before I lost her focus. My intention was to work towards developing a segment of time during future Theraplay sessions when I could substitute the children's book for a carefully written EMDR narrative.

Dyadic sessions continued with a focus on using Theraplay activities to create joyful moments of play and connection, co-regulation, and nurture with Olivia. As is commonly experienced during Theraplay, Olivia moved quickly from initial cooperation to more controlling behavior and boisterousness. She showed many fight or flight behaviors, such as running around the room, and grabbing and throwing props. We were in the "work" phase of Theraplay.

Pure Theraplay sessions, with regular parent-only sessions, continued so that we could provide Olivia with the experience of being regulated by us. Patience and faith in Theraplay were essential at this stage rather than rushing to include EMDR as some magical technique. Over time, Olivia responded well to activities that matched her energy level before guiding her into a more regulated state. It was crucial that Olivia was provided with the core foundations of Theraplay, which included clear physical positioning and sequences. The activities at the beginning and end of the session were kept the same (to aid predictability), while some different activities were included during the middle of the session to facilitate co-regulation and connection.

Sessions with Olivia were rich in the "unseen, deep, and hard-to-articulate" work of Theraplay; we were working at "relational depth" (Peacock 2020). While it is beyond the scope of this chapter to explore these, suffice to say that I experienced Olivia as re-enacting a dynamic internal script where she controlled and dominated Michelle and me. Theraplay activities provided the opportunity for Olivia to experience prediction errors so that her IWM of herself and adults could be nudged. Theraplay activities were strategically chosen to provide Olivia with experiences that ran counter to her IWM.

After initial pure Theraplay sessions, I added in more EMDR adaptations, including:

- Psychoeducation about EMDR (including simple information about BLS) with Olivia. This was spoken about during quiet, calm moments after the feeding activity. I also introduced the idea of mind, heart, and body (Gomez 2013).

- When Olivia engaged in Theraplay activities and showed genuine mastery, joy, and connection, I incorporated BLS by, for example, encouraging her to stomp her feet from left to right, or by holding the bean bag animal and inviting Olivia to watch it move from left to right (to elicit eye movements). Moments of mastery and joy were explicitly verbally named by me playfully calling out, "Olivia is brilliant" and "Olivia is having fun with her mum."

- Specific vocalized imagery of Olivia being in a calm, soothing place was added into the floating on a raft activity. When Olivia looked genuinely relaxed, this was installed using EMDR.

Over the course of Theraplay sessions, Olivia became more able to sit and focus on a short story during feeding. Michelle commented that Olivia had never sat for a story before but had become able to accept a short story at bedtime.

Using EMDR, I installed an "okay space" with Olivia. This was done through a "Build a fort" activity, using cushions and blankets. Then, while Olivia sat relaxed inside it, with Michelle alongside her, I installed this "feeling" using EMDR. Michelle added in BLS by using slow, gentle, alternating taps on Olivia's shoulders. It was important that I knew Olivia felt connected with Michelle while in the fort rather than Olivia using it as a space to hide and regulate alone. Olivia was encouraged to use her hands to show how "okay" she felt.

As sessions progressed, Olivia's "okay space" was developed by inviting her to imagine being in a place that felt okay. Olivia was told that, in her mind, she could choose the setting and the activity. For example, she could be still or busy doing something physical. Olivia created an imaginary "sweety land" in which she played ball with her bean bag animal. Slow BLS was added by Michelle tapping Olivia's alternate shoulders a few times.

Over subsequent dyadic Theraplay sessions, we moved into EMDR Phase 3: Assessment and Phase 4: Desensitization. During a parent session, Michelle and I co-created a story of Olivia's life. The story used a different character, rather than naming Olivia explicitly, and it began positively with a girl being born "lovable, strong, and healthy." The middle part contained themes about distressing events—for example, "As she was growing up, this little girl often felt alone" and "There was shouting and fighting." It ended with the girl moving to live with a lady who told her, "I'm going to help you have a good life. Even when things are difficult, I'll figure them out with you to make things better."

During the middle of a subsequent dyadic Theraplay session, I read this story to Olivia while Michelle added BLS by tapping Olivia's shoulders. After the story, Olivia was asked whether she wanted to change anything about the story. She replied, "No," but during the days following the sessions, Olivia experienced nightmares, and she mentioned a "nasty man" to Michelle. This became our next target memory.

At a subsequent Theraplay session, after the usual beginning Theraplay activities, I incorporated EMDR Phase 3: Assessment by inviting Olivia to draw the "nasty man." Olivia drew a "nasty man" throwing her into the air, while her mum was drawn as a tiny figure on the corner of the page. This image was processed using the standard EMDR protocol. Using visual props (pictures showing emotions;

cubes with simply worded positive and negative cognitions written on them), Olivia identified a negative cognition ("I am going to die"), positive cognition ("I am safe"), emotion ("scared"), and body sensation (heart pounding). Olivia used her hands to rate how much she believed the positive cognition, and how disturbed she felt. BLS involved Olivia watching me pass the bean bag animal from left to right as I tapped it onto her alternate hands. Desensitization progressed through to the installation and body scan phases. The session ended with enjoyable familiar Theraplay activities. During the post-session check-in with Michelle, I was told that Olivia had started to sleep better through the night.

Theraplay sessions continued with EMDR being used to process specific parts of Olivia's life timeline, including her move into foster care and her move to Michelle. We wrote a narrative about the loss and grief of her birth mother. Michelle added BLS by tapping Olivia's alternate shoulders during desensitization of this narrative. Olivia's processing became stuck, which I hypothesized as being due to a conflict of feelings and loyalty towards her birth mother and Michelle. An EMDR interweave was added by having Michelle gently tell Olivia, "Your heart has room for two mums." It was important that Michelle had been prepared for this during parent sessions prior to the EMDR session. It was crucial that Michelle could fully convey acceptance to Olivia that it was okay for Olivia to have feelings for her birth mother.

Parent sessions

During the initial stage of pure Theraplay, Michelle and I had typical parent sessions, which included viewing video segments from dyadic sessions. The main intention was to support Michelle in developing her use and understanding of Theraplay activities and Olivia's needs. We also used parent sessions to revisit psychoeducation about trauma, EMDR, and BLS, to ensure that Michelle was fully informed and to plan jointly for Olivia's EMDR.

The EMDR protocol was also used with Michelle to address the distressing memories that came up for her in connection to parenting Olivia. For example, when Olivia was working through her feelings of grief for her birth mother, Michelle began to experience intrusive memories of childhood separations from her own birth parents. These became memory targets using the standard EMDR protocol with Michelle. We also used EMDR to strengthen Michelle's positive memories (resourcing) of her parenting of Olivia. For example, Michelle shared an experience of feeling self-regulated and attuned while comforting Olivia (who had become distressed at home by a broken toy). This was an important parent resource to install using EMDR. A future template was installed within Michelle that comprised her feeling well regulated while at the same time being emotionally responsive to Olivia when she had an attachment need.

CHALLENGES ENCOUNTERED
While writing this case illustration, I have deliberately not stated exactly how many sessions were spent at each stage to avoid the reader taking this prescriptively. The time spent at each stage of the intervention, from the initial intake, MIM process, through to the dyadic sessions, needs to be flexible so that it can stay focused on what the child and parent need.

Case descriptions run the risk of showing therapeutic interventions in their best possible light. It's important to highlight that this intervention did not always move smoothly. There were gaps in sessions due to unexpected life events, and issues arose that needed attending to (e.g., when Michelle received distressing news about Olivia's birth mother). It is beyond the scope of this chapter to describe everything, but I want to emphasize that it was pure Theraplay that provided the core foundational intervention and stable base throughout the work.

OVERALL OUTCOME
Over the course of Theraplay, Michelle and Olivia's relationship improved. Michelle reported a greater understanding of Olivia's needs and relational patterns, and more confidence in knowing how to respond as her parent. Olivia's behaviors of concern reduced, and she began to share more of her inner thoughts and feelings with Michelle.

Theraplay re-oriented Michelle and Olivia onto a more connected and adaptive future path. Together, they found a way to be in the here and now. It would be erroneous to declare that all of Olivia's challenges were solved. Inevitably, there were ongoing obstacles for Olivia to work through. Still, Olivia's increased trust with Michelle and within herself gave her more resources for facing her inner and outer world.

Conclusion
Theraplay can effectively provide a child with reparative relational experiences with their parent while also supporting a child to develop their regulation capacity. Theraplay alone does not directly address past trauma memories, so additional trauma-focused interventions are necessary. EMDR is an evidence-based trauma intervention that can be smoothly and logically

incorporated into the Theraplay process. Using EMDR, a child's positive relational experiences and developmental capacities can be enhanced while disturbing experiences are processed in an adaptive way. EMDR can also be used to enhance a parent's capacities while also processing disturbing memories that have arisen as they parent their traumatized child. Together, Theraplay and EMDR provide an effective attachment and trauma-focused intervention that can be tailored for each child's unique needs. Many different EMDR protocols and procedures have been developed, which makes it widely adaptable to traumatized children of different ages and developmental abilities. This is sensitive yet rewarding work that draws on our capacities to be patient, curious, creative, and optimistic.

Key takeaways

- Theraplay and EMDR are compatible therapeutic models that are supported by theories of attachment and neurobiology.

- Do not under-estimate the power of pure stand-alone Theraplay as the means for providing a child with reparative relational, attachment, and co-regulation experiences.

- Integrate EMDR within Theraplay rather than vice versa.

- Become proficient and confident with Theraplay first before using EMDR within it. Make sure you get specialist training and supervision in both modalities.

- Developing and maintaining a therapeutic relationship with the child's parents is essential throughout the intervention.

References

Artigas, L., Jarero, I., Mauer, M., López Cano, T., & Alcalá, N. (2000). EMDR and Traumatic Stress after Natural Disasters: Integrative Treatment Protocol and the Butterfly Hug. Poster presented at the EMDRIA Conference, September, Toronto, ON.

Booth, P. B., & Jernberg, A. M. (2010). *Theraplay: Helping Parents and Children Build Better Relationships Through Attachment-Based Play* (3rd edn). Jossey-Bass.

Bowlby, J. (1969). *Attachment and Loss. Volume 1: Attachment.* Penguin.

Darker-Smith, S. (2020). EMDR Child & Adolescent Training, Level 2 (Advanced). https://childtraumatherapycentre.com/services/training/child-emdr-level-2-advanced

Gomez, A. M. (2013). *EMDR Therapy and Adjunct Approaches with Children.* Springer Publishing Company.

Hobday, A. (2001). Timeholes: A useful metaphor when explaining unusual or bizarre behaviour in children who have moved families. *Clinical Child Psychology and Psychiatry* 6(1), 41–47. https://doi.org/10.1177/1359104501006001005

Hughes, D. A., & Baylin, J. (2012). *Brain-Based Parenting: The Neuroscience of Caregiving for Healthy Attachment*. W.W. Norton & Co.

Logie, R., Bowers, M., Dent, A., Elliott, J., O'Connor, M., & Russell, A. (2020). *Using Stories in EMDR: A Guide to the Storytelling (Narrative) Approach in EMDR Therapy*. Trauma Aid UK.

NICE (National Institute for Health and Care Excellence). (2018). *Post-Traumatic Stress Disorder*. NICE Guideline NG116. www.nice.org.uk/guidance/ng116

Norris, V., & Lender, D. (2020). *Theraplay®—The Practitioner's Guide*. Jessica Kingsley Publishers.

Omaha, J. (2004). *Psychotherapeutic Interventions for Emotion Regulation: EMDR and Bilateral Stimulation for Affect Management*. W.W. Norton & Co.

Peacock, F. (2020). *A Necessary Life(Story): A Novella as a Research Process and Findings*. Peacock Counselling.

Porges, S. W. (2011). *The Polyvagal Theory: Neurophysiological Foundations of Emotions, Attachment, Communication, and Self-Regulation*. W.W. Norton & Co.

Purvis, K. B., Lyons Sunshine, W., & Cross, D. R. (2007). *The Connected Child: Bringing Hope and Healing to Your Adopted Family*. McGraw-Hill.

Schore, A. (1994). *Affect Regulation and the Origin of the Self*. Laurence Erlbaum Associates.

Shapiro, F. (1995). *Eye Movement Desensitization and Reprocessing: Basic Principles, Protocols and Procedures*. Guilford Press.

Shapiro, F. (2001). *Eye Movement Desensitization and Reprocessing: Basic Principles, Protocols and Procedures* (2nd edn). Guilford Press.

Siegel, D. J. (2012). *The Developing Mind: How Relationships and the Brain Interact to Shape Who We Are*. Guilford Press.

Siegel, D. J., & Hartzell, M. (2003). *Parenting from the Inside Out*. J.P. Tarcher/Putnam.

van der Kolk, B. A. (2005). Developmental trauma disorder: Toward a rational diagnosis for children with complex trauma histories. *Psychiatric Annals* 35(5), 401–408. https://doi.org/10.3928/00485713-20050501-06

van der Kolk, B. A. (2014). *The Body Keeps the Score: Brain, Mind, and Body in the Healing of Trauma*. Viking.

Walker, P. (2003). Codependency, trauma and the fawn response. *The East Bay Therapist*, Jan/Feb. www.pete-walker.com/codependencyFawnResponse.htm

WHO (World Health Organization). (2013) *Guidelines for the Management of Conditions Specifically Related to Stress*. www.who.int/publications/i/item/9789241505406

Chapter 8

Gestalt Play Therapy and Theraplay

A HYBRID MODEL OF WORKING WITH ADOLESCENTS

Hyunjung Shin and Felicia Carroll

 CASE ILLUSTRATION

When I (HS) met Sam, he was a 15-year-old boy who had been diagnosed with attention deficit hyperactivity disorder (ADHD). He had had difficulties with teachers and his parents with his hyperactivity since kindergarten. His teachers often told Sam's mother to have him seen by a doctor because of concerns about his inattentiveness and hyperactive behaviors. Since his mother had a full-time job and was very busy, it was difficult to make the needed appointments. Instead, his parents attempted to control his behavior with strict discipline, scolding him to be more attentive at school, and not to disturb the teachers or his classmates. This approach had not provided the support and understanding that Sam needed throughout his childhood. He did not develop the ability to co-regulate his excitement and energy with the demands of school and family activities. His parents had attempted to comply with many of the suggestions, including medication. They followed these recommendations inconsistently, and were not successful in helping him to adjust to the demands of his teachers. Eventually, his mother quit her job in order to be more available for his treatments and other activities.

When Sam entered middle school, his inattentive and hyperactive behaviors had not changed. In fact, he was becoming more aggressive toward his parents and others. He withdrew from his classmates. On more than one occasion, he was removed from the classroom and not allowed to participate in classroom activities. His parents, who had controlled his tantrums in his earlier childhood, were not able to contain his anger as he grew older and bigger. They felt threatened by his angry words and gestures.

Sam refused to go to school and became preoccupied with video games. He would stay up at night playing, and then sleep during the day, missing school. When his parents attempted to set limits on his gaming, he would become enraged, insult his parents, and ignore their efforts. When he was not enraged, he would become limp and lifeless. He would not eat and would lock himself in his room, where he would sleep. His parents were worried and felt powerless about how to help their adolescent son. Sam's interactions with his parents in our clinical interviews and on the Marschak Interaction Method (MIM) indicated that there was not a secure relationship with either parent. The attachment foundation for emotional regulation and social engagement was clearly disorganized. His parents' interactions were intrusive, dismissive, critical, and disorganized. I was concerned as to whether one or both of his parents could participate in the more sensory touch attachment-focused activities of Theraplay. I was uncertain if Sam, as a 15-year-old adolescent, would be willing to participate as well. Sam's internal working model (IWM) of self and his relationships with others had been shaped by his 15 years of strict, harsh, and unattuned parents.

Introduction

Adolescents with similar features to Sam are familiar to clinicians. Adolescents with ADHD usually cannot control their behavior and cannot regulate their emotions. They have difficulty building good relationships with others, including parents and siblings. Many therapeutic interventions do not help such adolescents. Their physiological, relational, and neurobiological states can become even worse over time, as was the case for Sam.

Sam was unable to regulate both his physical behavior and his emotions. His "window of tolerance" (Siegel 2012) was narrow, so he often was verbally or physically abusive to others or withdrew and isolated himself from others. He could accept neither interventions and advice nor instructions from others, such as parents and teachers. Shaming, admonishing, punishing, and hurtful discipline had caused him to defensively attack his parents and teachers who used such strategies. His lack of a secure attachment with his parents made it impossible for him to develop more interdependent relationships with other adults and peers, which are needed for healthful wellbeing in young adulthood.

After much consideration of Sam's age, dysregulated functioning, and initial rejection of many Theraplay activities, I decided to incorporate my training in Gestalt Play Therapy into his treatment plan. In addition to supporting Sam and his parents in forming a more trusting attachment, I knew Sam also needed to develop his self-functions and capacity for reflecting on his needs and interests. The following review of the basic principles of both Theraplay and Gestalt Play Therapy will provide my rationale for creating an integrative approach with Sam.

Comparison of Theraplay and Gestalt Play Therapy

Theraplay is an effective approach that supports children and adolescents in developing their capabilities to regulate their behaviors and emotions and build up social interactions, a good relationship with their parents, and an IWM of themselves (Booth & Jernberg 2010; Bundy-Myrow 2005; Munns 2008; Wettig, Coleman, & Geider 2011). Gestalt Therapy with children and adolescents is an established seminal approach to play therapy (Carroll & Orozco 2019) that provides a process to develop a child's contact functions (senses, body, movement), a sense of self (who I am, and who I am not), emotional regulation, and awareness of choice and actions (Oaklander 1978).

The theoretical principles of Gestalt Therapy are compatible and in agreement with those of Theraplay. Ann Jernberg, Phyllis Booth, and Violet Oaklander were contemporaries and had similar backgrounds as educators with young, emotionally disturbed children. Oaklander's initial book, *Windows to Our Children: A Gestalt Therapy Approach to Children and Adolescents*, was published in 1978. *Theraplay* followed in 1979 (Jernberg 1979). The Theraplay approach has theoretical roots in John Bowlby's attachment theory. The theoretical roots of Gestalt Therapy include Gestalt psychology and phenomenology (McConville & Wheeler 2001). Both approaches focus on the wellbeing of a child, and emphasize that a secure relationship that responds to the needs of a child is necessary for wholesome development. This need for a secure, supportive relationship with a therapist is one of the distinctive similarities between these two approaches. The integration of treatment modalities of Theraplay and Gestalt Play Therapy allows for unfolding a safe and secure base for therapeutic work.

Similarities and differences between these two approaches can have benefits when integrated into the therapeutic work with children and adolescents. One of the distinctive factors of Theraplay and Gestalt Play Therapy is the need for a supportive secure relationship that must be maintained among children, parents, and therapists. Regulation of children's behavior/emotion and gaining awareness/insight of their experiences can emerge based on a safe relationship. The integration of modalities between

Theraplay and Gestalt Play Therapy allows for scaffolding of the safe and secure base for therapeutic work.

As a Certified Theraplay Therapist for 15 years, I have often recognized the need for interventions other than those used in Theraplay that would deepen my understanding of the child or adolescent's life experience as well as support the strengthening of the relationship between parents and child. I attended several training sessions in "Gestalt Play Therapy with Children and Adolescents" focused on the approach developed by Violet Oaklander. Since that training, I have become a Certified Gestalt Therapist with Children and Adolescents focusing on the Oaklander Approach. In this study, I recognized that Gestalt Play Therapy and Theraplay shared many of the same foundational principles. Therefore, in the therapy process with Sam and his parents, I developed a hybrid approach using the theoretical perspectives and interventions of these two clinical models.

Table 8.1 outlines some similarities and differences between these two approaches. It represents a differentiation of these two approaches, which I integrated into my clinical work with Sam.

Table 8.1: Comparison of Theraplay and Gesltalt Play Therapy

	Theraplay	Gestalt Play Therapy
Purpose	• Restore secure bond or attachment between parent and child	• Restore child's integrated, energetic functioning within supportive environmental conditions
Similarities	• Organismic functioning and neurobiological underpinnings • Relationship-focused • Phenomenological/meaning-making • Use playful interactions as a vehicle to understand and process child's issues • Emphasis on using therapist's self in therapy process	
Differences	• Used for all ages but commonly for young children and parents	• Used for all ages, but relatively older ages
	• Focus on preverbal, non-verbal, sensory, touch-based	• Focus on processing and facilitating the integration of body, senses, emotions, and cognitions
	• Parent included in session (dyad therapy preferred)	• Parent not included in session (individual therapy preferred)

cont.

Theraplay	Gestalt Play Therapy
• Therapist-guided structured therapy	• Therapist-guided unstructured therapy
• Emphasis on strengthening parents' reflective functioning	• Emphasis on developing child's self-functions
• Focus on developing new experience through sensory/body interaction between parents and child	• Focus on the development of awareness of self-functions

Gestalt Play Therapy: Oaklander Approach with Children and Adolescents

Principles

The principles of Gestalt Play Therapy are rooted in the neuroscience of Gestalt psychology; organismic functioning within environmental situations in order to get needs, interests, choices, and values met; field theory understanding of the dynamics of relational and environmental variables; experiential arts of theater and dance (movement); and knowledge of lifespan human development (Lee 2011; Lee & Harris 2011). From the Gestalt perspective, the symptoms that bring a child into therapy are indications of their unfulfilled attempts for self-regulation and being supported in his world of family, school, and community (McConville & Wheeler 2001). The goal of the therapy process is to restore integrated aliveness—the networking of all organismic functions so that the adolescent's basic physical, developmental, social, emotional, and intellectual needs and wants are understood and organized (Oaklander 2006). Organismic integration emergence occurs when conditions of self/other support are present. The Gestalt approach is effective in supporting the developmental needs of children and adolescents (McConville 1995).

Another resource that the Gestalt approach offered to support Sam's adolescent development was the use in Gestalt Play Therapy of the phenomenological approach. The phenomenological method in working with projective techniques such as drawing, sandtray, clay, self-cards, games, etc., provides support in creating the meaning of Sam's experiences (Oaklander 1978) and of helping him develop an IWM of self and how he interacts in his world. The phenomenological approach is a non-analytical method that allowed Sam's "voice" to provide depth of meaning to the various projective modalities that he uses in sessions. As he explores the images through projection, he can identify and reclaim the meaning of the life experiences he associates with the images (McConville 1995).

Also, through playful, rough-and-tumble (Panksepp 2005) interactions with the therapist, and through games and "experiments" designed together to "test" old and new behaviors, Sam can find his energy mobilized towards understanding his emotions, moving out into the environment and developing his interests, and making contact with peers and activities in his world. The process of Gestalt Play Therapy supports the assimilation of experience and the learning of what is workable, desirable, and worthy of repeating. In this way, Sam can make choices of friends, activities, values, and a sense of direction for his future.

Sam's childhood experiences resulted in an IWM held together by shame and self-recriminations. He had internalized the attitudes of critical parents, teachers, and peers. This shame-based model of self/other relationships resulted in his withdrawal into video games, attacking peers, and his antagonistic stance towards his parents and teachers in particular and others in general. Oaklander (2006) developed what is called the "self-nurturing process." This provided a way for Sam to bring into his therapy an awareness of these internalized attitudes and his behaviors as ways to protect himself from his self-rejection and the hurt he felt by the criticism and rejection of others. It provided a way for Sam to become more accepting and caring towards himself. In Gestalt Play Therapy, this self-nurturing process is essential to the process of organismic integration and self-functioning. It establishes a more organized and resilient IWM model of self.

Elements

The Gestalt Play Therapy process (Carroll & Orozco 2019) has the following elements:

- Experiencing the ways that the child makes contact through the body senses.

- Use of sandtray, drawings, games, and play to strengthen the child's sense of confidence, knowledge about self, and feeling of self-support.

- Increasing one's understanding of emotions and the ability to utilize a range of emotional expression modailities, expressed through books, music, role-play, clay, and so on.

- The child develops an increased ability for self-acceptance and self-nurture using experiential play and art that may include puppet role-play, expressive drawings, clay, or other materials.

- Finding a variety of ways to have one's needs met and obtaining preferred objects and activities, a process that benefits from role-play and social experimentation.

- Healthy support is cultivated from parents, teachers, and other significant caregivers through parent consultations or team or caregiver consultations.

- Termination of therapy involves ending the process of formal therapy through rituals to acknowledge accomplishments, engaging with family and eliciting their support, and reflecting on important changes and growth experiences.

Because older children and adolescents can use symbols, they can utilize various methods for expressing and understanding emotions and behaviors. They need to integrate the whole brain for good development. Theraplay assists with mid-brain and limbic functions of sensory processing, emotional reactions, and attachment behaviour. The upper brain can work through narrative activities, drawings, or projection methods of Gestalt Play Therapy. Theraplay therapists can work the mixed intervention into one session or different sessions according to a child or adolescent's symptoms, situation, and the therapist's therapeutic plans. The Theraplay therapist also expands the child's social engagement system (SES) by utilizing touch, eye contact, posture, and gestures to create a safe environment and situation for them (Lindaman & Mäkelä 2018). The Gestalt therapist utilizes narrative, drawings, clay, sandtray, and other projective modalities to provide experiences that support therapeutic energy for the integration of all brain and neurological functions (Lee 2011; Oaklander 1978). The approach of Gestalt Play Therapy is more acceptable for adolescents who don't want to be treated like young or immature people (McConville 1995). Even though they need Theraplay interventions to meet earlier unmet developmental needs, they sometimes protest those activities as "childish." The challenge dimension of Theraplay is essential when working with adolescents (Booth & Jernberg 2010). Therefore, some Theraplay therapists, when they work with older children and adolescents, utilize the Theraplay activities along with the challenge dimension from Theraplay to interact with them (Booth & Jernberg 2010). Munns (2005) also suggested utilizing activities drawn from the structure and challenge dimensions of Theraplay with older children.

The developmental need of an adolescent is that they are able to function separately from their engagement with parents with a sense of self that could take on the challenges of the complex emotional and physical tasks of adulthood. Of course, a stable and supportive attachment relationship with caring adults, especially parents, is essential for the adolescent to navigate these developmental tasks successfully. Developmental theorists have written much about the shift in developmental focus during adolescence (Erikson 1950; Steinberg 2008). Along with addressing the primary concerns of the adolescent in therapy, the therapist needs to support the adolescent to face new responsibilities and privileges; to survive and thrive in an unpredictable social network of friends and others; to assimilate the physiological and cognitive changes; and to select partners or mates for establishing intimate, family relationships. In my clinical work, I found the approach and activities of Theraplay alone were insufficient to engage with an adolescent client in developing a solid sense of self and reconsidering the decisions and relationships of childhood.

The parent work with adolescent clients in Theraplay is as important as with a younger child (Norris & Lender 2020). Depending on the adolescent's problems, Theraplay therapists attune and manage the participation of the parents. Parents can be involved in many ways without directly participating in the adolescent session. Even if the adolescent may not permit their parents to participate in the session, the therapist can work cooperatively with the parents. An adolescent may sometimes prefer not to involve their parents because of privacy and confidentiality, and not want their parents to interfere in his process. Separating from parents is an essential developmental need of adolescents. Therefore, I developed a hybrid approach for Sam's therapy by utilizing the Theraplay processes of restoring an attuned attachment with parents and the Gestalt Play Therapy processes of integrated self-functioning with myself.

Hybrid approach to Theraplay and Gestalt Play Therapy

The hybrid approach combining Theraplay and Gestalt Play Therapy strategies with Sam began with Theraplay strategies that would build rapport and trust to establish a safe working relationship. These activities also served to relax him as we developed our connection. Our connection happened from check-ups, such as not using too many touches according to his needs, keeping a safe distance from each other, and accepting Sam as he is in a secure environment.

With our relationship established, I could transition to more Gestalt modalities using the phenomenological process to support him in learning more about himself, such as what he likes and what he doesn't like, and reflect on his choices. The purpose again was to deepen his awareness about himself (who he is, what he likes, what he doesn't like, what he wants, and what more he wants to know about his self-function).

I began my work with Sam realizing that I had three basic therapeutic purposes that needed to be addressed: (1) to provide a way for the parents to learn a more nurturing discipline style based on the principles of attuned attachment; (2) to establish a safe and secure relationship that supported Sam's acceptance of changes in his parents' interactions; and (3) to support the developmental tasks of adolescence of building a resilient sense of self in a world of complex relationships. This includes helping the adolescent achieve emotional understanding, make choices and mobilize their energy to carry out their choices, develop interests and friendships outside the family, and become self-compassionate and self-supportive while also enjoying support from others. The three purposes above would require a therapeutic program beyond the attachment focus of Theraplay for Sam to develop more interdependent relationships, which he would need for healthy and productive adulthood.

I planned specialized sessions for Sam to achieve these purposes. I divided each session into two parts. Generally, I started with Theraplay; after that, I used Gestalt Play Therapy interventions. As I mentioned before, I decided to do Theraplay first because Sam needed a check-up, sensory-attuned intersubjectivity, and engagement based on face-to-face play to activate his SES and to expand his "window of tolerance." After that, I provided an opportunity for Sam to express his feelings, develop a more self-nurturing process, and enhance his awareness of himself through the contact functions (senses and body), sense of self, and life narrative.

Sam did not want his parents' participation in his sessions, so I initially met his parents without him to support his need to keep a safe distance from them—I respected his boundary. Older children and adolescents frequently do not want their parents to participate. Respecting the adolescent's boundaries of confidentiality is primary to maintaining a safe and trusting relationship. Nevertheless, in Sam's case, he and his parents needed to have playful and enjoyable sessions together for the parents to create a more attuned understanding of Sam, and for them to receive support in respecting and nurturing his adolescent need for individuation. Sam's parents needed to participate in his therapy process in both conjoint sessions with Sam and their parent-only sessions.

As in Theraplay, parent involvement with adolescent clients is crucial in Gestalt Play Therapy (McConville 2011). The element of Gestalt Play Therapy is to create and sustain trust between the adolescent and their parents, and to promote safety and security in the relationship. The adolescent learns why they are brought to therapy so that they can participate in establishing consent, goals, expectations, and interventions (Carroll & Orozco 2019). Even though the approaches have minor differences regarding parent participation, I integrated both direct involvement and parent consultation in working with Sam's parents. This integration of both models supported them in learning to make changes to their everyday life.

Sam's parents needed to learn from me how to interact with Sam with less criticism and fewer demands for compliance. We focused on how to listen and develop a needed empathy for his adolescent development. To accomplish this, I did psychoeducation for good parenting and carried out a few Theraplay activities with Sam's mother to improve her reflective function. Even though Sam did not participate with his parents in every session, they gradually learned to relate together in a more interdependent, collaborative style.

Sam's parents cooperatively established a safe environment and helped him to co-regulate. With the established secure environment based on a healthy relationship with his parents and myself in the sessions, Sam could build a resilient sense of self and integrate his whole brain. The following objectives were achieved through our work together:

- safe and secure environment

- co-regulation

- resilient sense of self

- integration of the brain.

Description of Sam's progress

When Sam came to me at the first session after MIM, he seldom made eye contact and seemed annoyed. His hair was messy, his body was as stiff as wood, and he resisted making eye contact with me. He consistently yawned, lying on the floor even though we were both in the playroom. I wanted Sam to feel the interaction between us was safe, and tried to make it feel safe for him. I hoped he could have the experience of taking charge of himself with an adult. For instance, I reflected that I saw him lying on the floor as a way of giving him recognition and acceptance. I also told him we would meet once a week, sometimes doing childhood play with his parents. I reassured him that he could feel free to do as he liked here, as long as he felt safe.

Each time Sam came to the therapy room, he would lie on the floor. In one session, I checked up on his changes, even subtle things. I felt that I wanted to activate his healing energy, so I kept a distance and softly hit a balloon towards him. He did not want me to get close, so I kept a distance from him. I understood this was related to his felt safety. I told him, "I will touch your elbow with this balloon." I hit the balloon lightly toward his elbow. He didn't move when the balloon hit his elbow. I then said, "I will touch your feet with this balloon. You can feel it." And I hit and sent it toward his feet. When it arrived at his feet, he hit it with his foot lightly. The balloon was moving in the air. I didn't miss the chance: "I will send it to you, and you send it back. We will hit it together as much as we can. Let's see how many we can hit."

I hit it toward him lying on the floor, and he moved like a worm on the floor. However, the more he was active, his energy level rose. He did not want to interact with me and did not permit me to get close. I had wanted him to move by himself to have his boundary and power to do something by himself through co-regulation with me. So this balloon game was a start.

Sam also lay down after a special handshake at the next session. He consistently wanted to lie on the floor. He needed to co-regulate with me not to be withdrawn. I blew bubbles toward lethargic Sam. Repeating blowing the bubbles like that, I caught one bubble and let the bubble pop at his elbow. Sam gazed at my move. Even though he was lethargic, repeatedly lying down on the floor during sessions, with rapport being established, he could interact with me, step by step. If Sam lay down, I made him sit and stand, like hitting balloons together or playing bubble tennis. When he hit the balloons with a racket, he was stiff with tension. He could not integrate his body movements even though he was a teenager. I was respectful of his inconsistent experiences. As time passed, Sam could soothe his resistance and became more cooperative. When sometimes he still lay down during sessions, I sent him a balloon, asked him to return it to me, and he fortunately followed my request. Sam's energy level increased when he used many body parts to send the balloon back to me. It was from self-motivation, not from therapist pressure to perform. After watching our interaction through a one-way mirror for a while, Sam's parents joined us. The parents and Sam followed my guide, cooperatively hitting the balloon back and forth. They laughed together, not criticizing each other.

Sometimes Sam and I had a balloon fight. We respectfully bowed to one another as we began and set the time to "fight." Through this rough-and-tumble play, Sam could release his energy in a safe environment. Sam and I were enthusiastically involved in this play. After that, we sat together and laughed, taking deep breaths. We both felt energized. Experiencing Theraplay and Gestalt Play Therapy activities improved his capacity for co-regulation significantly. I used physical touch, bubbles, and balloons to interact well with him in face-to-face play, utilized a calm voice to give him relaxation, and smiled with a respectful attitude. Sometimes I planned sensory/body activities for him to experience his contact functions and co-regulation. After active movement and deep breaths, he could work to express his emotion and strengthen self-support and his sense of self through drawing, clay, and role-play.

Theraplay's activities and care made Sam relaxed. After that, he took a deep breath to become aware of himself and participated in Gestalt Therapy activities.

After the Theraplay activities, I asked Sam to color his feelings as happy, embarrassed, sad, angry, nervous, annoyed, etc. As shown in the image below, Sam's primary emotion was annoyance. Many parts of his emotion were absent. He could not feel it as well as express his feelings well, and he even could not color them. For example, he picked a peach color as an annoyance; however, he could not choose a color except this peach color, even though emotions matched other colors (e.g., sad-blue color, happy-yellow color). Sam could not be aware of his emotion and could not describe it. So we tried to let him notice it through the visual work expressing his emotions, and integrating those.

I had to work with Sam's parents to help him. His parents sometimes joined Theraplay to establish a good attachment relationship and a positive IWM. They came to the playroom at my request, when Sam agreed to them joining the session, and they all did Theraplay activities such as hand stack and balance on pillows. Through these activities, they developed a better relationship. Instead of negative interaction patterns such as criticism, dispute, and taunting, his parents practiced and became accustomed to a different approach, step by step.

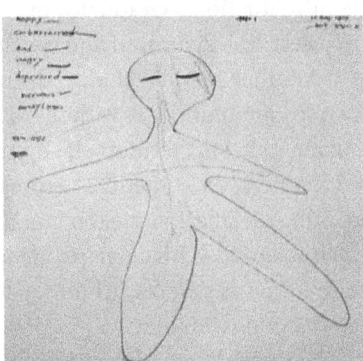

Figure 8.1. Sam's emotion drawing

Sometimes, when Sam did Gestalt Play Therapy strategies after Theraplay activities, he could express conflict with his parents to me by narrative or using drawings instead of his powerless lying down or acting out. He told me his parents used to do everything without his agreement. Sam could express his negative feelings in more organized ways through Gestalt Play Therapy. He could activate and regulate his arousal through physical, psychological, sensory, and neurobiological integration, be aware of his states, and gradually talk about himself through Theraplay and Gestalt Play Therapy.

Sam needed to recognize and activate his sense of self. I had to support him in discovering more about who he is and his sense of self. So Gestalt Play Therapy was very effective for Sam developing more self-awareness. He also needed to console and care for himself without others' help. Gestalt Play Therapy could do this for him. He projected aspects of himself and was gradually able to express them through drawings as well as narratives. He became aware of many facets of self as he identified previously unassimilated experiences. Sam became more competent through the challenge dimension of Theraplay, and felt the joy of interaction through its engagement. He accepted my touch more comfortably.

The picture below was created during the self-nurturing work of Gestalt Play Therapy. The color and the lines Sam drew were more apparent compared to previously. In the drawing, there was a powerless person stuck inside a whale. This story of what was happening in the picture was also more relational and organized than in the past. According to Sam, the fairy in the picture was finally able to rescue the person who had no hope in the dark whale's belly. He told me the tale through the projection technique of Gestalt Therapy. As he talked as the projected hopeless person, we began to recognize that it was Sam himself. He reflected on how he felt hopeless in school and family situations. Gradually, over the next few weeks, he could nurture the hopelessness in himself and became more confident in his relationships.

Another marked change during this time was that Sam would keep his therapy appointments without being late, which was different from the past six months. Furthermore, he began to talk about changes in his relationship with others. He sometimes expressed respect toward his parents, was aware of using his smartphone too much, tried to reduce his time-wasting, and once even abandoned his smartphone spontaneously. Importantly, he could accept care from his parents. And they were being more consistent in their caring interactions with him.

Nevertheless, some minor difficulties persisted. On one occasion, Sam broke an appointment without consideration for me or for others. Sometimes

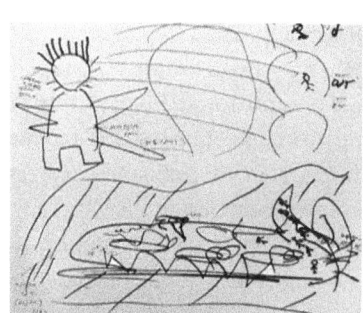

Sam's self-nurturing work

he could not follow the rules, although he could accept the evaluation of his behavior without significant resistance, and apologize for his faults. He could reflect on his own behavior and its effect on others. His study habits changed, and he was more committed to getting high scores at school. Sam and his parents had a more comfortable relationship, and were happy to share experiences together. His parents expressed that they were both surprised and grateful for these changes. Sam could regulate his body and emotion when upset in a safe environment based on his parents' cooperation at the closing of our work together. Sam was a brilliant boy, but did not recognize his potential. Throughout our work together, he developed a sense of self and awareness of how to use all of himself to be more resilient in challenging situations. Integration of his brain through the approaches of Theraplay and Gestalt Play Therapy made him aware of himself and his functioning in relationships. At school, he was able to make many friends. He had a good sense of humor, but nobody had noticed this about him in the past. Sam's change enabled him to build better relationships with his parents, friends, and school teachers. As a result, Sam became popular in school!

Conclusion

The effects of integrating Theraplay and Gestalt Play Therapy are considerable because of their similarities, such as organismic functioning/neurobiological, relationship-focused, phenomenological/meaning-making through intersubjectivity and playful therapeutic interventions. At the same time, they are complementary to each other. For example, Theraplay focuses on the right brain functions, the development of younger ages, preverbal state, and sensory interaction such as building up secure attachments, relationships, and a good IWM. On the other hand, the Gestalt approach stresses the integration of the brain, organismic function, sense of self, self-nurturing, and awareness.

Similarities and differences between the two approaches can help many children, especially older children and their parents. Children can feel safe in a secure therapeutic environment of Theraplay and Gestalt Play Therapy. Based on a safe relationship with the therapist, the adolescent is supported in developing unique values, a healthy IWM, and a healthy attachment with their parents, peers, and others in their life. In this process, the adolescent can activate their SES, expand their "window of tolerance," and develop a sense of intersubjectivity through attunement, co-regulation, playfulness, and sharing joy with another person.

In order to respect their privacy, the older child or adolescent may not want their parents' participation. Before establishing a secure, attuned relationship with parents and the therapist, the adolescent may need to keep their emotional distance to protect themself from others. If they don't want their parents' involvement from the beginning, the therapist has to respect their choice and their reasons for that choice. After building rapport and trust with the therapist, they may be more able to accept their parents' participation in the sessions. However, the therapist must work with the parents in a supportive and cooperative way, to make this possible.

Theraplay and Gestalt Play Therapy can be combined and modified depending on the child's situation and difficulties. In Sam's case, Theraplay and Gestalt Play Therapy were combined in the same session, but in other cases the two approaches can be applied at different times. For example, Theraplay activities can be done first, with Gestalt Play Therapy strategies later. Optimal treatment planning depends on the needs and readiness of each child and parent.

References

Booth, P. B., & Jernberg, A. M. (2010). *Theraplay: Helping Parents and Children Build Better Relationships Through Attachment-Based Play* (3rd edn). Jossey-Bass.

Bundy-Myrow, S. (2005). Theraplay for Children with Self-Regulation Problems. In C. Schaefer, J. McCormick, & A. Ohnogi (Eds), *International Handbook of Play Therapy: Advances in Assessment, Theory, Research, and Practice* (pp.35–64). Jason Aronson.

Carroll, F., & Orozco, V. (2019). Gestalt Play Therapy. *Play Therapy*, September, 46–49. www.a4pt.org

Erikson, E. H. (1950). *Childhood and Society.* Norton.

Jernberg, A. M. (1979). *Theraplay: A New Treatment Using Structured Play for Problem Children and Their Families.* Jossey-Bass Publishers.

Lee, R. G. (2011). Shame and Belonging in Childhood: The Interaction between Relationship and Neurobiological Development in the Early Years of Life. In R. G. Lee & N. Harris (Eds), *Relational Child, Relational Brain: Development and Therapy in Childhood and Adolescence* (pp.55–74). Gestalt Press.

Lee, R. G., & Harris, N. (2011). *Relational Child, Relational Brain: Development and Therapy in Childhood and Adolescence.* Gestalt Press.

Lindaman, S., & Mäkelä, J. (2018). The Polyvagal Foundation of Theraplay Treatment: Combining Social Engagement, Play and Nurture to Create Safety, Regulation and Resilience. In S. W. Porges & D. Dona (Eds), *Clinical Applications of the Polyvagal Theory: The Emergence of Polyvagal-Informed Therapies* (pp.227–247). W.W. Norton & Co.

McConville, M. (1995). *Adolescence: Psychotherapy and the Emergent Self.* Jossey-Bass.

McConville, M. (2011). Relational Modes and the Evolving field of Parent–Child Contact: A Contribution to a Gestalt Theory of Development. In R. G. Lee & N. Harris (Eds), *Relational Child, Relational Brain: Development and Therapy in Childhood and Adolescence* (pp.175–195). Gestalt Press.

McConville, M., & Wheeler G. (2001). *The Heart of Development: Gestalt Approaches to Working with Children, Adolescents and Their Worlds. Vol. II.* Gestalt Press.

Munns, E. (2005). Theraplay with Adolescents. In L. L. Gallo-Lopez & C. Schaefer (Eds), *Play Therapy with Adolescents* (pp.30–46). Rowman & Littlefield.

Munns, E. (2008). Theraplay with Zero- to Three-Year-Olds. In C. E. Schaefer, S. Kelly-Zion, J. McCormick, & A. Ohnogi (Eds), *Play Therapy for Very Young Children* (pp.157–170). Jason Aronson.

Norris, V., & Lender, D. (2020). *Theraplay®—The Practitioner's Guide.* Jessica Kingsley Publishers.

Oaklander, V. (1978). *Windows to Our Children: A Gestalt Therapy Approach to Children and Adolescents.* The Gestalt Journal Press.

Oaklander, V. (2006). *Hidden Treasure: A Map to the Child's Inner Self.* Karnac Books.

Panksepp, J. (2005). *Affective Neuroscience: The Foundations of Human and Animal Emotions.* Oxford University Press.

Siegel, D. J. (2012). *Pocket Guide to Interpersonal Neurobiology: An Integrative Handbook of the Mind* (Norton Series on Interpersonal Neurobiology). W.W. Norton & Co.

Steinberg, L. (2008). A social neuroscience perspective on adolescent risk-taking. *Developmental Review 28*(1), 78–106. doi: 10.1016/j.dr.2007.08.002

Wettig, H. G., Coleman, A. R., & Geider, F. J. (2011). Evaluating the effectiveness of Theraplay in treating shy, socially withdrawn children. *International Journal of Play Therapy 20*, 26–37. http://doi.org/10.1037/a0022666

Chapter 9

Music from the Harp of Chaos

USING GROUP ANALYTIC THEORY TO ORCHESTRATE
THERAPLAY GROUPS FOR CHILDREN WITH MODERATE
TO SEVERE MENTAL HEALTH DIFFICULTIES

Fiona Peacock

 CASE ILLUSTRATION

It was like being taken unexpectedly by a whirlwind. The eight children arrived with high energy that spilled in all directions. I could see from the face of the teaching assistant that this was not unusual behavior. "Can you do some Theraplay with them?" I had been asked. "Just to help them regulate themselves in the classroom a bit." Nothing in the information I'd been given raised the thought of relational or developmental trauma. Nothing indicated these were anything other than ordinarily developing Year 1 children aged around five and six. They seemed a bit younger for their age than I was told. And here they were, rampaging around me. Games with bean bags were ignored. Cooperative cotton ball blowing resulted in cotton wool being pounded into the carpet. I kept the lotion and bubble mix well away. I left with a renewed admiration for our educators, quite a sweat from vacuuming the cotton wool out of the carpet, and an extreme case of self-doubt about how to create something therapeutic out of such chaos.

Introduction

This chapter demonstrates how Group Analytic Psychotherapy (GAP) and Theraplay can be used together in conducting therapeutic groups for children and young people who are displaying moderate to severe mental health difficulties.

It could be argued that all Theraplay is group therapy—families are, after all, a group. It seems natural, therefore, to consider ways in which the Theraplay model can be adapted for other group settings. In the early years of Theraplay development, Phyllis Rubin (Rubin, Tregay, & DaCosse 1989) pioneered Group Theraplay for entire classrooms or small groups of children displaying special needs as part of the US Head Start and elementary school programs. Sunshine Circles (Schieffer 2011) have been developed to enable the non-clinical population in classrooms to access the benefits of an attachment-enhancing model, providing teachers with tools for attachment-based group regulation, peer connection, and nurturing play in the school group setting. Evangeline Munns (2009) outlines many ways that Theraplay can be utilized with different populations through groups. Often these approaches follow the Theraplay technique of working with the child and primary caregivers, but locate this in a group context. Other group Theraplay approaches identify specific populations, such as children and young people with autism spectrum disorder (ASD), who might benefit from the relationship rehearsal inherent in the Theraplay model.

When I first trained in Theraplay, there was no acknowledgment of group analytic concepts. Having undertaken GAP training to postgraduate certificate level, I was intrigued by what seemed to me the strong synergy between the orientations. However, Theraplay practitioners seemed unaware of group analysis, and group analysts seemed unaware of Theraplay.

Theraplay and GAP

It is outside the scope of this chapter to address all the issues around psychotherapeutic groups for children and young people. One of the fallacies to address about groups is that they are cheaper and quicker than providing individual therapy. To the non-clinically trained professional, seeing six to eight children in one therapeutic session instead of individual children for six to eight sessions could appear to be a more efficient option. Careful management is critical to ensuring the group is truly therapeutic. From my experience, the multiple relationships created in the group create an intensity that requires a depth of understanding of group processes to ensure that those relationships work to the benefit of each member as well as the group as a whole. This requires meticulous preparation and rigorous post-session thinking about the work. Each child needs to be considered as an individual alongside the infinite number of relationships that are created between group members. This pre- and post-session work can be time-consuming.

Given the challenges of group therapy, you might ask why we would choose to provide therapy in a group format. The answer is that, beyond the family group, adults expect children to function in groups on a daily basis by requiring them to be in school. Adults then label children as problems if they are unable to manage the challenge of the group setting. Providing therapeutic treatment in a group setting can create a restorative experience (Yalom 1995). For children who do not feel they have a problem, the relational experiences that happen in a well-conducted therapeutic group can show a child that their way of being is out of step with the norm (Whitaker 2001). By activating their attachment desires, the child may become motivated to change so they fit in with their community (Foulkes 2002; Holmes 2001). The child benefits as their sense of belonging is affirmed, and they have the developmentally appropriate experience of peers becoming co-regulators of behavior.

Evaluating the efficacy of group therapy is difficult. Neither GAP nor Theraplay is a particularly good fit for what could be seen as the medical model gold standard of an evidence-based randomized controlled trial (RCT). For a complex relational model, controlling variables would be extremely difficult. However, there is a wealth of evidence that relationship is the factor that enables healing in therapy (Norcross 2011; Wampold 2015; Yalom 1995). The evidence base for GAP, therefore, lies more within the realm of practice-based evidence. Practice-based evidence for GAP with children and adolescents is more limited than for adults or individual therapy. Behr and Hearst (2005), Lanyado and Horne (1999), Anthony and Foulkes (1965), and Evans (1998) have all published on the topic of child GAP, and, as you can see, many of the references are now outdated. Practice-based evidence through case studies is needed to promote theory and technique (Stiles 2007). Using GAP theory with Theraplay practice is, therefore, innovative. By combining the two models, two things can be accomplished at once. First, the depth of clinical formulation for the presenting difficulties of the group is greatly deepened. Second, conducting the group in a playful and developmentally appropriate manner for children is strengthened. Theraplay is the technique, and GAP is the framework. In sharing my experience, the hope is to stimulate interest in this combined model and create a basis for this modality toward evidence-based practice.

The history of Group Analytic Psychotherapy (GAP)

S. H. Foulkes, a German-British psychiatrist and psychoanalyst, developed GAP. As a psychiatrist trained in Germany and of Jewish extraction, he was relocated to the UK and set up practice in Devon. He said he "discovered" group analysis when he was running behind with appointments and came into the waiting room to find his patients talking about their difficulties (Foulkes 1990). His theory and practice were further refined while working with war veterans at Northfield Hospital, taking over from Wilfred Bion, an influential English psychoanalyst (Pines 1983). In shifting the therapeutic technique from "couch to circle" (Schlapobersky 2016), Foulkes also needed to adjust the theory from the dominant psychoanalysis of his time (Weinberg & Rolnick 2020). The core technique for GAP is that six to eight group members sit together with a group conductor. By using "free-floating conversation," what could be seen as verbal "play" within the context of a well-conducted therapeutic group, the way each member responds gives a platform where it becomes possible to see, feel, and make conscious attitudes and expectations that have previously driven behavior unconsciously. These mirroring and resonating processes can then enable therapeutic transformation. Thus, seeing the link between GAP and Theraplay techniques may not be immediately apparent.

Foulkes' view was that suffering arises from the feeling of not belonging (Foulkes 1990). Healing of the emotional distress that comes from this dislocation comes from learning to belong to a group again. This is similar to Bowlby's assertion that distress arises from unwanted losses of relationship (Bowlby 1999). Both Bowlby and Foulkes also challenged the dominant psychoanalytic position that emotional disturbance was located purely in the inner world of the individual, their intrapsychic functioning. Both attachment and GAP theory see people in the context of their interpersonal connection, as well as their intrapsychic experience. For both Bowlby and Foulkes, meaning develops from the deepening insight that comes from the shifting perspective between these interpersonal and intrapsychic phenomena.

Despite these similarities between attachment and GAP theories, there is little writing that explicitly looks at GAP with children and young people through a joint lens of attachment and group analysis. There is, however, some literature that integrates attachment theory into GAP thinking for adults (Barwick & Weegmann 2018; Weinberg & Rolnick 2020). With developing literature around the connections between attachment and GAP, it becomes easier to see the links between GAP and Theraplay as an attachment-enhancing method of therapy.

Structuring the group for safety

 CASE ILLUSTRATION

Following that awful first session, I asked for some more information about each of the children. Each child faced multiple Adverse Childhood

Experiences (ACEs). Goodman's Strengths and Difficulties Questionnaire scores indicated all were at risk of developing symptoms that would warrant a mental health difficulty (Goodman *et al.* 2000). When these scores were shown to the school with a query about whether Child and Adolescent Mental Health Services (CAMHS) referrals had been considered, they just laughed. The view was that it wasn't even worth suggesting to parents to seek a CAMHS referral or make one themselves. They had so many children in school with that level of need that only those who were actively likely to harm themselves or others stood a chance of obtaining help for their mental unwellness from statutory services. "That's why we asked you to come and do some Theraplay for six weeks," they said.

To put the presentations of these children into an attachment context, using a traditional attachment theory model, we would consider anxious avoidant (A-type) or anxious ambivalent (C-type) attachment styles (Ainsworth *et al.* 2015; Main & Solomon 1986). Using Crittenden's Dynamic-Maturational Model of attachment, we would conceptualize the children falling in the A5/6 to C3/4 range of presentations—that is, children where there is a compulsion to avoid depth of relationships either through superficial engagement (A5), excessive self-reliance (A6), or aggression and/or feigned helplessness (C3/4) (Crittenden n.d.; Holmes & Farnfield 2014). These are children with enduring mental health difficulties who may have been exposed to multiple ACEs (Felitti *et al.* 1998), but not where their difficulties could be classified as relational and developmental trauma (Peacock & Holliday 2021). Their difficulties typically have a moderate to severe impact on their lives by creating lifelong deprivation through limiting access to education and causing diminished capacity for rewarding and enriching relationships.

The out-of-control nature of the group immediately put me in mind of the Theraplay dimension of structure. Structure makes for safety. Structure is represented in group functioning under the Theraplay rules of "No hurts," "Have fun," and "Stick together." First, I had to find my own structure and work out how I could contain my own anxieties about what I could offer to this group in such a short space of time. GAP theory gave me this, enabling me to feel a sense of safety through understanding the nature of the difficulties within the group and, therefore, how I could create sequences of Theraplay activities that would address those core difficulties.

The route map of complexity

 CASE ILLUSTRATION

Mumtaz literally stood out in the group, using his physical presence to communicate rather than language. After the second session, I found myself making my notes of the session knowing there were eight children but only being able to call seven to mind. Noah seemed to be the opposite of Mumtaz, timid to the point of invisibility, hence him dropping out of my mind. Noah was the oldest in his family, expected to care for his three siblings while his single-parent father worked all hours at three different jobs to keep the family together. His mother had left without any explanation. My hypothesis was that Noah was required to be overly responsible at home. In the group, it seemed he wanted to shrink away, Mumtaz's size and exuberance being more than he could bear. Mumtaz had survived a challenging time to arrive in the country. He and his mother had been unintentionally separated from his father in fleeing to the UK to escape persecution in their country of origin. Mumtaz could not let himself fall out of anyone's mind for fear of losing even more connection.

One of the key concepts in GAP theory is that of a group matrix—think about each member of the group being like an anchor point for a set of musical strings. Some of those are fixed deep down in a person's functioning, unconscious and unknown. Some are quite near the surface. What is deeply unconscious for one may be near the surface for another. As those connections are formed, these strings play out their tune, and the notes may be "heard" in the way in which people see themselves through others' eyes (mirroring), and in the way the group stirs up individual feelings (resonance). These connections happen at many different paces and levels in the group, and can appear discordant or harmonious. This is the power of the therapeutic group, and the challenge for the group conductor is to steer the process toward harmony.

Capturing the concept of the group matrix visually, as in the diagram below, makes it easier to think about the complexity of multiple potential meanings of group activity. By thinking about how one activity may activate different aspects of individuals, the group conductor can modify the activities to enable the group as a whole to support each individual as they develop healing relationships.

Group matrix diagram

The people in the group are marked by the shape of a cylinder, and relationships are indicated by a line. Feelings that people are aware of are drawn from the top of the person's marker. They may be received unconsciously by another, shown by a connection lower down.

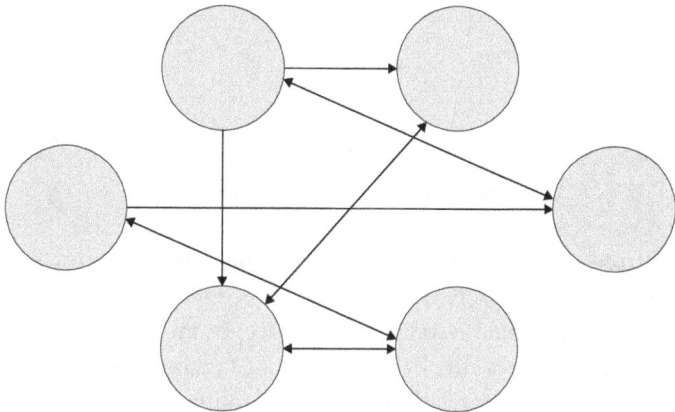

Group matrix viewed from above

In this diagram, the matrix between six group members can be viewed from a variety of angles. The perspective they are viewed from makes the connections more or less complex. Choosing from which angle to view the complexity of the matrix is akin to choosing what depth of engagement you are seeking to elicit in the group. Picking the right depth of engagement is an aspect of selecting the right kind of group for the right kind of child at the right time. Theraplay, as a method, can be used to activate and create healing opportunities at all levels of group members' development, depending on the skill level of the practitioner and what is ethically appropriate for the context they are working in, their professional accreditation, and employment status.

Viewed from above, the depth of connections is evened out, and some become invisible. I would see this perspective on group functioning as working at a cognitive or behavioral level. Such engagement is effective for children who have achieved a developmental stability and are able to connect thoughts, feelings, and behaviors, and where there are fewer disturbing and unconscious drivers to their behavior.

Viewed from the side, some complex interconnections are obscured or even confused. It is not always clear which communication joins with which. However, the diagram indicates an awareness of how different members of the group can impact the inner process of others when a conscious action of one person activates something unconscious in another. This perspective on the matrix is suitable for children where the roots of their difficulties are reasonably clear, but the children may require different levels of support. Groups with a single presenting issue may be one example of this, for example children who are young carers or who are bereaved.

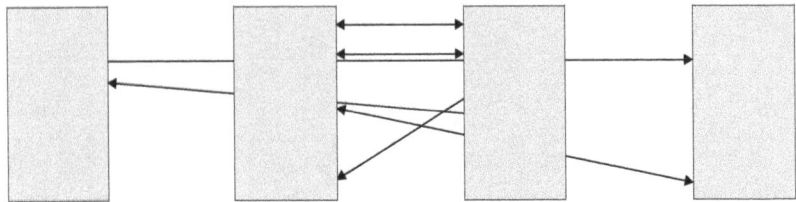

Group matrix, viewed from the side

Viewed three-dimensionally, you can see the most complex but most illuminating representation of the matrix. It becomes clear how the surface levels of experience could resonate with the deeper, more unconscious levels of experience for others (the Z1–Z2 and Z1–Z3 connections). At the same time, you can see where relationships create mutual recognition between individuals through connections at a similar level of functioning (the Y1–Y2 connections). This illustration represents groups for children where there are multiple presenting issues, the roots of which are not clear, and where there are profound difficulties for all group members. As the conscious and unconscious resonances are mapped out, it becomes easier to consider the needs of individuals and how specific dyads within the group as well as the group as a whole can work together towards experiences of belonging.

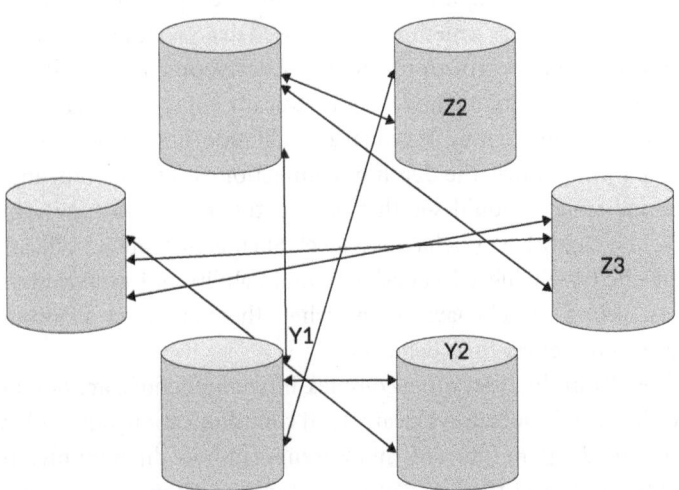

Group matrix viewed from three dimensions

Seeing the matrix this way makes it easy to imagine it is a stringed musical instrument where the plucking of a connection can produce different notes depending on the nature of the connection between people. Plucking the conscious connection in one person can resonate at a deeper level for another. When conducting a group for children with moderate to severe mental health difficulties, you don't want to blunder into twanging a string that would be fine for one child but would activate another in a way that may challenge the integrity and safety of the group. Hence, the functioning of a group matrix is an important concept to consider in any therapeutic group process.

However, by orchestrating this "harp of chaos" intentionally, carefully, and reflexively, it becomes possible to use the group-as-a-whole functioning to harmoniously ease out the deep-level conflicts of group members without having to move those conflicts to the spoken realm. The techniques of play in Theraplay, when combined with this understanding of the concept of a matrix, become a very powerful tool in considering what interventions may enable the group as a whole to progress towards stronger attachment connections.

Conducting the group

 CASE ILLUSTRATION

I viewed the video of the session in great detail. Some children flitted across the screen with such speed I could barely register them. Mumtaz used his height and strength to stand in the middle of the room. It seemed like he had taken possession of the camera. As others ran past, he cuffed them. How come I hadn't seen that in the group itself? Mrs. Smith continued to stand at the door with a warm smile on her lips and a faraway look in her eyes. As the children bashed into her, she caught them, turned them around, and fired them back into the chaos. My first thought on watching the video was that everyone in this room needed to be seen, including Mrs. Smith and me.

Foulkes (2002) talks about "conducting" groups, not leading, facilitating, or convening. The conductor is as much within and part of the group as every other member. The term "conductor" immediately suggests notions of an orchestra where the role of the conductor is to draw out the harmonies to tame the cacophony. Other aspects of conducting bring to mind the need to be a bus conductor, telling people when to get on or off, and how. Or that of a lightning conductor, rerouting destructive powers to protect the main structure. All these three ways to conduct will enable the group conductor to think about what is happening within the group, and consider how best to form an intervention to bring about harmonic energy.

CASE ILLUSTRATION

In one session, I paired Noah and Mumtaz. Noah had an uncanny way of communicating without words. It was no surprise he cajoled his two-year-old brother through the day's routines as a carer at only six years of age himself. When Mumtaz started to become explosive, as he couldn't understand my verbal instructions, I indicated to Noah to guide Mumtaz. Noah taught him the game. They made a great pair. I then teamed them together against D'ryce and Alice in balloon volleyball. Mumtaz lifted Noah high to bat the ball back. "Good job, Mumtaz," I called out, "let's keep everyone's feet on the floor, so we are all safe!"

Again, I thought he was going to blow. He picked up from my voice that he'd done something, and I was saying he needed to do something else. I quickly formed everyone into a circle. We needed some lightning conduction here. I stamped a rhythm with my foot, made sure Mumtaz wasn't opposite me and indicated D'ryce to copy my rhythm, and then everyone joined in. The sticky moment where D'ryce could have lost it, as she didn't like being beaten, was averted. Mumtaz could process his sense of rejection and "I've got it wrong-ness" by being carried along by the stamping rhythm of the group. I improvised an activity where we moved from stamping a rhythm to sitting down and tapping a rhythm quietly. Everyone was now settled on the floor for feeding. Wow, bus to lightning to orchestrating in a few short activities! This was the hardest piece of group analysis I'd ever done. Tony put a chocolate button in my mouth quite naturally, as we fed each other in the circle—therapy by the group, of the group, for the group, including the group conductor (Foulkes 2002). I think Foulkes would have been proud.

In a GAP session, as conductor, I might talk about the fearfulness of being nothing and invite people to explore their stories around that. In the Theraplay group, that would translate into planning activities that create a safe structure within which the children could feel safe to be seen and then safe to be lost and found. Through strong bus conducting to hold the boundary of "No hurts," and lightning conducting to ensure "Sticking together," then, maybe then, the cacophony could be orchestrated.

Dynamic administration to create safety

To feel safe inside the room, I had to attend to the networks surrounding the group.

"Dynamic administration" refers to imbuing every step of the group process with therapeutic meaning—all communications with all aspects of the child's system: parents, school administrators, the senior management team, the class teachers and assistants, the dinner ladies who will be around in the non-structured time after the session. I needed to let all of them know about the purposes and process of the Theraplay. The GAP term "dynamic administration" affirms that the work done outside the therapy session is as therapeutic as the session itself. Such work outside of the actual therapeutic session creates the right kind of space for children to flourish. I view it as the equivalent of parent preparation in dyadic Theraplay. If we invest in the adults around the child in the dyadic model, why would we not do so in the group model as well?

No matter how regulated children may become in session, if that isn't affirmed and supported in the other group systems that the child inhabits, gains are unlikely to stick. Talking to groups of adults about GAP concepts, such as group matrix and resonance phenomena, isn't very user-friendly. Theraplay's four dimensions and seven core concepts, illustrated with video material, is a more accessible way to talk with the whole school community about what we were seeking to achieve in the sessions, and why seemingly simple activities could bring about change.

Deciding to intervene

The adult structures Theraplay to enable children to access reparative relational experiences. This makes Theraplay stand out as a deeply child-centered therapy even though it is not child-led in the same way as non-directive therapy groups that involve play (Lanyado & Horne 1999). I prepare carefully for Theraplay groups with children with moderate to severe mental health difficulties. However, the complexity of the matrix and the potential to unintentionally "twang" a discordant note by using an activity that activates a child at levels that are too deep for the group context mean that the decision to intervene often needs to be made at the moment to respond to unexpected situations.

GAP thinking has developed a useful set of questions to ask yourself when trying to intervene, as shown below (Kennard, Roberts, & Winter 1993, p.16).

What is the state I am observing?

↓

What processes are contributing to it?

↓

Do I judge it constructive, destructive, or neutral?

↓

Would it be advantageous to change this state?

↓

Is it possible to change it?

↓

What interventions might influence the constituent process and state?

↓

Are the necessary interventions in my repertoire?

↓

Is the time ripe for an intervention?

Clinical supervision is vital even before the group begins to meet. Maybe I could have avoided that terrible first meeting if I had engaged in this process sooner. It is also a place to tease out tricky issues of ethics and challenging issues of selecting activities based on understanding the stories emerging via the matrix.

The quest of "decision to intervene" can be used to reflect on the appropriateness of each of the Theraplay activities chosen. My overall aim for the remaining sessions was to enable the group to get to the point where they could play hide and seek, regulate each other with a feather-blowing partner activity, and sit down together for a shared snack. This would show the group's capacity to co-regulate, tolerate up and down energy levels, as well as nurture and vulnerability. For such activities to be successful, group members would need to process the experiences I felt they'd missed out on—first to be seen, and then to be able to tolerate disappearing and returning. Essentially, we were working on building resilience by using play to rehearse the rupture-and-repair cycle in relationships.

Drawing on Kennard *et al.*'s (1993) definitions of intervention types has helped me deepen my thinking process in constructing plans for Theraplay groups and responding at the moment to issues that arise. Table 9.1 below summarizes Kennard's interventions and how I see them corresponding to Theraplay groups for children with moderate to severe mental health difficulties.

Table 9.1: Kennard's interventions and Theraplay

Intervention types		
	Kennard's definition	Theraplay equivalent
1. Maintenance	Clarifying or reaffirming a boundary of time, place, task. Maybe aimed at the group as a whole or an individual	Theraplay rules: "Have fun," "Stick together," "No hurts"
2. Open facilitation	An intervention that helps the group move forward in some way, not based on a particular hypothesis of the conductor, and not working with unconscious material	Interventions that are aimed at being together in the room in a way that is predictable and fun—things such as opening and closing rituals
3. Guided facilitation	Remarks that indicate the conductor has a hypothesis in mind and is trying to guide the group to self-discovery through questioning, prompting, and observing	Group activities that are devised to address specific group needs such as working towards hide-and-seek or using a specific feeding activity to extend a group's "window of tolerance"
4. Interpretation	A verbal intervention by the conductor that makes manifest feelings or meanings that are close to the surface for either the group as a whole or an individual	This would be a departure from the Theraplay model that would keep the discovery in the realm of play. I would see the closest equivalent being extending the "window of tolerance" of an individual or the group as a whole in activities, so enabling group members to enjoy more of the benefits of group membership
5. No immediate response	A significant part of the group conductor's response is to silently observe the group. The conductor may reserve the right to intervene at a later time, depending on further development of the situation	This is such a useful intervention, reminding me that if the boundaries are set well and structure is good, I can trust the group to address many of the issues that may arise—when group members remind each other of the "No hurts" rule, you can see the co-regulatory processes are moving towards internalization in the peer relationships and away from these having to be adult-initiated

cont.

Intervention types		
	Kennard's definition	Theraplay equivalent
6. Action	Any kind of physical activity that the conductor might engage in inside the group, which involves them leaving their chair and touching another group member	An intervention that we do a lot of as Theraplay group conductors, one of the major differences in the method of the group
7. Self-disclosure	A declaration by the conductor about the content of their inner world, or outer world, that doesn't fit any other category of intervention	I would see this as the Theraplay practitioner being fully present and voicing their enjoyment and pleasure of being with the children. Beyond that, I see no reason for self-disclosure due to the nature of the developmental stage of the children. It may, however, be appropriate in an adolescent group
8. Modeling	Any activity on the part of the conductor that contains an implicit intention that it should be identified with and become part of the repertoire of the group's behavior	Again, being a bit more action-based, this form of intervention is significant in the Theraplay therapy group

 ## CASE ILLUSTRATION

Last session. Each child took turns hiding in the room, behind a chair, using a blanket, behind Mrs. Smith. She obligingly held her arms out wide and draped a blanket over them to make extra space for the hider. All the other children whispered quietly, entirely without direction, as if they knew that was the best way to seek out the hider. I was worried it would be either a riot or damp squib as they "found" the other child. In previous weeks, I had seized opportunities to "find" lost children in the room to serve as a model. I wanted this last session to go well so much. It took a lot of self-control to hold back and let the group manage its process. I felt my heart swell with pride in them as they spontaneously gathered around the found child and gently hugged or high-fived them. Even Sarah, our quietest member, responded to Mumtaz's high-five, and he was noticeably gentle with her.

We moved on to playing sleeping lions. Mumtaz actually fell asleep. The group quietly talked about what they should do. They decided to have their snack while he slept, but made sure his snack was saved. At the end of the session, they gently woke him up. He sleepily rubbed his face and said, "Thank you" when Noah passed him a paper towel they had used to improvise a plate for his crisps. I hugged each of them as they left, amazed and heartened at how they had embraced the healing power of the group. I had learned so much from them. Mrs. Smith beamed at me wholeheartedly as she closed the door behind them all.

Conclusion

In this chapter, I have drawn some parallels between Theraplay and GAP as a way to deepen the containment of a Theraplay group process for children with moderate to severe mental health difficulties. There is little literature that gives accounts of such work. This may be because such group work is challenging to set up and maintain, and does not lend itself to quantitative, evidence-based methods of evaluation. Through giving an account of practice-based evidence, the combined model of GAP theory and Theraplay practice for working with children can be shared. Hopefully, through case accounts, the material can be diligently gathered in order to extend the process of generating theory through case studies.

References

Ainsworth, M. D. S., Blehar, M. C., Waters, E., & Wall, S. N. (2015). *Patterns of Attachment: A Psychological Study of the Strange Situation*. Routledge.

Anthony, A., & Foulkes, F. (1965). *Group Psychotherapy: The Psychoanalytic Approach* (2nd edn). Karnac Books.

Barwick, N., & Weegmann, M. (2018). *Group Therapy: A Group Analytic Approach*. Routledge.

Behr, H., & Hearst, L. (2005). *Group-Analytic Psychotherapy: A Meeting of Minds*. Whurr.

Bowlby, J. (1999). *Attachment and Loss: Attachment* (2nd edn). Basic Books.

Crittenden, P. M. (no date). DMM Model. Family Relations Institute. https://familyrelationsinstitute.org/dmm-model

Evans, J. (1998). *Active Analytic Group Therapy for Adolescents*. Jessica Kingsley Publishers.

Felitti, V. J., Anda, R. F., Nordenberg, D., Williamson, D. F., Spitz, A. M., Edwards, V., Koss, M. P., & Marks, J. S. (1998). Relationship of childhood abuse and household dysfunction to many of the leading causes of death in adults. *American Journal of Preventive Medicine* 14(4), 245–258. https://doi.org/10.1016/S0749-3797(98)00017-8

Foulkes, S. H. (1990). *Selected Papers: Psychoanalysis and Group Analysis*. Karnac Books.

Foulkes, S. H. (2002). *Group Analytical Psychotherapy: Methods and Principles*. Karnac Books.

Goodman, R., Ford, T., Simmons, H., Gatward, R., & Meltzer, H. (2000). Using the Strengths and Difficulties Questionnaire (SDQ) to screen for child psychiatric disorders in a community sample. *British Journal of Psychiatry 177*(6), 534–539. https://doi.org/10.1192/bjp.177.6.534

Holmes, J. (2001). *The Search for the Secure Base: Attachment Theory and Psychotherapy.* Brunner-Routledge.

Holmes, P., & Farnfield, S. (Eds) (2014). *The Routledge Handbook of Attachment: Theory.* Routledge.

Kennard, D., Roberts, J., & Winter, D. A. (1993). *A Workbook of Group-Analytic Interventions.* Jessica Kingsley Publishers.

Lanyado, M., & Horne, A. (Eds) (1999). *The Handbook of Child and Adolescent Psychotherapy: Psychoanalytic Approaches.* Routledge.

Main, M., & Solomon, J. (1986). Discovery of an Insecure-Disorganized/Disorientated Attachment Pattern. In T. B. Brazelton & M. W. Yogman (Eds), *Affective Development in Infancy* (pp.95–124). Ablex Publishing.

Munns, E. (Ed.) (2009). *Applications of Family and Group Theraplay.* Jason Aronson.

Norcross, J. C. (2011). *Psychotherapy Relationships that Work: Evidence-Based Responsiveness.* Oxford University Press. https://doi.org/10.1093/acprof:oso/9780199737208.001.0001

Peacock, F., & Holliday, C. (2021). Relational and Developmental Trauma and Schools. Education, Oxford Bibliographies. https://doi.org/10.1093/obo/9780199756810-0270

Pines, M. (Ed.) (1983). *The Evolution of Group Analysis.* Routledge & Kegan Paul.

Rubin, P. B., Tregay, J., & DaCosse, M. A. (1989). *Play with Them—Theraplay Groups in the Classroom: A Technique for Professionals Who Work with Children.* C.C. Thomas.

Schieffer, K. (2011). *Sunshine Circles: Interactive Playgroups for Social Skills Development and Classroom Management.* The Theraplay Institute.

Schlapobersky, J. R. (2016). *From the Couch to the Circle: Group-Analytic Psychotherapy in Practice.* Routledge.

Stiles, W. B. (2007). Theory-building case studies of counselling and psychotherapy. *Counselling and Psychotherapy Research 7*(2), 122–127. https://doi.org/10.1080/14733140701356742

Wampold, B. E. (2015). *The Great Psychotherapy Debate: The Evidence for What Makes Psychotherapy Work* (2nd edn). Routledge.

Weinberg, H., & Rolnick, A. (2020). *Theory and Practice of Online Therapy: Internet-Delivered Interventions for Individuals, Groups, Families, and Organizations.* Routledge.

Whitaker, D. S. (2001). *Using Groups to Help People* (2nd edn). Brunner-Routledge.

Yalom, I. D. (1995). *The Theory and Practice of Group Psychotherapy* (4th edn). Basic Books.

Chapter 10

Music, Rhythm, and the Safe and Sound Protocol in Theraplay

Cindy Mitchell Perkins

Introduction

From the moment we take our first breath, we are rhythmic beings. Our heartbeat, breathing, and almost everything we do has an innate rhythm. The shh, shh, back and forth rhythm of my kayak paddle as I move out to sea, walking, running, and even crawling all have a rhythmic nature that we need to keep ourselves organized. An infant lies against your chest, and you feel your hearts connect. The baby calms when they are able to hear your heartbeat. Heart-to-heart connection generates emotional engagement and nurturing attunement. It also aligns with a dimension of natural musicality.

Theraplay is, by its very nature, musical. Awareness of rhythm within each activity, the session, and the overall body of work is important to success as a Theraplay therapist. Understanding rhythms and how to use them is a large part of using Theraplay to meet the goals of each client. This chapter shares my personal and professional journey in using music within the Theraplay model. You are invited to try these methods within your sessions.

Power of music in Theraplay

Every time a therapist or a caregiver speaks, the tone and rhythm of their voice convey a message as powerful as the words to the child. Rhythm and regulation are stressed during the course of Theraplay training and supervision. One of the most powerful tools to help a child regain composure is for the adult to maintain a calm rhythm that the child can engage in. This is the basis of co-regulation of affect (Norris & Lender 2020). The Theraplay dimensions of nurture and engagement require that the caregiver and the child be attuned to each other for the child to regulate (Booth & Jernberg 2010). Rhythm is a powerful way to enhance these dimensions and to help the child accept the nurturing and engage in a trusting relationship.

Music has been used in all cultures to create bonding among group members (Hart 1990). Drums have been used to communicate between villages in Africa or historical native groups in the Americas. Song lyrics and rhythms can bond the most unusual groups of people and appears to be a universal experience across world cultures (Levitin 2006, 2016). Drumming and other instruments have been used as armies advance in war. Music has been used to protest wars.

Speaking the same verbal language is unnecessary when coming together with music. The language of music is universal. Watch and listen to animals sing back and forth to each other. Observe two toddlers dancing along to the same rhythm as they discover their bodies joining the music—what a delight as we watch this being discovered, and how hard to resist our own bodies joining in the dance.

Music powerfully affects mood states (Campbell 1997; Leeds 2001). A magical experience is singing or humming a lullaby to a baby or young child and feeling them fall asleep in your arms. This is what we mirror at the end of a Theraplay session when we have the parent feed the child (all ages) and often sing a lullaby they know and/or we teach them our variation of *Twinkle Twinkle Little Star*.

In my high school band, I loved the energy I felt when my flute blended perfectly into the music my bandmates played. When a drumming friend invited me to play the bass drum in our parades, I learned the bass drum was the heartbeat of the marching band. These activities are ways we experience the Theraplay dimension of engagement within a group culture. Band, choral, and orchestra members are attuned to others through their music. They are experiencing the shared joy so important for human connection. The learning in Theraplay is preverbal, and the attunement of music does not have to be explained verbally in order to be shared and experienced together. The caregiver and baby do not need to process the calming of the lullaby or the comfort of a heartbeat.

When my son was young, his therapist suggested that he get a hand drum to help him with a recent trauma. I read about how drumming could help and found that it helped him. This was the beginning of my journey using music and rhythm to help regulate clients. Tapping to one's own heartbeat can be very soothing. Doing this individually and then with another can be a compelling experience. Each client, couple, family, or group can find their heartbeat and quietly tap it on their leg or an object. Have everyone in the room keep quietly tapping and focusing on their heartbeat. At first, the tapping will be chaotic and disorganized as everyone in the room finds and taps their heartbeat. However, it will only take a few minutes for the entire group to become synchronized and begin tapping a very regular and even rhythm. Having done this exercise in large groups at conferences with as many as 100+ participants, the entire room is soon very rhythmic and calm, all tapping the same rhythm. They become regulated by simply tapping the beat of their own heart, which synchronizes with the others. Beats with patterns of three are powerful and calming. In 2013, at the Annual Conference of the American Music Therapy Association, 50–60 beats per minute were recommended for relaxation.

Entrances and exits set the tone of a Theraplay session by coming in or going out with structured rhythmic activity. The entrance sets the tone of each session and is a critical part of a Theraplay session. It also ensures that the adults are focused on the child from the moment they are greeted in the waiting room. Each entrance activity used has a rhythm incorporated into it. These include movements such as hopping, skipping, dancing, and tiptoeing. The entrance structure can be enhanced by allowing the child to move when the adult taps the drum or claps until the child is at the place where the session will start. Having the adult lead into the office in this way naturally has the adult keeping the rhythm of the walk, dance, or hop. The entrance activity is a method of saying "hello." The exit activity (often a repetition of the entrance) is how we say "goodbye."

Integrating music and Theraplay

 ## CASE ILLUSTRATION

This child was like many of my clients, who would often have individual sessions before I was able to get permission for a trusted adult caregiver to be part of the sessions. Many of the young people I saw were in foster groups or pre-adoptive or adoptive homes, so I worked with the agencies they were involved with to get a trusted consistent adult to be part of their sessions.

The child would come into the sessions agitated, and it often would take a large part of our session to regulate them enough to engage in even simple Theraplay activities. Their mood could quickly escalate into raging behaviors. These could include yelling and throwing things. Episodes could quickly become unsafe if adults were unable to help them find a strategy to regulate themself, if the adults started to become dysregulated themselves, or if the adults tried to interact too much verbally. On one particular day, the child could not settle down. I had tried to bring them in with a very regulated entrance of stomping in and counting our elephant steps. However, on this day, it failed. Their presentation was very stressed and on the verge of tantrum decompensation. Mindfully staying regulated myself, I considered my options. I judged that if I used a commanding "You-need-to..." voice, they would have quickly escalated to kicking, hitting, throwing, and other unsafe behaviors.

Previously, we would do call and repeat rhythms on the djembe, which would usually calm and regulate the child enough to move to the rest of the activities for that day. Today, I made sure safety was maintained as they expressed rage and anger by pacing around my office. They verbally let me know that participating in any "stupid" games today was not going to happen. I invited them to join me by tapping my rhythm of 1, 2, 3 on the djembe. "No way!" Words were clearly going to cause an escalation, so I just began tapping out two side taps and one center bounce on the djembe. Periodically, I would motion for them to join me. I tapped a rhythm with the center beat that varied from louder to quieter, matching their energy as they paced around the room. By matching their energy, I hoped to resonate with their felt affect, creating a sense of empathic connection.

This was based on the match and regulate principle, beautifully described in *The Happiest Baby on the Block* by Harvey Karp (2012). The objective is to meet the baby where they are when trying to calm them. This is demonstrated in a mother holding her crying infant and "Shhhshing" her with a louder "Shhhhhh" to match the crying of the baby and then modulating her voice down to a very quiet and soothing "Shhhh." The effect is to match the baby's affective intensity and then regulate it downward.

This eight-year-old child began making demands as a method of gaining control of themselves. While this could have been interpreted as defiance, I recognized it as the child's attempt to keep their world safe and manage their emotional intensity. I reassured them that as soon as we did a little drumming together, we would be able to do the activity that they wanted, an activity I had already planned and knew we would get to later. By letting them know I had already planned what they wanted, I reassured them that I knew them well and would keep them safe. In Theraplay, this falls under the structure dimension.

I continued to tap the beat consistently on the drum. Gradually, the child started to engage. At first, they stomped on the floor to the beat, which had the effect of entering a process of emotional regulation.

Next, they clapped very hard once. Following that clapping, once or twice they would look to me for a reaction. The expectation was that I would correct this. I just continued tapping the beat on the drum. They remained safe but agitated, with moments of calming, for 20 minutes. They then came over and sat down across from me at the drum and stated, "I'm not doing the stupid drum." I nodded and kept drumming. They then quickly banged the drum very hard with a very irregular beat. I just kept the beat going, 1, 2, 3. They then tried doing the 1, 2, 3 very loud and said, "There, I did it." I nodded and kept the rhythm going. After several more tries, they joined me with the rhythm—at first loud, which I matched once we had the rhythm, and then led with rising and then falling volume, and then a few minutes of quieter drumming, just like shhhshing the baby!

We were then able to do bubbles as they had wanted to, followed by more Theraplay activities, ending the session with a weather report and feeding time, which was how we always ended our sessions. As we always did, we finished with our exit, counting our big steps to the transition person. This was the "goodbye" of our sessions. They left that day very regulated due to the integration of the rhythmic drumming that I brought into the session before we continued with Theraplay as planned.

This scenario has been repeated in many variations over the years in my office when a child comes in agitated and unable to regulate enough to continue with a planned Theraplay session. Many clients and I began our sessions with drumming and then moved into a planned Theraplay session with check-in, four dimension activities, and wrapping up with weather report and feeding. "Hello" and "goodbye" continued with an entrance and an exit activity. These children who presented with trauma, attachment issues, anxiety, loss, and other presentations were able to begin trusting the adults in their lives through the combination of Theraplay and music. Experiencing regulation through musical activities helped them to learn that they could regulate their emotions. This helped them be more available for the relationships they needed in their lives.

Music has become a core component of my Theraplay sessions. A review of 25 years of clinical cases has demonstrated the value of this added modality when done with intentionality and used in coordination with concepts of attunement, emotional engagement, playfulness, and reciprocity. The outcomes have consistently shown that young people have increased their ability to trust the adults in their lives to keep them safe, learning to regulate their bodies and emotions, and proceeding to engage in relationships with a greater sense of calm and intimacy building.

Musical activities in Theraplay

Over time, the activity with a small table drum or the djembe drum has become a regular part of my Theraplay sessions in addition to traditional Theraplay songs (The Theraplay Institute 2018). An adult (clinician or caregiver) drums a rhythm on the drum, and the young person repeats the same rhythm. The intensity of the drumming goes up and down with a regulation pattern similar to the Theraplay game peanut butter and jelly, loud/soft, fast/slow, until the therapist brings the client to a regulated state. This can be done in a group where the rhythm is passed around the circle or within a family, where adults take turns leading the activity.

Theraplay uses music and rhythm in this fashion to help the child experience a regulated state. The back and forth of the activity keeps them engaged, and they experience shared joy with the caregiver or the clinician. These skills can easily be incorporated into the home without appearing to be a task.

The obvious music activities in Theraplay are the ones where a song is used. When applying lotion, the caregiver may sing the lotion song, "Lotion, oh lotion, on [name of child]'s hands, lotion, oh lotion, it feels so grand." This simple song has a calming rhythm, much like a waltz, which has a quiet rhythm when dancing.

While feeding, the Theraplay version of the *Twinkle* song can be incorporated as the caregiver feeds the child. This quiet, child-focused song keeps the feeding in a more quiet lullaby tone instead of what can become more playful and upregulating. I often sit to the side and play *Twinkle Twinkle Little Star* on a ukulele or a guitar while the caregiver is led through the singing of the song. This song is easy to learn even if you have never played a ukulele before. This background music to the feeding activity sets a tone for calmness, and helps organize the child for the exit and a calmer transition to their next activity.

Hand-clapping games incorporate many aspects of relationship building within a Theraplay session. These include eye contact, touch, and the engagement dimension of Theraplay. These games are older child versions of "Patty Cake," and have the same result for promoting engagement. Cooperative hand-clapping games promote relationship building, and caregiver–child shared joy and calming effects within the rhythm and regulation of the rhymes. There are many of these partner hand-clapping games across many cultures. One strategy is to begin with a few simple ones and then send the caregiver and child home with "homework" to find a new one to bring back and demonstrate in therapy the following week. It is important to maintain the adult as the leader, as many children will want to increase speed, soon going so fast they are dysregulated and outside their "window of tolerance" (Siegel 2012). By having the adult be the leader, the speed and tone can be regulated so that the child is successful and co-regulation is facilitated. Maintaining the up-and-down regulation of fast and slow within the clapping games will give the child the experience of becoming up- and downregulated successfully without escalating and losing control. The adult in charge keeps things successful, facilitating the child's learning to trust that the adult will keep them safe and yet still have fun. Shared joy is promoted through this process.

Integrating the Safe and Sound Protocol

The most recent musical addition to my Theraplay practice is the Safe and Sound Protocol (SSP), developed through decades of research by Stephen Porges. In 1994, he introduced polyvagal theory (Porges 2011), which is the basis of the Safe and Sound Protocol under his development.[1] This was launched through collaboration with Integrated Listening Systems in 2017.

The SSP impacts the vagus nerve functioning through a listening intervention. The core of this program is 10 half-hour listens to music that is filtered in order to regulate the autonomic nervous system. This regulating has the impact of helping the person listening (the child or adult) be better equipped to access their coping strategies and remain in a regulated state. I have found this valid for most of the caregivers and children who have used this program.

I recommend practitioners partake in the experiential program for themselves first so that they experience the program firsthand in order to better understand the process. Many people experience significant benefits (including myself), such as waking more rested, focusing more consistently with less distractibility, and having an increased ability to access coping strategies when faced with stressors. Based on personal experience and training in the method, it has become a helpful adjunct to my Theraplay practice. Many families and young people have found it to accelerate progress. It can be powerful to have a child listen with a caregiver and participate in a joint activity while listening. Activities for the caregiver and child can include coloring, building blocks, tossing a ball back and forth, Zentangle™, and

---

1   http://integrated listening.com

mirroring activities, as used in Theraplay. This reinforces the dimensions of Theraplay while participating in this protocol.

Exploring the use of SSP in Theraplay

Many of the children in my practice experienced setbacks during the COVID-19 pandemic in 2020. Dustin had experienced high levels of school anxiety, rage, panic, and emotional reactivity since a medical trauma when he was four years old. Transitions and separating from parents were extremely difficult after his lengthy hospitalization and many intrusive procedures. Being in school was very difficult for him. His anxiety often was expressed through behavior or within his nervous stomach. He had support programs set up through his school to visit the school nurse as needed, and regular interventions with the school counselor.

Through the work of his dedicated parents and Theraplay, he was beginning, by second grade, to move through these transitions without the rage, reactivity, shutdowns, and even dissociation that he had experienced prior to coming for Theraplay treatment. When COVID-19 hit in March 2020 (toward the end of his second-grade year), most of our schools in Maine went to remote learning via the internet. Classrooms became virtual, and Dustin and others like him were not required to separate from their caregivers. Remote learning worked for many of these children with trauma and attachment issues. Dustin's highest anxiety issues of having to be in classrooms with lots of overstimulation from others, in addition to separating from the adults he was learning to trust, were removed. He loved remote learning. He loved being at home. The rage incidents become almost non-existent.

The fall of his third-grade year began with a mixed schedule. He was in school two days a week and home learning remotely the rest. He was in a panic, saying, "I'm not going," "I will die," and "You can't make me." Many times a week, he had raging incidents with his parents. He was back to being unable to eat any breakfast due to his nervous stomach. This was his way of trying to be in control of himself to feel safe. He was losing trust in his parents, teachers, and other adults in his life.

Working with the school, we came up with a plan where he would be met at the drop-off circle by a school counselor or administrator to start his day. This person would help him transition to the classroom. He had to check in with the school counselor on a regular basis. Asking to see the nurse or counselor up to 8–12 times per day was not unusual. He would begin his panic the night before. Bedtime became a time for meltdowns and worry.

In therapy, we were working virtually continuing with Theraplay and Dyadic Developmental Psychotherapy (DDP). At this time, I have added the SSP.

CASE ILLUSTRATION

I had Dustin's mother listen to the SSP first and then begin with him. I listened to the first few sessions with Dustin and his mother via telehealth. The first day, he said his stomach was uncomfortable, so we stopped for five minutes. He took a break and came back in five minutes. He said he would like to finish. His stomach was okay, so we finished the half-hour session. We did many familiar Theraplay activities quietly while listening. I would put a Beanie Baby on my head and mouth out "1, 2, 3", and then we would virtually pretend he had caught the toy. We copied hand and facial expressions. We would also draw together. After a few listens together with me, I turned over the listening and the engaging Theraplay activities to his mother, who listened with him for the rest of the protocol. She continued with some of these activities and incorporated ball tossing.

At this point, I had been riding along (via FaceTime) in the car to drop off with him to support the transition to school. After two half-hour listens, his mother texted me the night before school to say bedtime had gone remarkably well. There was no mention of school that night, just reading their stories and saying "Goodnight, Mom and Dad." Both parents and I were expecting the usual meltdown in the morning.

Mom and Dad were in the kitchen with his younger sister when there was a FaceTime call from Mom's iPad upstairs, asking her to come up. Mom and Dad gave each other with the "here it comes" look. When Mom got upstairs, Dustin wanted to know what he should wear to school. Mom helped him get ready with no mention of not going to school.

Downstairs at the breakfast table, Dustin ate his usual one pretzel (as that was all he could normally put in his nervous morning stomach) when he looked over at the scrambled eggs everyone else was having and said, "Can I have some eggs?" Mom calmly replied, "Of course," even though, inside, she was both waiting for the other shoe to fall and wanting to jump for joy.

As they headed to the car, she asked if he would like to call me, as that had become the routine. He said, "Sure" in a very matter-of-fact tone as opposed to the usual panic. So the call went something like this:

Me: "Good morning, how are you doing this morning?"

Dustin: "I'm good."

Me: "What do you need today?"

Dustin: "I just wanted to say 'hi.'"

Me: "So you know your plan?"

Dustin: "Yup."

Me: "Okay. Have a great day."

Dustin: "Okay, bye."

Dustin transitioned to his classroom easily, asked to see the counselor one time (not nine times), and his teacher reported he had one of his best days ever. This continued through the rest of the school year. He had only one more strong rage a few days later. In May, his school went to full classroom size and full in school. Again, he transitioned to this easily. He could process any worries verbally, find solutions, and go with minimal anxiety.

Through the summer, Dustin engaged more socially with other kids than before, joined teams without anxiety, and participated in neighborhood activities at a typical developmental level. His behaviors are now typical of a child his age, and interactions with his parents and sister are normal. He started the new school year, and his teacher made sure to check in on how his day was going, and that is all he needed for support for the rest of that school year. By the end of that school year and continuing on, he has not needed therapeutic support.

Incorporating Theraplay activities while listening with myself or the caregiver ranged from dramatic shifts like the child described above in just a few listens to subtle changes that have lasted since the listening was stopped many months or, for some, a year or more ago. These children have progressed from severe tantrums to no more rages or only an occasional tantrum. They are better able to access their coping strategies. They are also able to access their verbal and executive brain and let caregivers know what they need and why. Some children have repeated the listening protocol after three months or more have passed from their first listen, with continued or more improvement in presenting issues. The improvents are consistent with theory and research on the healing effects of music (Campbell & Doman 2012) and research and theory by Stephen Porges (2017).

For some, the shift happened very early into the listening. For others, it was more subtle, and the children slowly stopped having rage outbursts or resisting going to school or out to play with other children. One child moved from not wanting to leave their home to wanting to be out in the neighborhood with friends most of the time. The plan for this child was a mix of homeschooling and a shortened day at school. They moved to a full school day and reported liking school, including lunch and recess, which were originally anxiety-producing times. For the rest of the school year, many of these children needed minimal intervention for support and no longer needed help transitioning. Participation outside of school activities and visits to friends' houses without meltdowns now occur on a regular basis.

A current review of caregivers in my practice who have used this protocol has found minimal stress regarding the return to school for the fall of 2021 and 2022. The children who have completed the SSP in my private practice are back to functioning as they were pre-COVID-19 or are often stronger. Many are functioning much closer to their chronological age level. Several have moved to no longer needing therapeutic support.

Music and Theraplay are natural partners in the healing process. This is true in both individual and family work and group work. Incorporating musical activities into the Theraplay practice produces powerful results that amplify the effects of the Theraplay process. Be inspired to use your creative spirit and incorporate music in new and beautiful ways that work for your children and families.

References

Booth, P. B., & Jernberg, A. M. (2010). *Theraplay: Helping Parents and Children Build Better Relationships Through Attachment-Based Play*. Jossey-Bass.

Campbell, D. (1997). *The Mozart Effect: Tapping the Power of Music to Heal the Body, Strengthen the Mind, and Unlock the Creative Spirit*. Avon Books.

Campbell, D., & Doman, A. (2012). *Healing at The Speed of Sound: How What We Hear Transforms Our Brains and Our Lives*. Plume.

Hart, M. (1990). *Drumming at the Edge of Magic: A Journey into the Spirit of Percussion*. HarperCollins.

Karp, H. (2012). *The Happiest Baby on the Block: The New Way to Calm Crying and Help Your Newborn Baby Sleep Longer*. William Morrow.

Leeds, J. (2001). *The Power of Sound: How to Be Healthy and Productive Using Music and Sound*. Healing Arts Press.

Levitin, D. J. (2006). *This is Your Brain on Music: Understanding a Human Obsession*. Dutton.

Levitin, D. J. (2016). *The World in Six Songs: How the Musical Brain Created Human Nature*. Dutton.

Norris, V., & Lender, D. (2020). *Theraplay®—The Practitioners Guide*. Jessica Kingsley Publishers.

Porges, S. W. (2011). *The Polyvagal Theory: Neurophysiological Foundations of Emotions, Attachment, Communication and Self-Regulation*. W.W. Norton & Co.

Porges, S. W. (2017). *The Pocket Guide to the Polyvagal Theory: The Transformative Power of Feeling Safe* (Norton Series on Interpersonal Neurobiology). W.W. Norton & Co.

Siegel, D. J. (2012). *The Developing Mind: How Relationships and the Brain Interact to Shape Who We Are*. Guilford Press.

The Theraplay Institute. (2018). *The Theraplay Song Book*. https://theraplay.org/product/theraplay-song-book

Chapter 11

Integrating Principles of the Neurosequential Model© into Theraplay Practice

Mary J. Ring and Christie Mason

Introduction

In his introduction to *The Boy Who Was Raised as a Dog* (Perry & Szalavitz 2017), Dr. Bruce Perry shared that in the early 1980s, the dominant belief was that children were inherently resilient. The impact of childhood trauma was poorly understood and under-appreciated. Perry found in his lab research that stressful experiences caused young animal subjects to have lasting damage to the development and functioning of their brains, and thus their behavior. In his clinical practice, he saw that children who came from chaotic, neglectful, and violent settings presented with difficult behaviors and struggled to interact successfully with others. He began to understand these challenges in light of neuroscience, and used this understanding to inform interventions with children served by the clinical team he led. Out of this work, the Neurosequential Model of Therapeutics© (NMT) and the broader, more generalizable Neurosequential Model© (NM) were developed to integrate concepts of neurodevelopment into clinical problem solving (NMT), education (NME), caregiving (NMC), and sport (NM Sport).

The NMT is "a developmentally sensitive, neurobiologically informed approach to clinical problem solving" (Perry & Dobson 2013, p.249). Its focus is on identifying the earliest developing areas of the brain significantly impacted by trauma, and then intervening in ways that will help regulate and reorganize those brain regions. The NMT is not specific to any therapeutic technique or intervention; rather, interventions are chosen from many existing options to stimulate the areas of the brain in need of development via brief, repetitive, patterned activities that occur within the context of safe relationships (Perry 2006). Theraplay is one such intervention.

Because the NMT includes a focus on how the brain develops during the primary bonding experience with a caregiver, and the foundation of Theraplay is the caregiver–child attachment connection, the two models are compatible for treatment of those children and families with traumatic experiences. Bruce Perry and Ann Jernberg shared goals of restoring functional relational health to those who experienced trauma in the earlier stages of life and creating a model that many could use. Theraplay concepts were initially published by Ann Jernberg in 1979, focusing on methods to create change through playful social interactions between a caregiving or therapeutic adult and a child. As noted by Eliana Gil (quoted in Sori & Schnur 2014), NM principles are useful in understanding how Theraplay activities can result in improved relationships. As such, the following NM principles are described in brief to provide some limited information about how they correspond to Theraplay practice.[1]

Theraplay and the Neurosequential Model
Sequential development

A key principle of the NM is that the brain organizes and develops in a sequential and hierarchal manner, with lower brain regions primarily developing early in life and the highest (cortical) brain regions not reaching maturity until early adulthood. The key illustration (i.e., the primary heuristic) used in the NM to assist clinicians in understanding brain functioning is an upside-down triangle with four distinct regions: brainstem, diencephalon, limbic, and cortex (bottom to top). The following figure illustrates the sequence of brain organization, from lower, earlier developing regions to higher, later developing ones.

Alongside this image is a list of functions mediated by each of these brain regions; disruptions in these functions suggest under-development or disorganization in the corresponding area of the brain, providing the clinician guidance on which brain areas to target for intervention (Perry 2006).

Neurodevelopment begins in utero and continues through infancy into childhood and young adult life. Ultimate organization and function are determined by a complex admixture of genetics, epigenetics, early life attachment experiences, and, ultimately, the nature and timing of all experiences. A key driver in this process is the collection of regulatory networks that originate in the lower brain regions. When development goes well, these provide the foundational signals to increase the probability of

---

1   When a practitioner enlists in the NMT certification model, all readings, training videos, and application enable a more solid understanding of NMT principles and how to consider their use in treatment planning and application exercises.

healthy development and functioning in the higher brain regions that include the limbic system and cortex (Beeghly, Perry, & Tronick 2016; Perry 1999, 2006, 2009). When the lower regions are disorganized or under-developed, this makes it difficult not only for an individual to perform the functions associated with the lower regions (e.g., regulating heart rate, immune functioning, sleep, arousal, etc.) but also for the higher brain regions to develop and optimally mediate their functions (e.g., emotional reactivity, attachment, reflective cognition). Thus, dysregulation at the lowest areas of the brain can disrupt functioning throughout the entire brain.

The lower regulatory networks that develop early in life are likely to be altered by exposure to adversity, such as maternal stress during pregnancy, exposure to alcohol or drugs, problems with attachment to caregivers, or any experiences of chaotic life situations. The chief implication of this information is that practitioners who wish to help children to become regulated and develop healthily after exposure to early life adversity must select interventions that target the lowest areas of the brain that have been significantly dysregulated by the adversities they have experienced (Perry & Hambrick 2008). Not coincidentally, these areas of the brain are best regulated by relevant, rewarding somatosensory input delivered in the context of a safe, predictable, responsive relationship—a description consistent with Theraplay practice.

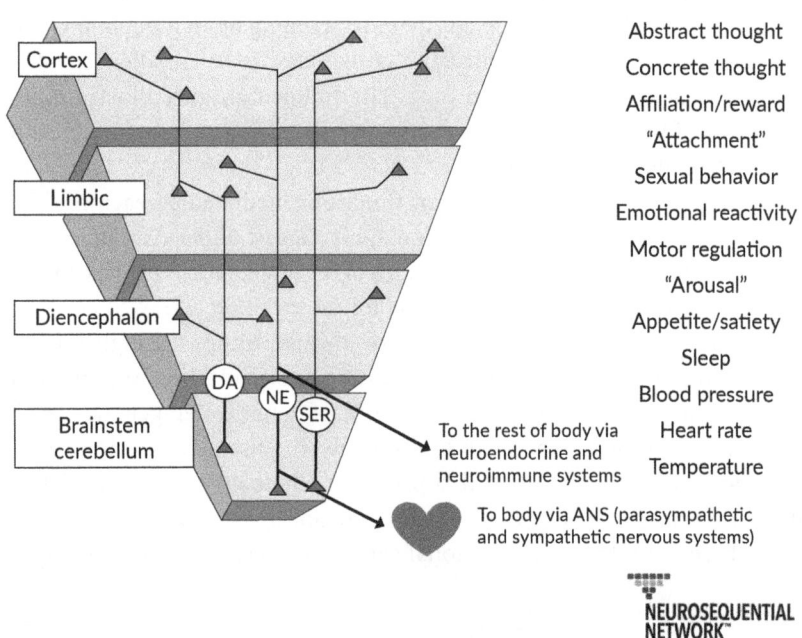

Sequence of brain organization
SOURCE: © 2002–2020 BRUCE D. PERRY

Use-dependent development

Another of the principles underlying the NM is that part of the brain can only be changed when it is consistently activated. Thus, any attempt to change a child's behavior or functioning must include repetitive, patterned activation of the area of the brain that mediates that behavior or functioning. This NM principle of use dependency, in part, describes the need for caregivers to provide the appropriate predictable and reciprocal interactions during infancy and childhood to support brain development that will provide a solid foundation for future functioning (Ludy-Dobson & Perry 2010; Perry 2009), a concept that corresponds with the emphasis on the core dimensions of structure, engagement, nurture, and challenge within Theraplay. It also describes the need for practitioners to facilitate these experiences when a child's brain development has been disrupted by adversity, something Theraplay practitioners do whenever they implement a treatment plan for a client. When a practitioner understands what neural functions need to be improved, the treatment plan can include the repetitive and patterned Theraplay activities that activate and regulate the neural system responsible for problematic trauma-based symptoms to the point needed for a particular neuronal system to change (Gaskill & Perry 2017; Perry 2017; Perry & Hambrick 2008).

Relationship, reward, and regulation

According to the NM, core regulatory neural networks are organized in the human brain by the rhythmic, predictable, patterned, and attuned interactions of caregivers with young infants. When the child is repeatedly regulated by an adult caregiver, they learn to develop healthy self-regulation over time. In addition, these attuned interactions facilitate the necessary neural development for later meaningful interpersonal relationships (Beeghly *et al.* 2016). According to the NM principles, these intense moments of personal adult-to-child focus create a neurobiological interweaving of relationship, reward, and regulation (Ludy-Dobson & Perry 2010; Neurosequential Network 2020c; Perry & Hambrick 2008). In Theraplay, practitioners want the interaction with the caregiver to be the most interesting experience in the room, thereby facilitating these same intense moments of personal focus. The caregiver is coached to attune to the child and help regulate them through upregulating and downregulating activities across the Theraplay domains, especially engagement and nurture.

Neuroarcheology of associations and attachments

As noted above, the NM asserts that, very early in life, infants come to experience human relationships as sources of reward and comfort when they develop associations between nurturing touch and relief from distress, such as hunger or cold. Positive nurturing care and touch from caregiver to child are considered essential in the theoretical basis of both Theraplay and the NM (Booth & Jernberg 2010; Perry 1999). If, instead, early caregiving experiences involve neglect, abuse, or any other form of trauma, what should have been a positive, pleasurable interaction can become associated with a state of fear or alarm when others enter their personal space, especially key attachment or caregiving figures (Perry *et al.* 2018). Both the NM and Theraplay recognize the importance of providing new, safe, and responsive experiences of caregiving to update internal models of attachment figures rooted in negative early experience. These sorts of interactions are evident in activities from the Theraplay dimension of nurture, including feeding, rocking, checking for hurts, and applying lotion.

State-dependent functioning and sensitization

One of the most widely applicable concepts from the NM is that of state-dependent functioning. When someone is in a calm state, they have access to their maximum capacity for brain functioning (resulting from age, biological capacity, experience, etc.). However, as stress increases, their access to the higher brain regions decreases (Neurosequential Network 2020b). Someone who feels highly threatened may have minimal access to advanced cortical functions such as speech, planning, judgment, and impulse control, and rely instead on faster yet more primitive brain regions. Behavior arising from these lower brain regions may appear to be oppositional, overreactive, aggressive, or disengaged.

Unsurprisingly, when children have consistently experienced threatening caregivers or traumatic experiences, they become acutely attuned to cues that they are under threat. Their state of arousal can change quite quickly from calm to fear. This rapid move up the stress response continuum is referred to as sensitization, and a person whose stress response is sensitized frequently responds in this manner to new situations or experiences that register as threatening, based on having adapted to a higher baseline level of arousal (Perry *et al.* 2018). According to the NM, repeated proactive opportunities for regulation have the potential to decrease this sensitization, resulting in a more typical, gradual move up the stress response continuum corresponding to the level of stress being experienced. Theraplay activities can provide just those sorts of regulating experiences. The goal of Theraplay treatment sessions is to plan the session, so patterned up- and downregulating activities take place in such a manner that a safe and tolerable experience happens for the child and caregiver and results in co-regulation, as described by Beeghly *et al.* (2016). Over time, as treatment continues, the goal is to widen the "window of tolerance" (Siegel 1999), and to strengthen the capability of the child to have trust and pleasurable expectations for interacting with caregivers and others (Ludy-Dobson & Perry 2010; Theraplay 2010).

In addition to proactively regulating clients during a Theraplay session, the practitioner needs to remain aware of any stress response exhibited during the session, and adjust the activity accordingly to maintain regulation (Neurosequential Network 2020a). Gaskill and Perry (2017) have written about some of the core elements of NMT useful in guided play activities in order to limit the level of stress response for clients during structured play, many of which are similar to Theraplay interventions.

Intimacy barrier and internal template

The "intimacy barrier" is the term for an NM principle that describes how comfortable a person is with emotionally close interactions. Clients who have trauma histories often become more easily triggered by a lesser amount of emotional closeness than someone who has a more typical developmental history (Neurosequential Network 2020c). Early relational experiences determine how reactive a person can become, and how easily their intimacy barrier gets triggered during interactions with others. Practitioners are encouraged to be mindful of this and take care not to cross the client's intimacy barrier unless invited, as that will dysregulate the client. Nurturing and playful activities within the Theraplay session need to be carried out with an awareness of what the child and/or caregiver has experienced in their early life with caregivers. The practitioner may need to provide more space or adjust the nurturing approach to create a subjective experience of safety. The goal is to provide new experiences of care with the dosing and spacing needed for the child or caregiver to create a new internal template of relationships (internal working model (IWM)).

Dosing and spacing

Dosing and spacing (Neurosequential Network 2020d) is an NM intervention principle that guides the practitioner to consider how to structure therapeutic experiences for maximum therapeutic benefit. In order for changes to occur in the child's brain, these therapeutic experiences need to be of sufficient intensity, duration, and frequency. Much like lifting weights regularly to build muscles, therapeutic experiences must be repeated in a pattern for the brain to be altered. Dr. Perry mentions basic research studies that demonstrate that very brief activations of neural networks (Neurosequential Network 2020), which are seconds long and repetitive in nature, can bring about change. For the change to become lasting, a pattern of these brief activations (a minimum of four activations over an hour) needs to occur and then be followed by repetition at some point for integration of the experience (Neurosequential Network 2020d). This description fits what can happen during Theraplay sessions and afterward, as activities are repeated at home by caregivers and the children. In NM terms, the goal of Theraplay is to create positive relational experiences between children and caregivers with sufficient frequency and patterning to alter a child's template of relationships (Booth & Jernberg 2010; Neurosequential Network 2020d).

Table 11.1: Theraplay theory or dimension with corresponding NM principles

Theory or dimension	Description	Matching NM principles
Theoretical tenets of attachment and connection in Theraplay	Attunement + co-regulation = intersubjectivity (Trevarthen 1993; Siegel 1999; Siegel & Hartzell 2004)—consistent and focused caregiving in early life leads to secure attachment (Bowlby 1988)	• Sequential development of the brain • Use-dependent development • Relationship, reward, regulation • Neuroarcheology of associations and attachments
Structure dimension	Predictable, patterned, rhythmic interactions led by adult. Development of neuroception of safety (Porges 2011)	• Intimacy barrier and internal template • State-dependent functioning and sequential development
Engagement dimension	Felt safety, inner state regulation, attunement, social engagement system (Porges 2011), attachment experiences	• Intimacy barrier and internal template • Neuroarcheology of associations and attachments • Relationship, reward, regulation
Nurture dimension	Self-worth, stress reduction, downregulation, development of neuroception of safety (Porges 2011)	• State-dependent functioning and sensitization • Intimacy barrier and internal template • Relationship, reward, regulation
Challenge dimension	Competency, confidence, self-efficacy	• Use-dependent development • Dosing and spacing

Using the NMT metric and Marschak Interaction Method (MIM) for assessment

While the description of how NM principles support the use of Theraplay as an intervention offers an introduction to integrating the two models, for maximum benefit it is essential that practitioners complete thorough intake interviews and develop a treatment plan specific to the needs of the child client. For Theraplay, this means conducting a Marschak Interaction Method (MIM) observation, which provides the practitioner with information about which of the Theraplay domains of structure, engagement, nurture, and challenge need to be emphasized in treatment. For the NMT, this means gathering information from parents and collateral contacts about a child's exposure to adversity and quality of relational support from conception to the present, as well as using psychometric tools and reports about the child's current functioning to determine how well developed specific regions of the brain are relative to age-typical peers (Ludy-Dobson & Perry 2010; Perry & Hambrick 2008). This information can then be used to find the lowest area of the brain that has problems with functioning in order to develop a treatment plan that will include interventions to activate that area to facilitate further development and organization of that brain region (Perry & Hambrick 2008). Certification in the NMT is needed to gain access to its assessment tool so Theraplay practitioners interested in using the NMT to inform their Theraplay practice are encouraged to either pursue certification in the NMT[2] or partner with a clinician who is already certified to complete the NMT assessment process for a client.

One of the outcomes of the NMT assessment process is a brain map, which provides both a visual and numeric illustration of a client's brain functioning by evaluating them on 32 items known to be mediated by specific brain regions. Collectively, this information results in a comparison of the client's functioning, represented as a percentage of age-typical functioning in four domains: sensory integration, self-regulation, relational, and cognitive. These domains of functioning roughly correspond to the regions of the brain identified in the upside-down triangle model used to help clinicians understand the brain. For treatment planning purposes, a functional domain rated as less than 65 percent of age typical is considered "essential" for intervention, 65–85 percent as "therapeutic," and above 85 percent as "enrichment." Treatment begins with interventions that will activate the lowest functional domain rated "essential." Once that area of the brain has been better developed or organized, treatment can proceed with the next

---

2   See www.neurosequential.com

lowest area rated essential, until no domains are rated essential when an updated brain map is completed.

When a practitioner provides caregivers with the brain map report and the results of the other assessment measures along with sharing the MIM video of caregiver–child interaction, caregivers often develop a deeper appreciation for the struggles the child is experiencing. Because the practitioner can provide a rationale for intervention based on the most recent research in the neurosciences, caregivers may have increased confidence in therapy and a greater willingness to be part of the healing journey for the child.

As mentioned earlier, the NMT does not dictate particular intervention methods. Rather, it provides information on the kinds of therapeutic experiences that will help develop or organize specific functional domains. As an attachment-based play model, Theraplay strengthens the relational supports that are a prerequisite for individual brain growth, and provides experiences that develop and organize the functional domains rated as essential for intervention.

CASE ILLUSTRATION 1

Mark presented with struggles in the caregiver–child relationship, particularly with his foster mother. An MIM was done, and because authorization for therapy had not yet been given, psychoeducation in Theraplay-type activities was provided to guide his foster mother on how to use activities with the child at home to strengthen the mother–child relationship while waiting for court approval for treatment. Six months later, bonding improved, but regulation difficulties became more apparent. A second MIM was done, along with an NMT assessment. The NMT report revealed that treatment in the domain of sensory integration was "essential." The family was referred to a local occupational therapist to address sensory needs. When occupational therapy was completed, the family returned for Theraplay treatment. A third MIM was done, and a full course of Theraplay treatment was provided with both foster parents involved. The goal, in this case, was to follow the principles of neurosequential development by addressing deficits in the lower functional domain of sensory integration before focusing on the relational domain via Theraplay.

CASE ILLUSTRATION 2

Julian came home to his adoptive family at 10 months old. He developed a strong bond with his foster parents and had regularly received speech and occupational therapy since being in preschool, though he continued to become dysregulated when encountering new experiences. At age seven, he sustained a serious injury requiring six months of bed rest, which further restricted his access to new experiences, and led to over-reliance on screens for reward and regulation. Because numerous factors in his background were likely to have negatively influenced his neurodevelopment, an NMT assessment was completed. The domain of sensory integration was rated at the "therapeutic" level of need. Therefore, a major focus in the beginning Theraplay sessions was the inclusion of sensory activities. To allow him to feel safe with the novelty introduced by Theraplay, activities were done first by the therapist and mother in proximity to Julian while he observed, and then he and his foster father repeated the activity. In addition to participating in Theraplay, his foster parents intentionally stopped most of his screen usage. After four months of treatment, his foster parents reported that Julian was interested in playing with the neighborhood children. After eight months, Julian was referred to a neuro-movement specialist for some additional treatment in patterned movement. A second MIM indicated marked improvement with regulated interpersonal interaction at one year. Focusing treatment at the lowest level of neurological dysfunction was key for Julian, and Theraplay was able to address that need while also restoring his pleasure in interpersonal relationships, which ultimately helped him benefit from other treatment modalities.

As these cases indicate, the NMT can be incorporated into Theraplay to determine whether a client is ready for the relational aspect of Theraplay intervention, what activities to emphasize during sessions, and how a client's neurodevelopment is progressing as a result of intervention. In turn, Theraplay can be incorporated into NMT via the selection and sequencing of activities to promote growth and development in specific functional domains identified as essential or therapeutic for intervention. Additionally, the NMT assessment process results in visual and numeric representation of a child's brain functioning, such that parental empathy and patience may be enhanced, frustration decreased, and expectations altered to match the child's developmental rather than chronological age. It also offers a neurobiological rationale for Theraplay intervention that may be an asset in motivating caregivers' investment in Theraplay treatment with their children. As with many other theoretical models on which Theraplay draws, the NMT adds depth and validity to a model many know to be invaluable in promoting secure attachment relationships between caregivers and children.

Table 11.2: Theraplay activities related to NMT functional domain

NMT functional domain	Description	NMT-recommended activities	Corresponding Theraplay activities
Sensory integration	A set of functions that integrate, process, store, and act on sensory input from outside and inside the body. Many of the neural networks involved in sensory integration originate in, or engage, lower areas of the brain	*Characteristics*: patterned, repetitive somatosensory activities provided multiple times each day for approximately 7–8 minutes at a time. *Examples*: massage, music, movement (swimming, walking/running, jumping, swinging, rocking), yoga/breathing, and animal-assisted therapy that includes patterned, repetitive activities such as brushing	Hand-clapping games Lotioning Slippery, slippery, slip Blanket swing Eye signals *Row, Row, Row Your Boat* *This is the Way the Baby Rides*
Self-regulation	A broad set of functions that modulate and regulate the activity of other key systems in other parts of the body and brain. This includes the three main forms of self-regulation: bottom-up somatosensory regulation, top-down cerebromodulation, and dissociation. The neural networks involved in self-regulation originate in many areas of the brain, but all ultimately influence activity in the lower and middle areas of the brain	*Characteristics*: structure and predictability provided consistently by safe, nurturing adults across settings. *Examples*: developing transitioning activity (using a song, words, or other cues to help prepare the child for the change in activity), patterned, repetitive proprioceptive occupational therapy activities such as isometric exercises (chair push-ups, bear hugs while child tries to pull the adult's arms away, applying deep pressure), using weighted vests, blankets, ankle weights, various deep breathing techniques, building structure into bedtime rituals, music and movement activities, animal-assisted therapy, and Eye Movement Desensitization and Reprocessing (EMDR)	Animal entry Wheelbarrow Wiggle in-and-out Zoom-erk Hand stack Toilet paper bust-out Weighing Soft and floppy Balancing activities Crawling race Newspaper punch Feather blow Pillow push Tug-of-war Motor boat

Domain	NMT description	Therapy characteristics and examples	Theraplay activities
Relational	The complex set of relationship-related functions such as bonding, attachment, attunement, reward, empathy, and related emotional functions. Neural networks that influence these functions arise in all areas of the brain; however, the primary mediating networks are concentrated in the corticolimbic areas	*Characteristics*: include interactions with multiple positive and healthy adults who are invested in the child's life and in their treatment *Examples*: art therapy, individual play therapy, Parent–Child Interaction Therapy (PCIT), dyadic parallel play with an adult, and, when mastered, dyadic parallel play with a peer, small group activities may be added, animal-assisted therapy, and targeted psychotherapy	Eye signals Hide something on child and find it Beep and honk Check-ups Mirroring Pop cheeks Special handshake Progressive pass around Decorate the child Feeding Face painting Lotion prints Manicure *Twinkle* song Cooperative cotton ball race Straight face challenge
Cognitive	The myriad functions involved in complex sensory processing, speech, language, abstract cognition, reading, future planning, perspective taking, moral reasoning, and similar cognitive capabilities. The neural networks primarily responsible for these functions appear to be located in the cortex, although neural networks from other areas can influence and modify these functions (such as is seen with threat or stress-related changes in cognitive functions)	*Characteristics*: take place in the context of safe, nurturing relationships with invested adults *Examples*: speech and language therapy, insight-oriented psychodynamic treatment, Cognitive Behavioral Therapy (CBT), and family therapy	Not an explicit focus of Theraplay, but regulation of the lower brain regions in Theraplay likely contributes to increased availability of the cortex for learning

Note: NMT description and activities are drawn from an unpublished NMT metric report © Bruce D. Perry, MD, PhD 2009–2021. Identification of Theraplay activities (drawn from the 3rd edn of Theraplay by Booth et al. 2010) as corresponding to the NMT domains reflect the authors' judgment.

References

Beeghly, M., Perry, B. D., & Tronick, E. (2016). Self-Regulatory Processes in Early Development. In S. Maltzman (Ed.), *The Oxford Handbook of Treatment Processes and Outcomes in Psychology: A Multidisciplinary, Biopsychosocial Approach* (pp.42–54) [Oxford Handbooks Online]. Oxford University Press. www.oxfordhandbooks.com/view/10.1093/oxfordhb/9780199739134.001.0001/oxfordhb-9780199739134-e-3

Booth, P. B., & Jernberg, A.M. (2010). *Theraplay: Helping Parents and Children Build Better Relationships Through Attachment-Based Play* (3rd edn). Jossey-Bass.

Bowlby, J. A. (1988). *A Secure Base: Parent–Child Attachment and Healthy Human Development.* Basic Books.

Gaskill, R. L., & Perry, B. D. (2017). A Neurosequential Therapeutics Approach to Guided Play, Play Therapy, and Activities for Children Who Won't Talk. In C. A. Malchiodi & D. A. Crenshaw (Eds), *What to Do When Children Clam Up in Psychotherapy: Interventions to Facilitate Communication* (pp.38–66). Guilford Press.

Jernberg, A. M. (1979). *Theraplay: A New Treatment Using Structure Play for Problem Children and Their Families.* Jossey-Bass.

Ludy-Dobson, C. R., & Perry, B. D. (2010). The Role of Healthy Relational Interactions in Buffering the Impact of Childhood Trauma. In E. Gil (Ed.), *Working with Children to Heal Interpersonal Trauma: The Power of Play* (pp.26–43). Guilford Press.

Neurosequential Network. (2020a). 1. Patterns of stress & resilience. Neurosequential Network Stress & Trauma Series, March 23 [Video series]. www.youtube.com/watch?v=orwIn02h6V4

Neurosequential Network. (2020b). 2. State-dependent brain functioning. Neurosequential Network Stress & Trauma Series, March 26 [Video series]. www.youtube.com/watch?v=PZg1dlskBLA

Neurosequential Network. (2020c). 13. The intimacy barrier. Neurosequential Network Stress & Trauma Series, March 30 [Video series]. https://youtu.be/7crm3JcVfJs

Neurosequential Network. (2020d). 6. Dosing and spacing in education & therapeutics. Neurosequential Network Stress & Trauma Series, April 3 [Video series]. www.youtube.com/watch?v=5ATSl8XhF-k

Neurosequential Network. (2020). The Neurosequential Model of Therapeutics: NMT as an Evidence-based Practice. Unpublished manuscript.

Perry, B. D. (1999). Bonding and attachment in maltreated children: Consequences of emotional neglect in childhood. *CTA Parent and Caregiver Education Series 1*(3). ChildTrauma Academy Press.

Perry, B. D. (2006). Applying Principles of Neurodevelopment to Clinical Work with Maltreated and Traumatized Children: The Neurosequential Model of Therapeutics. In N. B. Webb (Ed.), *Working with Traumatized Youth in Child Welfare* (pp.27–52). Guilford Press.

Perry, B. D. (2009). Examining child maltreatment through a neurodevelopmental lens: Clinical application of the neurosequential model of therapeutics. *Journal of Loss and Trauma 14*, 240–255. https://doi.org/10.1080/15325020903004350

Perry, B. D. (2017). Trauma and Stress-Related Disorders. In T. P. Beauchaine & S. P. Hinshaw (Eds), *Textbook of Child and Adolescent Psychopathology* (3rd edn) (pp.683–705). Guilford Press.

Perry, B. D., & Dobson, C. (2013). Application of the Neurosequential Model (NMT). In J. Ford & C. Courtois (Eds), *Treating Complex Traumatic Stress Disorders in Children and Adolescents* (pp.249–260). Guilford Press.

Perry, B. D., & Hambrick, E. P. (2008). The Neurosequential Model of Therapeutics. *Reclaiming Children and Youth 17*(3), 38–43.

Perry, B. D., & Szalavitz, M. (2017). *The Boy Who Was Raised as a Dog and Other Stories from a Child Psychiatrist's Notebook: What Traumatized Children Can Teach Us about Life, Loss, and Healing* (2nd edn). Basic Books.

Perry, B. D., Griffin, G., Davis, G., Perry, J. A., & Perry, R. D. (2018). The Impact of Neglect, Trauma, and Maltreatment on Neurodevelopment. In A. Beech, A. Carter, R. Mann, & P. Rotshtein (Eds), *The Wiley Blackwell Handbook of Forensic Neuroscience* (pp.813–835). John Wiley & Sons.

Porges, S. W. (2011). *The Polyvagal Theory: Neurophysiological Foundations of Emotions, Attachment, Communication, and Self-regulation.* W.W. Norton & Co.

Siegel, D. J. (1999). *The Developing Mind: How Relationship and the Brain Interact to Shape Who We Are.* Guilford Press.

Siegel, D. J., & Hartzell, M. (2004). *Parenting from the Inside Out: How a Deeper Self-Understanding Can Help You Raise Children Who Thrive.* Penguin Group.

Sori, C. F., & Schnur, S. (2014). Integrating a neurosequential approach in the treatment of traumatized children: An interview with Eliana Gil, Part II. *The Family Journal: Counseling and Therapy for Couples and Families* 22(2), 251–257. https://doi.org/10.1177/1066480713514945

Trevarthen, C. (1993). The Self Born in Intersubjectivity: The Psychology of Infant Communication. In U. Neisser (Ed.), *The Perceived Self: Ecological and Interpersonal Sources of Knowledge* (pp.121–173). Cambridge University Press.

Chapter 12

Neuro-Physiological Psychotherapy (NPP)

A MODEL OF SOMATIC EXPERIENCE IN THERAPLAY

Jay Vaughan

Introduction

This chapter focuses on the use of body-based approaches in the Neuro-Physiological Psychotherapy (NPP) model in relation to Theraplay, and in particular highlights how the work of Peter Levine and his Somatic Experiencing® model (Levine 1997, 2010; Levine & Kline 2007) can enhance Theraplay for traumatized children. The model highlights that in order to be in a relationship, we need to be calm and regulated enough to relate. In this way, Theraplay's regulation of the body and brain is an essential part of the process. This focus on regulation is essential for traumatized children where the trauma has been part of their early relationships, and it is the relationship with their new family that terrifies them. With children who are terrified, it is not words and assurances that can make things better. This chapter outlines how this Somatic Experiencing model can be helpfully applied to therapy and Theraplay.

Development of NPP

Family Futures is a UK-based, Ofsted-regulated and inspected, not-for-profit Adoption and Fostering Agency specializing in the assessment and treatment of traumatized children placed into foster, special guardianship, or adoptive families. Family Futures has a therapy model entitled Neuro-Physiological Psychotherapy (NPP), an integrative therapy model, including Theraplay as a key intervention. The team at Family Futures is interdisciplinary and consists of therapists, psychologists, sensory integration therapists, social workers, and teachers as well as specialist consultants. Family Futures research published in 2016 consisted of two peer-reviewed articles on research into the NPP therapy model (McCullough *et al.* 2016; Vaughan, McCullough, & Burnell 2016). This research showed statistically significant positive outcomes for the children and young people who had the full treatment intervention at Family Futures. In addition, McCullough and Mathura (2019) conducted an experimental study comparing individuals who received NPP and those who did not. The conclusions were shocking, highlighting how vital it was for traumatized children to have a wraparound intensive therapy provision that is interdisciplinary, such as NPP.

The main clinical issue for this population of children and young people is that early childhood trauma impacts all aspects of their development. It impacts how they feel about themselves and the world, and how their whole neuro-physiological system is wired to manage the world. This means that their ability to regulate their senses, heart, or body temperature to feel safe to trust others is impaired (Brown & Ward 2013; Felitti *et al.* 1998; van der Kolk 2009). Children from the care system make up a substantial number of adults in psychiatric hospitals, prisons, and the homeless. It is also increasingly recognized that this population of children and young people need a long-term intervention that can support them at different stages of their lives. Without support, the long-term impact of their history will impact their adult lives and outcomes.

The Family Futures NPP model is based on the triune brain and an assessment process that assesses a child's therapy needs and what is the appropriate therapy modality. All Family Futures multidisciplinary assessments involve a Theraplay Marschak Interaction Method (MIM) assessment as part of the assessment process. It is based on making sense of how much the child is in primitive brain fight, flight, or freeze, to decide if the child can do limbic brain relationship-based therapy, or if they can manage cortical brain reflective thinking. In this way, Theraplay is a key part of intervention modalities for children who are sufficiently regulated to be helped to be in a relationship with their parent or caregiver and develop a more secure attachment relationship. It is important to mention that the NPP approach recognizes that for all children and young people, the progression from primitive brain work to limbic brain work to cortical brain work is not always linear. Some children can move between these areas all within one session, or cycle between the levels of the brain and body in one session. In this way, it is not necessarily a smooth linear process, but a complex integrative process requiring a range of therapeutic skills.

I first began working as a Dramatherapist with traumatized adopted and foster children 30 years ago. There was a phrase around at the time for both parents and professionals struggling to engage positively with a child, that you just needed to "fake it until you make it." At this point, this didn't necessarily seem a helpful message for some parents and professionals struggling with what we now call "blocked care" (Baylin & Hughes 2016; Hughes & Baylin 2012). Now, looking back at all the research into neuroscience and how we read each other, this seems ridiculous—completely missing how we work as human beings and the power of our non-verbal communication to the child. Our ability to read each other's non-verbal communication means that the slightest flick of an eye, frown, or tensing of the body means how we feel can be read by the other person. And as we know, the ability of the traumatized child or adult to read non-verbal communication is acute. The "reading" can be complicated, but in essence, we are nervous systems communicating with other nervous systems. We can gather an array of information to work out these very nuanced non-verbal communications and the underlying feeling.

As Levine says in his book *In an Unspoken Voice* (2010), we are in essence animals, but animals that speak. However, the language we use is of little value when we are distressed, and then the soothing of our nervous systems is a physical touch-based soothing, and it is not the words we utter but the tone of our words that provides comfort for our distress.

Components of NPP

Theraplay is a modality that requires absolute authenticity because it relies on such close proximity and intimate interactions. So exactly what we feel and communicate with our bodies is even more imperative. There is no escaping with Theraplay that the other person will be "reading" us, and they are going to pick up on everything we are communicating at that moment. In this way, it is vital in Theraplay for the communication to be "real." Theraplay requires the practitioner to be authentic and present in the moment in order to support the vital connection and subtle interaction between parent and child. It is only by being genuinely present and authentic in your interactions as the Theraplay practitioner that you can truly help parent and child in that delicate process of developing a more attuned dance of attachment with each other. The role of the practitioner in Theraplay is to facilitate the "right brain to right brain" interaction between parent and child. Of course, this means that you are not working so much with the words but with all the non-verbal ways of being. It is "not what you say, but how you say it" with Theraplay.

Somatic Experiencing is training based on Peter Levine's work. It focuses on understanding the impact of trauma on the nervous system, and how to track dysregulation in the nervous system and the body in order to help the body heal. Theraplay requires the practitioner to really notice what is happening to the parent and child, but it is also vital for the practitioner to notice what is happening to their own nervous system. You then have to wonder what the "fake it until you make it" advocates of 30 years ago were communicating about their own nervous system and picking up about the client's nervous system.

Theraplay is an unusual intervention where there is no distance between the client and practitioner, no blank screen, and no time to pause and reflect on gaps in the conversation. It is an intervention that is very much in the moment and requires the closeness and intimacy of non-verbal communication. The voice is used to soothe and lull the parent and child as much as imparting instructions or occasional reflections. The engagement of the whole person in the intervention is crucial. What Theraplay brings as a therapeutic modality is unusual because it requires such closeness and intimacy, which is not necessarily always the way with other modalities. What Somatic Experiencing can bring to Theraplay is a very particular way of tracking what is happening in the nervous system for both parent and child and the practitioner. Somatic Experiencing teaches practitioners to track the arousal in the nervous system and to look for signs of sympathetic and parasympathetic activation.

Somatic Experiencing ROSE model

This ROSE model, devised by Raja Selvam for teaching, has four parts:

- the *resonance* that is communicated between the client and therapist
- the *observations* by the therapist of the client's body, and signs of sympathetic and parasympathetic activation
- what the client *self-reports* about the body *symptoms* to the therapist
- psycho*education* of the client by the therapist about these communications.

It is important when considering dyadic Theraplay to emphasize that there are two client nervous systems in the therapy—the child's nervous system and the parent's nervous system. So, in Theraplay sessions there are three nervous systems in the room (including the Theraplay practitioner's), all of which are continually communicating with each other largely outside our awareness.

1. Resonance

"Resonance" in the Collins English Dictionary is described as "the sound which is produced by an object when it vibrates at the same rate as the sound waves from another object." Resonance in Somatic Experiencing is the body-based communication that is transmitted from one nervous system to another. As practitioners, we are used to thinking about transference and countertransference, and we all know how feelings can be projected onto us. But the idea that body-based feelings can be communicated and enacted in our bodies is vital when working with such an intimate and non-verbal modality as Theraplay. Perhaps with some therapies where touch and intimacy are not such an issue, the concept of resonance is not so crucial (although the Family Futures NPP model would say it is), but for Theraplay, it is crucial. If we can think as Theraplay practitioners about our own bodily states and track what we are feeling and where in our body, this will give us a resource and help us take care of our own bodies. If we can then use this communicated bodily sensation, this resonance, and track if this bodily sensation is ours or if it belongs to the child or parent, that will heighten our ability to help all parties in the Theraplay session regulate. Tracking the somatic resonance between practitioner and both clients (caregiver and child) gives vital information about the clients, which will enhance the Theraplay work. The Theraplay practitioner in this way needs to use their own body as a reference point and for sensing vital information about the client's inner experience.

If we want to track how our body and the client's body are managing in a session, the most helpful way of differentiating this is to think about the autonomic nervous system and the sympathetic and parasympathetic areas of the nervous system. The role of the Theraplay practitioner can be enhanced by tracking the following in their own nervous system:

- heart rate

- body temperature

- breathing rate

- digestion

- sensation.

If we accept that trauma impacts the whole of the system, not just how we think and feel, then we need to think about how the body is impacted. If we accept that trauma can be communicated body to body, then we need to think about how we are impacted by working with vicarious trauma. If we can care for our own nervous systems, we are also caring for our client's nervous systems and gathering vital information about the level of arousal. If we want to be authentic and attuned, we need to have heightened awareness of what our body is experiencing in the interaction. We cannot think our way out of it because we have to be aware and track our bodies. The concept of resonance and the tracking of our own nervous system and awareness of the client's nervous systems in Theraplay with traumatized children is the foundation on which all other healing and relationship-building is based.

2. Observations

The next part of the Somatic Experiencing ROSE model is observation. In order to help the client's regulation, we need to heighten our awareness of what we are observing in the client. For Theraplay, this will be for both parent and child. This will not only protect us from the impact of providing Theraplay for traumatized children (and sometimes traumatized parents too), but also provide another rich source of information to enhance our practice. The good news is that most of us are already doing this instinctively. The gift for us all from the body work world is to recognize that we have this skill and can use it to look after ourselves and deepen our work.

There is a difference between noticing non-verbal cues and tracking the nervous system. It is really a matter of practice, not only tracking our own nervous system but also the client's. The signs to look for in the client are:

- heart rate increasing or decreasing

- body temperature heating up or cooling down

- skin looks pale and clammy

- skin becomes blotchy and patchy

- breathing becomes faster and more rapid or slows down and is more in the belly

- digestion, and if eating and digesting are not possible and there is activation for fight or flight

- bodily sensations and if hairs are on end or the skin or body is struggling with touch.

Of course, not all of these things are easily seen, but once we are aware, they are easier to spot—the body gives off clues to its stress system being activated. All of this will impact Theraplay and the ability to be soothed and enjoy an intimate relationship. How can we have an intersubjective experience of being enjoyed as a child if we are not regulated enough to be in the moment and our body calm enough to allow for that connection to occur? We are literally tracking the resonance and our observations are attuning to the child's and parent's nervous systems and tracking the level of regulation in sessions.

3. Self-report

There are two ways the Somatic Experiencing ROSE third element of self-report can be used. The first is in Theraplay sessions to inform interactions so that observations are fed back and responded to. For the traumatized child or young person, having their stress responses noticed means that it is then vital to negotiate skin-to-skin interactions through waving fans, offering cold water, or reducing distance or touch. Theraplay is good at knowing that intimacy and interaction have to be modified for the traumatized child; within this context, we need to think about the autonomic nervous system symptoms and calming the body. A key part of the NPP model is to think, whatever modality is being used, about the body, and to track the nervous system and reduce the physiological stress responses. Many children and young people's bodies are wired to stress, so their physiological response to normal parent–child interactions is easily tipped into overwhelm, and their primitive brain of fight, flight, or freeze is activated. In Theraplay, we have an opportunity to do something different and adjust not just the games but also the physiology of what we are doing in sessions, to track the nervous system from a dysregulated to a regulated state.

Second, information about the bodily responses to Theraplay can be helpfully reflected on in parent sessions. These can then provide a forum for parents to begin to notice their child's autonomic nervous system responses and their own. The Theraplay practitioner can give feedback to the parent on their observations of both the child and the parent. The Theraplay practitioner can also self-report their own physical experiences and wonder about what they were picking up in the resonance for the child and the parent. Untangling what belongs to who would be such a valuable part of the usual Theraplay process. This work in parent sessions will help teach the parent to track their own nervous system to look after themselves and heighten their ability to notice what is happening to their child's nervous system. The value of this process is that it promotes awareness of what is happening at a body-based level, which is helpful to work in sessions, and importantly life at home too.

4. Education

The final part of the Somatic Experiencing ROSE model is psychoeducation. This is already a valuable and important part of Theraplay, and something that once again can be further deepened by adding the body to this process. Parents can learn about Theraplay and gain an understanding of their child.

Most importantly, they can understand their child's nervous system, how to soothe the nervous system, and how to notice when it is activated by stress.

CASE ILLUSTRATION

Fiona was furious and began to rip the room apart while her adoptive mother looked on horrified, unsure what to do. The cotton wool balls were scattered all over the room, the banana snack was lying under a chair, and all the contents of the Theraplay bag were ransacked. The therapist breathed deeply and put a reassuring hand on the parent's arm. They breathed together. Fiona continued her frenzied attack on the room until everything from the bag lay visible on the floor around her. She was hot and sweaty, breathing fast, her eyes wide in horror. The therapist could feel her heart beating faster and realized she was breathing higher in her chest, so she breathed out long and hard, very quietly deepening her breath. The adoptive mother followed her lead, and they breathed out together. They reflected later that they could feel Fiona's panic in their own bodies, and had to work hard to calm their impulses to move into action instead of staying calm and waiting.

Fiona did not see her adoptive mother as she stared across the room, nor the therapist. Fiona saw something else that no one could see apart from her. The air was hot and a strange smell drifted across the room. Fiona had wet herself, and a puddle appeared at her feet. The therapist spoke in a quiet voice, very gently saying, "It's okay, Fiona; it's okay. You're safe now." Fiona did not seem to hear at first and seemed frozen, hot with sweat and yet also clammy now, with cold urine. She began very gently to shiver and tremble. The therapist could feel her own nervous system ripple with sadness, and the hairs on her arm stood on end. She touched the adoptive mother's hand, which rested on the floor next to hers, and noticed her own tears reflected in the mother's eyes.

The therapist repeated, "You're safe now, Fiona. We will keep you safe now." Fiona gave the smallest look in the direction of her adoptive mother, and her mouth opened in what looked like fear. The therapist could feel her own breathing and the adoptive mother's breathing settle as they both noticed the fear in Fiona. Fiona watched them both closely out of the corner of her eye, and as their breathing settled, her chest was now no longer moving rapidly. Fiona's breathing settled lower in her belly.

Picking her moment, the therapist took the blanket thrown on the floor, with gentle murmurings of "It's okay, we will look after you and wrap you in the blanket." She slowly got up and gathered Fiona up in the blanket. The therapist began to sing very quietly, "My Fiona lies over the ocean, my Fiona lies over the sea, oh bring back my Fiona to me," and carried Fiona to her adoptive mother's lap. Fiona let out a small sigh and a little shiver as she settled into her adoptive mother's arms. Fiona's adoptive mother and the therapist continued their gentle singing, and Fiona was rocked and soothed. Fiona's breathing calmed a little bit more, and her skin tone developed an even warm glow rather than the blotches of stress. The therapist could feel the warmth in her own cheeks and see the flush of love in the adoptive mother's eyes as she rocked her daughter, humming to her.

Fiona was then offered a cold drink that she gulped back and let out a loud burp. Her adoptive mother gently patted her back and praised her for the burp, saying, "Better out than in, good girl." Fiona beamed and snuggled into her arms proudly. The singing continued, and some snacks (secreted in the therapist's large jacket pocket) appeared. Fiona's adoptive mother fed her little bits of banana. Fiona munched them happily and stared with sparkling eyes up at her adoptive mother, surveying her face. The therapist encouraged the adoptive mother to admire and count Fiona's freckles. Fiona giggled with delight at this. The therapist quietly explained that it would soon be time to go home, after the *Twinkle* song, adding in the explanation that "Today, as you worked so hard, we can carry you to the car in your blanket." The therapist reassured the adoptive mother with a kind smile and touch of the arm that the blanket could return to the therapy room next week. Fiona left in her adoptive mother's arms, calm and snuggled.

Later, the adoptive mother and the therapist talked on the phone and reflected on the session. They agreed it was not the session that had been planned, but an important session nonetheless. The therapist and the adoptive mother were both struck by the intensity of feeling they both felt in their bodies to Fiona's profound terror and abject pain, so that viscerally they were with her every step of the way. They were also both struck by how hard they had to work to calm their own body responses, feeling what Fiona felt, but not themselves being tipped into overwhelm, just bearing the pain.

The adoptive mother reported that it was the first time Fiona had allowed her to show her some tenderness and loving care. She went on to explain that when they got home, Fiona had allowed her to bathe her and soap her body, as she might have done if she had been her baby. The therapist and adoptive mother both knew that Fiona had been beaten in the birth family when she wet herself, and had some very scary things happen to her. It felt like the beginning had been arrived at with the wetting session, and an important message about how the stress in the past was being reenacted in the here and now. There was no doubt in this session that Fiona was physiologically activated in her trauma, and that taking time and tracking her physiology and stress response would be key going forward.

In time, Fiona learned that she did not need to take apart the Theraplay bag, and that she could trust good fun things would be inside. Most importantly, Fiona learned that she could risk being enjoyed and loved by her adoptive mother, and the glazed look of terror came over her face less often. The adoptive mother learned that regulating herself was key to helping her daughter regulate. She also learned that the trauma was held in her daughter's body, and she had to find ways to read this bodily information and support them both. It was a beginning, Fiona had a long way to go, but the trust and a sense of safety had begun.

Conclusion

In the NPP model, we use pure Theraplay with this body work emphasis as well as Theraplay in a more general way for family sessions' beginnings and endings. We also use Theraplay dimensions of structure, nurture, engagement, and challenge as a vital part of our thinking.

What Family Futures know is that traumatized children and young people need to learn to be in relationships and trust their parents, in order to feel safe in the world. However, in order to feel safe, we need to think about the body and the nervous system. Finding ways to support all the little nuances of non-verbal communication is key to getting into a right brain to right brain dance of attachment. In the end, we are all animals and communicate nervous system to nervous system. This understanding of the non-verbal nervous system communication can be taken to another level by incorporating Somatic Experiencing principles into Theraplay work with traumatized children and young people to help them heal. As Gabor Maté says in Levine (2010), in order to heal from trauma, we need to listen to the unspoken voice of our bodies, and only then can the rage and terror of trauma be survived.

The Family Futures NPP model integrates this unspoken voice of the body into all aspects of the NPP model to help the child, parent, and therapist listen and not be overwhelmed by the depth of rage and terror trauma leaves reverberating to all those in its wake. Theraplay is a unique and powerful modality taking everyday parent–child communication and teaching the parent and child this dance with slow and gentle, but powerful, steps. Peter Levine's work can help bring this dance to another level as the subtle signs of nervous system activation are tracked and calmed in NPP Theraplay practice.

This integration of Theraplay and Peter Levine's Somatic Experiencing model support not just the child but also the parent and therapist, enabling them to truly listen and both survive and recover from the unspeakable, pervasive impact of trauma.

References

Baylin, J., & Hughes, D. (2016). *The Neurobiology of Attachment-focused Therapy: Enhancing Connection and Trust in the Treatment of Children and Adolescents.* Norton.

Brown, R., & Ward, H. (2013). *Decision-Making Within a Child's Timeframe: An Overview of Current Research Evidence for Family Justice Professionals Concerning Child Development and the Impact of Maltreatment.* Working Paper 16. Childhood Wellbeing Research Centre. https://assets.publishing.service.gov.uk/government/uploads/system/uploads/attachment_data/file/200471/Decision-making_within_a_child_s_timeframe.pdf

Felitti, V. J., Anda, R. F., Nordenberg, D., Williamson, D. F., Spitz, A. M., Edwards, V., Koss, M. P., & Marks J. S. (1998). Relationship of childhood abuse and household dysfunction to many of the leading causes of death in adults. The Adverse Childhood Experiences (ACE) Study. *American Journal of Preventive Medicine 14*(4), 245–258. doi:10.1016/s0749-3797(98)00017-8

Hughes, D. A., & Baylin, J. (2012). *Brain-Based Parenting: The Neuroscience of Caregiving for Healthy Attachment.* Norton.

Levine, P. (1997). *Waking the Tiger: Healing Trauma: The Innate Capacity to Transform Overwhelming Experiences.* North Atlantic Books.

Levine, P. (2010) *In an Unspoken Voice: How the Body Releases Trauma and Restores Goodness.* North Atlantic Books.

Levine, P., & Kline, M. (2007). *Trauma Through a Child's Eyes: Awakening the Ordinary Miracle of Healing.* North Atlantic Books.

McCullough, E., & Mathura, A. (2019). A comparison between a Neuro-Physiological Psychotherapy (NPP) treatment group and a control group for children adopted from care: Support for a neurodevelopmental informed approach to therapeutic intervention with maltreated children. *Child Abuse & Neglect 97,* 104128. https://doi.org/10.1016/j.chiabu.2019.104128

McCullough, E., Gordon-Jones, S., Last, A., Vaughan, J., & Burnell, A. (2016). An evaluation of Neuro-Physiological Psychotherapy: An integrative therapeutic approach to working with adopted children who have experienced early life trauma. *Clinical Child Psychology and Psychiatry 21*(4), 582–602. doi:10.1177/135910451663522

van der Kolk, B. A. (2009). Developmental trauma disorder: Towards a rational diagnosis for children with complex trauma histories. *Praxis der Kinderpsychologie und Kinderpsychiatrie 58*(8), 572–586. doi:10.13109/prkk.2009.58.8.572

Vaughan, J., McCullough, E., & Burnell, A. (2016). Neuro-Physiological Psychotherapy (NPP): The development and application of an integrative, wrap-around service and treatment programme for maltreated children placed in adoptive and foster care placements. *Clinical Child Psychology and Psychiatry 21*(4), 569–581. doi:10.1177/1359104516635222

Chapter 13

Building Security In and Out of the Tray to Help Children and Families Heal

COMBINING THERAPLAY AND SANDTRAY THERAPY

Mandy Jones-Fischer and Marshall N. Lyles

Introduction

This chapter explores the benefits of combining Sandtray Therapy and Theraplay for traumatized children. Studies indicate that Theraplay treatment alone can reduce both internalizing and externalizing symptoms of children struggling with emotional and/or behavioral issues (Salo *et al.* 2020). Similarly, it has been shown to reduce anxiety in both mothers and children (Smithee *et al.* 2021). Anecdotally, practitioners around the globe have seen the benefits of using Theraplay treatment with children who have survived trauma. However, a major shortcoming of Theraplay as a treatment modality for children (and parents) who have survived trauma is that it does not allow for explicit trauma processing. For most, the opportunity for non-verbal processing of traumatically stored memories is essential for integrating trauma and optimal healing. Acknowledging that Sandtray is a treatment modality that offers such opportunities for trauma processing, this chapter presents how to combine Sandtray with Theraplay when working with traumatized children. We will begin with the theoretical underpinnings of both treatment modalities, highlighting the sense of safety that comes from containment. Next, we illustrate how to craft a session by bookending with Theraplay using Sandtray for trauma processing from an expressive part of the brain. Lastly, applying Theraplay and Sandtray in treating traumatized children will be contextualized in a case study.

Sandtray Therapy

Since its introduction to the mental health field almost 100 years ago by Margaret Lowenfeld (1993), Sandtray Therapy has become a well-established modality within the greater field of expressive arts and creative therapies (Homeyer & Sweeney 2005). Purposely designed to be transtheoretical (Lowenfeld 1993), it offers a canvas for different clinical theories and approaches to make use of according to their various theoretical constructs. Featuring the use of a tray holding sand (or a suitable substitute where sand is not an option), water, and miniature figures (Homeyer & Sweeney 2017), Sandtray Therapy's materials make for a sensory-rich and symbolic exploration of the inner world.

The processes inherent to Sandtray Therapy begin by inviting a client into a relationship with the materials. Interacting with the sand by pushing, raking, burying, adding water, etc., all occurring within a boundaried space, allows for the body to experiment with making safe contact with self (McCarthy 2006). The client has the opportunity to externalize often-confusing parts of self into this contained space through the safe distance offered by the metaphorical representations of sand, water, and miniatures (Gil 2014; Gomez 2012). This is accomplished as clients are invited to create a world in the sand; the therapist, as a strong witness, holds space during that creation process; and co-constructed meanings are made during the processing of the client-created world (Gallerani & Dybicz 2011).

Homeyer and Sweeney (2017) define Sandtray Therapy as a type of expressive therapy that uncovers the issues within the self or with another using a non-verbal method of communication. The focus on safety, communication (largely non-verbal), and active work has been shown to make Sandtray Therapy an effective offering for those working through trauma (Kosanke 2013), including the trauma of unresolved attachment wounds (Green, Myrick, & Crenshaw 2013). However, as Homeyer and Sweeney's definition asserts, effective Sandtray Therapy needs to be conducted by someone who is well trained in the approach.

Early in the development of Sandtray Therapy, Lowenfeld realized that the worlds created in the sand gave therapists access to a client's thought life (Urwin & Hood-Williams 2014). This provides the client and therapist with a method for taking inventory of a lifetime of stored assumptions about self and the world. Because of the many elements that awaken the right brain hemisphere, Sandtray Therapy can tap into preverbal and even dissociatively held pockets of information (Badenoch 2008). It even offers integrative opportunities as the lower and upper regions of the brain, and left and right hemispheres find their way to a rhythm of cooperative communication (Kestly 2014), making meaning of inner experience (Rogers, Luke, & Darkis 2020).

The sandtray offers a place where all streams of attachment can manifest and become understood because it integrates unconscious experience and conscious awareness (Badenoch 2017). By providing access to sensory, emotional, and cognitive parts of self (Rae 2013), memory networks can come safely online, even if the material remains metaphor-based throughout processing (Homeyer & Lyles 2022).

Sandtray Therapy has been shown to be effective with multiple issues and populations, including the treatment of trauma (Lyles 2021), use with adoptive families (Lyles & Homeyer 2015), application to orphans following a natural disaster in the cross-cultural environment (Jeppsen 2012), use with attachment-wounded refugee children for assessment and treatment (Stauffer 2008), and adolescents living with attachment struggles (Green *et al.* 2013).

Theraplay and Sandtray Therapy

Theraplay was initially conceptualized as an approach to support children on the autism spectrum who were struggling with connection and social skills (DesLauriers & Carlson 1969). As the concepts began to be utilized by Ann Jernberg in the Head Start program, the modality as we know it today began to take shape. Children who received individualized attunement and co-regulating experiences created stronger relationships that led to improvements in their overall functioning (Jernberg 1979). As parents in Theraplay treatment today gain the skills to better understand what underlies their child's behaviors (i.e., mentalization), they are better equipped to respond in an attuned manner, thus allowing for physical and emotional containment of the child's needs (Fonagy *et al.* 1991).

Both Theraplay and Sandtray Therapy have the ability to provide containment. Within Theraplay, the parent plays the role of containing the child. They do this through structure, engagement, nurture, and challenge that meet the child where they are. The practitioner sets up a weekly course of play-based treatment that allows the parent to learn how to identify the underlying need that is leading to the problematic behavior. The practitioner and parent then use their vitality affect to create a co-regulated state within the therapy room. The body's movements allow the child's polyvagal system to experience a state of regulation and felt safety, thus leading to a sense of containment. When the parent becomes skilled at providing this co-regulation and reinstating felt safety on a regular basis, the child begins to rely on the parent to provide containment, even if the parent is unaware of what ultimately caused the child's dysregulation. The ebb and flow of interaction between parent and child allow for continual containment when safety is threatened. Once this has been established, the parent and child are in a position for the child to begin processing. Trauma processing has the potential to create dysregulation as the child experiences intense emotions and flooding of memories as they process whatever they endured. Because of Theraplay, the parent is then in a position to respond to the dysregulation.

The following highlights the opportunities inherent in attachment and trauma healing when following a treatment plan that features both Theraplay and Sandtray Therapy.

CASE ILLUSTRATION

Charlotte was referred to me (MJ) because of my work as a post-adoption therapist. Her parents had seen me present at a local conference for adoptive parents and knew their child would benefit from therapeutic support with a specialty in adoption. They had tried other types of therapy. They had been to a behavioral specialist and engaged in non-directive play therapy for several years. While Charlotte typically connected easily with her therapists (she did have a deep desire to please), her parents were discouraged by the lack of progress.

Charlotte was eight years old when I first met her. Her parents wanted help with her tantrums, anxiety, and processing her adoption story. Charlotte was adopted at the age of two-and-a-half from Russia. Charlotte's adoptive parents, Kate and Chris, had three biological children who were now in their teens. Kate and Chris knew there was a lot for Charlotte to process related to the trauma that had led to her adoption.

As with all of the families I serve, I began by conducting a Marschak Interaction Method (MIM) assessment. During the course of the MIM, what the parents described as "controlling" behaviors were demonstrated. For example, Charlotte would take the next envelope before her adoptive parents had instructed her to do so, and tried her best to direct each of the activities. Her parents displayed a lack of structure in that many of their directives were given as questions rather than statements, and they provided few physical boundaries. The family was able to easily engage, appeared comfortable with touch, and were generally at ease in each other's presence. There was significant eye contact and plenty of laughter. Charlotte was a "mover and a shaker," meaning that sitting still for more than a moment or two was hard for her. She fidgeted with her hands, rolled across the floor, bounced around the room, and experienced a general sense of dysregulation. The parents spoke about this during the parent feedback session as distracting and contributing to their frustration with her not listening.

The parents were receptive during the parent feedback session. Kate expressed relief that someone had finally seen her child's regulation challenges and identified Charlotte's sensory needs. They were highly affectionate and supportive of one another, including touching and hand holding. They appeared on the same page with many of their parenting skills. They wanted their child to be provided with many choices. Both exuded much praise for their daughter's accomplishments. Their desire to parent in a cohesive manner was evident in the parent work. Both participated in the parent demonstration session and easily nurtured one another in order to have the experience of being cared for. It was my recommendation that we start by focusing on structure and nurture in the Theraplay sessions to help Charlotte establish security with her parents. She had experienced so little safety during her early years, first with her birth family, and then during her time in the orphanage. Additionally, due to Charlotte's sensory needs, she required a great deal of containment. She needed physical touch and plenty of boundaries to further increase her sense of felt safety.

Our Theraplay sessions progressed beautifully. Charlotte easily engaged with both parents. The parents became more comfortable with implementing a structure, particularly during their morning and bedtime routines. Charlotte's tantrums decreased and her resistance toward Chris, particularly at bedtime, lessened substantially. The parents reported a lightness in Charlotte that was not previously present. She easily snuggled into them on the couch for movies and became less distractible at school. Of note is that during our Theraplay play sessions, the typical resistance phase of treatment was minimal. Charlotte was consistently eager to please me, engage, and go along with each session exactly as I had planned it out. Her dysregulation was present in small ways, but provided that I front-loaded the session with plenty of proprioceptive and vestibular input, Charlotte easily remained within her "window of tolerance" (Siegel 2012).

After approximately eight months, it became clear that the family relationship had greatly improved. As a result, I raised the question of whether to terminate treatment or move onto something that would offer to process the stored trauma. I suggested sandtray to the family as a place for Charlotte to process her adoption story and anxiety.

We prepared Charlotte for the transition to sandtray, noting that some parts of our sessions would remain the same, and that she would spend time playing only with me. I presented this information two weeks before transitioning to the sandtray work. The routine of our sessions transitioned to the following:

1. Structure entrance (generally leap frog to pillows)

2. Check-in/lotion

3. Slippery slip

4. A structured, downregulating activity such as hand stack or parent and child decorating one another

5. Parent leaves the room or sandtray with just Charlotte and myself

6. Sandtray is covered with a cloth and parent returns to the room

7. Blanket swing

8. Burrito

9. Feeding.

I was unsure what to expect as to the initial themes in the sandtray. I prompted Charlotte to "create a world in the sand." She generally created scenes with much disarray and chaos. The worlds she created were filled with lots of people, numerous buildings, and many animals. They appeared to be going in different directions without much of a central theme, although she was always present in the world, and she always knew where her family members were. Her mother and one brother, in particular, were central to her trays. In the beginning, she experienced difficulty creating narratives for the world she had created. Over time, the trays became more organized, and she was able to tell coherent, age-appropriate stories filled with direction and far fewer miniatures. Her narratives ebbed and flowed as to how to present her family in the tray. Often her narratives took on a fantastical nature, usually with a character being "saved." That character was never identified as herself, but it seemed clear that she was processing the experience of being removed from a negative experience and placed into a healthier, more positive one. While the fantastical nature of the stories was not true to her lived experience, the tray allowed her a place to process how she was integrating what had happened to her. The trays were often filled with various contrasting emotions, which seemed indicative of her adoption story.

By following the Theraplay treatment plan, Charlotte's inner world became more regulated, and her sense of accessing connected relationships grew. This enabled her to be prepared to move into the non-verbal and externalized trauma processing that Sandtray Therapy offers. When integrated by a clinician grounded in both approaches,

Theraplay and Sandtray Therapy can empower a client by creating increased attachment security and mastery over the lived experience of trauma.

References

Badenoch, B. (2008). *Being a Brain-Wise Therapist: A Practical Guide to Interpersonal Neurobiology* (Norton Series on Interpersonal Neurobiology). W.W. Norton & Co.

Badenoch, B. (2017). *The Heart of Trauma: Healing the Embodied Brain in the Context of Relationships* (Norton Series on Interpersonal Neurobiology). W.W. Norton & Co.

DesLauriers, A.M., & Carlson, C. F. (1969). *Your Child is Asleep: Early Infantile Autism: Etiology, Treatment, and Parental Influences.* Dorsey Press.

Fonagy, P., Steel, M., Steele, H., Moran, G. S., & Higgitt, A. C. (1991). The capacity for understanding mental states: The reflective self in parent and child and its significance for security of attachment. *Infant Mental Health Journal 12*(3), 201–218. doi:10.1111/j.1467-8624.1991. tb01578.x

Gallerani, T., & Dybicz, P. (2011). Postmodern sandplay: An introduction for play therapists. *International Journal of Play Therapy 20*(3), 165–177. https://doi.org/10.1037/a0023440

Gil, E. (2014). The Creative Use of Metaphor in Play and Art Therapy with Attachment Problems. In C. A. Malchiodi & D. A. Crenshaw (Eds), *Creative Arts and Play Therapy for Attachment Problems* (pp.159–177). Guilford Press.

Gomez, A. M. (2012). *EMDR Therapy and Adjunct Approaches with Children: Complex Trauma, Attachment, and Dissociation.* Springer Publishing Company.

Green, E. J., Myrick, A. C., & Crenshaw, D. A. (2013). Toward secure attachment in adolescent relational development: Advancements from sandplay and expressive play-based interventions. *International Journal of Play Therapy 22*(2), 90–102. https://doi.org/10.1037/a0032323

Homeyer, L. E., & Lyles, M. N. (2022). *Advanced Sandtray Therapy: Digging Deeper into Clinical Practice.* Routledge.

Homeyer, L. E., & Sweeney, D. S. (2005). Sandtray Therapy. In C. A. Malchiodi (Ed.), *Expressive Therapies* (pp.162–182). Guilford Press.

Homeyer, L. E., & Sweeney, D. S. (2017). *Sandtray Therapy: A Practical Manual* (3rd edn). Routledge [Kindle edition].

Jeppsen, M. L. (2012). *Sand Tray Therapy: Utilizing Indigenous Objects with Traumatized Haitian Orphans.* Regent University.

Jernberg, A. M. (1979). *Theraplay: A New Treatment Using Structured Play for Problem Children and Their Families.* Wiley & Sons.

Kestly, T. A. (2014). *The Interpersonal Neurobiology of Play: Brain-Building Interventions for Emotional Well-Being.* W.W. Norton & Co.

Kosanke, G. C. (2013). The Use of Sandtray Approaches in Psycho-Therapeutic Work with Adult Trauma Survivors: A Thematic Analysis. Unpublished Doctoral dissertation, Auckland University of Technology.

Lowenfeld, M. (1993). *Understanding Children's Sandplay: Lowenfeld's World Technique.* Sussex Academic Press.

Lyles, M. (2021). Room for Everyone: Family-based Play Therapy in the Sandtray. In A. Beckley-Forest & A. Monaco (Eds), *EMDR with Children in the Play Therapy Room: An Integrated Approach* (pp.75–108). Springer.

Lyles, M., & Homeyer, L. E. (2015). The use of sandtray therapy with adoptive families. *Adoption Quarterly 18*(1), 67–80. https://doi.org/10.1080/10926755.2014.945704

McCarthy, D. (2006). Sandplay Therapy and the Body in Trauma Recovery. In L. Carey (Ed.), *Expressive and Creative Arts Methods for Trauma Survivors* (pp.165–180). Jessica Kingsley Publishers.

Rae, R. (2013). *Sandtray: Playing to Heal, Recover, and Grow*. Rowman & Littlefield.

Rogers, J. L., Luke, M., & Darkis, J. T. (2020). Meet me in the sand: Stories and self-expression in sand tray work with older adults. *Journal of Creativity in Mental Health 16*(2), 1–13. doi:10.1080/15401383.2020.1734513

Salo, S., Flykt, M., Mäkelä, J., Lassenius-Panula, L., Korja, R., Lindaman, S., & Punamäki, R. (2020). The impact of Theraplay® therapy on parent–child interaction and child psychiatric symptoms: A pilot study. *International Journal of Play 9*(3), 331–352. https://doi:10.1080/21594937.2020.1806500

Siegel, D. J. (2012). *The Developing Mind: How Relationships and the Brain Interact to Shape Who We Are*. Guilford Press.

Smithee, L. C., Krizova, K., Guest, J. D., & Pease, J. D. (2021). Theraplay as a family treatment for mother anxiety and child anxiety. *International Journal of Play Therapy 30*(3), 206–218. https://doi.org/10.1037/pla0000153

Stauffer, S. (2008). Trauma and disorganized attachment in refugee children: Integrating theories and exploring treatment options. *Refugee Survey Quarterly 27*(4), 150–163. https://doi.org/10.1093/rsq/hdn057

Urwin, C., & Hood-Williams, J. (2014). *Child Psychotherapy, War and the Normal Child: Selected Papers of Margaret Lowenfeld*. Sussex Academic Press.

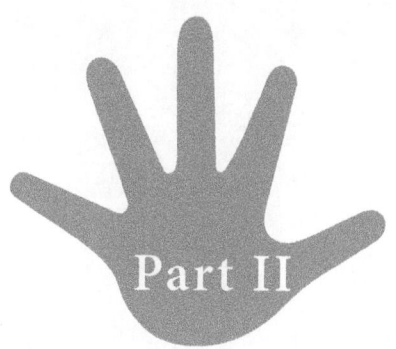

Part II

Specific Populations, Ages, and Settings

Chapter 14

Music in Theraplay for Children with Autism

Angela Siu and King-Chi Yau

Introduction

As described in the Fifth edition of the *Diagnostic and Statistical Manual of Mental Disorders* (DSM-V) (APA 2013), autism spectrum disorders (ASDs) denote a group of neurodevelopmental disorders characterized by impaired social interaction, self-regulatory issues, limited interests, and rigid behaviors. Children with ASD have difficulties in using and interpreting non-verbal social behaviors such as interpreting others' facial expressions and gestures and demonstrating reduced frequency in eye-to-eye gaze. These children also demonstrate repetitive patterns of behaviors such as clapping hands, twisting fingers, and rocking the body. The worldwide prevalence of autism is reported to be 1–3 percent (Maenner *et al.* 2020; Ofner *et al.* 2018). Dimian, Symons, and Wolff (2021) examined the effects of delay of early intensive behavioral intervention on outcomes for children diagnosed with ASD aged three to five years old. They revealed that an increase in average months of delay to intervention was correlated with decreased probability of placement in general education, increased need for special education and related services, and lowered math achievement scores. They suggested that children with ASD receiving treatment at early years would have better educational outcomes than their counterparts. In addition, delay to treatment for children with ASD also influences their families and caregivers. Parents of children with ASD are often accused of being "bad parents" due to their children's frequent behavioral problems caused by their impairments in social interaction and communication, increasing parental stress and causing entrenched cycles of psychological distress for parents (Elder *et al.* 2017; Hudson, Dallos, & McKenzie 2017). Early intervention is indispensable for both individual children with ASD and their parents, by nurturing children's proximal development and sustaining the harmony of families.

Music and ASD

Music is a way of relating, expressing communicating, learning, and being in a relationship (Small 1998). Studies have identified the relationships between music training and structural differences in the brain (Gaser & Schlaug 2003; Habibi *et al.* 2018), indicating that music is influencing our body. On a biological level, Kreutz (2014) and Keeler *et al.* (2015) show that when people sing together, the social bonding hormone oxytocin is released in a higher quantity. Haslbeck *et al.* (2020) also found evidence of the effects of music on higher brain connectivity underlying the socio-emotional functioning of young children. Music-making has an actual physiological effect on our bodies, enhancing social connectedness. On a psychological level, specific songs shared by an adult and a child serve as powerful and intimate symbolic reminders of the adult and their child's shared love and relationship. Music can be used for children to learn to cope with feelings and manage their own behaviors. We can use music to calm, energize, relieve boredom, focus, or redirect the attention. Adults can sing, hold, or even dance with a child, and join with the rhythm of their mood. We can slowly modulate or change the rhythm in order to help the child change mood, calm, or energize the body, co-regulate with feelings, and redirect attention. Corbeil, Trehub, and Peretz (2016) suggest that music can help to increase children's ability to regulate their feelings. Singing (exaggerated pitches and repeated phrases) could help them maintain a calm state for a longer time than control groups (directed speech but no singing).

Through music, ASD children can become better communicators. Music helps to enhance their social interactions. The shifting combinations of pulse, rhythm, melody, timbres, and expression (e.g., tempo and dynamics) in music provided communication venues as social interactions are created through vocalizing, facial expressions, gestures, and movements. A meta-analysis of a Cochrane Review found evidence of music intervention enhancing social interaction, verbal communication, socio-emotional reciprocity, and behavior of children with ASD (Geretsegger *et al.* 2014).

Joint attention occurs when a child notices something in the environment and points to that object, thereby engaging others in what has caught their attention. The reward for such action is the interaction with the caregiver as they both attend to the object that is of interest to them (Jones & Carr 2004). Children with ASD usually lack joint attention, and joint attention practice is a key to the intervention for ASD, helping the children in engage with others. Music helps children with ASD to facilitate communication without the need for verbal interactions. Some children initiate eye contact as they laugh and smile while making music with their caregivers. They would lean forward, nod, and reach out for preferred objects during musical activities (Corke 2002). In fact, interaction with these children through music (move, sing, listen, play instruments) provides numerous ways to develop the joint attention necessary for children to engage with others. Kern, Graham, and Aldridge (2006) investigated the impact of music on children's joint attention. Results showed that children were attracted to music instruments; however, such activity did not increase children's communication. On the other hand, when personal songs were sung to children by their teachers, there was positive interaction. The role of adults is to provide children the opportunities to practice social skills in a nurturing environment. In addition, there was evidence showing the role of motifs in music in enhancing a child's joint attention in a single case study (Yau & Fachner 2019). Moreover, music serves as an "auditory frame of reference for movement" (Ockelford 2000, p.204). Engagement through music has the potential to bridge the gap between children with ASD and their significant others. It is well noted that children with ASD enjoy interactions with others through and with music (Wan *et al.* 2010).

"Affect attunement" refers to the sharing of internal states, a phenomenon when infants synchronize their inner state with the caregiver, which enables a mutual and intersubjective sharing of feeling without the use of language (Raglio, Traficante, & Oasi 2011). The matching of social dialogues in a caregiver–infant interaction is essential for attunement, and this kind of matching is more than the direct imitation of sound, gestures, or facial expressions; it is the integration of cross-modal qualities such as intensity of voice, movement, and timespan of interaction. Based on the observation of early dyadic interaction between mothers and infants, Stern ([1985] 2018) analyzed the phenomena of affect attunement in terms of intensity, timing, and shape, and further divided those dimensions into six categories of matching: (a) absolute intensity (dynamic, level of intensity); (b) intensity contour (adjustment of intensity over time); (c) temporal beat (tempo changes in time); (d) rhythm (pattern of pulsation); (e) duration; and (f) shape (feature in time and space). Music attunement, a concept that develops from affect attunement, refers to the process of musical communication in a practitioner–client relationship, allowing for moments of synchronization that facilitate the client's sensory integration and affect regulation. This process creates a shared narrative and musical agenda for improvisation in the clinical session between practitioner and client child (Kim, Wigram, & Gold 2009; Mössler *et al.* 2020).

Theraplay and ASD

The goal of Theraplay is to model the attachment by establishing an empathic and attuned relationship between parent and practitioner, which serves as a model for the relationship between caregiver and child (Booth & Jernberg 2010). Theraplay seeks to work directly with the caregiver–child dyad in order to change the child's internal working model (IWM) and improve the overall attachment relationship between caregiver and child. The healthy attachment, as framed by Theraplay, includes several dimensions, namely, structure, engagement, nurture, and challenge (Booth & Jernberg 2010), as well as playfulness (Mäkelä & Hart 2011). *Structure* activities allow the child to practice complying with rules and limitations from adults. *Engagement* refers to the sharing of joyful in-the-moment experiences during which the adult is deeply attuned to the child's emotions and state of alertness. *Nurture* involves the adult's caring of the child's basic needs, and calming the child's distress and anxiety. *Challenge* refers to the child's feelings of mastery and motivation to grow and learn. All these dimensions occur in a context of playfulness and joy. The aspects of Theraplay that are appropriate for caregivers of children who have ASD include joint attention, attunement, regulation, synchrony, communication, parental insight, and processing of sensory information (Booth & Jernberg 2010). Hiles Howard *et al.* (2018) reported that there was significant improvement for ASD children on social interaction after using Theraplay.

Integration of music and other play approaches to work with children

An "integrative approach" is the idea of combining aspects of different schools of thought for the wellbeing of a person. This term is often used in psychotherapy to describe the way some practitioners perform their work. A review in the literature indicated that there is effective integration of music and other play approaches in work with children. A promising effect of the use of music and rhythm in Theraplay for children with ASD has been suggested previously (Siu 2021). During a session, children were asked to listen and respond to the music (musical matching) that created a context for two-way communication. Such interaction enhanced children's responsiveness to others in a natural setting, and in turn facilitated their social competence in developing connections. Lense and Camarata (2020) proposed that musical engagement experiences provided children with ASD with essential and active ingredients for treating ASD, including "(1) predictability; (2) reinforcement; (3) emotional regulation; (4) shared attention and (5) social play context" (2020, p.2), in which they comprise the PRESS-Play framework. The use of music in PRESS-Play creates a context for social engagement not only for children with ASD, but also their interaction partners, facilitating joint engagement. It also serves as an avenue for children to deliver social and linguistic information, scaffolding their social skills.

The Musical Contour Regulation Facilitation (MCRF) model was designed with the intention that the contour and temporal structure of a music therapy session alternate between high- and low-arousal states in a way that theoretically mirrors the changing flow of the caregiver–infant interaction. Based on the principles of MCRF, Williams (2018) has conducted studies using different play activities with musical elements to immerse children in a dynamic musical experience. The children receive stimulation through a relaxed or arousing rhythm or beat, then respond with a series of coordinated gestures involving sensory motor skills, bodily movement, and auditory and self-regulatory functioning; this is a process of sensorimotor synchronization.

There are seven components within the 30-minute session, beginning with neutral arousal (e.g., a welcome song), then fluctuating between low and high arousal facilitated by musical characteristics, ending the session with neutral arousal (such as a goodbye song or listening to soothing music). Examples of high-arousal activities include using shakers and bells to tap different parts of the body and move. Examples of low-arousal activities include soothing and soft music using the Ocean Drum®.

How music can be incorporated into Theraplay

Theraplay is an attachment-focused model that helps caregivers to understand and relate to their child. Based on a sequence of play activities that are rooted in neuroscience, it offers a fun and playful way for caregivers and children to connect. Music is perfectly designed for use to connect and communicate with children, especially those who are preverbal, or who have language and communication difficulties. Music can convey emotion and increase attention without using language, to help connect with and focus young children.

Practitioners can increase opportunities to make connection with children, and to enhance flexibility and variation in engaging children through the use of songs or musical instruments. Especially since children with ASD are reluctant or less sensitive to human interaction, musical elements (through singing or percussion instruments) may provide an additional means to connect with the children. In music, we talk about "move," "sing," "listen," and "play (instruments)." These strategies can be applied in Theraplay when working with caregiver and child dyads. Using movement can enhance engagement through action songs, facing each other singing and doing action, holding hands and singing the song, or moving to beat. The last musical phrase or word can be followed by something ticklish or silly. While using different elements (such as fast/slow, high/low, strong/weak, etc.) to "sing" a song, activities relating to structure can be further enhanced or modified for variety. Creating a personal song and singing to the child to "listen," or listening to what the child is singing can be something nurturing. "Playing" percussion instruments (such as a musical mat or piano mat) or using tuned and un-tuned music devices encourages cooperation. Producing music as a group is a good way to have fun together.

Below is a discussion on how elements of music can be integrated into Theraplay. Application of elements of music for working with children who have social impairment is emphasized.

Welcome

Song is an excellent way to signal the beginning of a session. When we hear music, it can sound and feel as if it is actually inside our heads and bodies. This helps build the bonding feeling with whom we want to share musical experiences. Examples of such songs include good morning songs or hello songs that are commonly used in kindergarten and preschool. Specific songs that the adult and child share serve as powerful and intimate symbolic reminders of the shared love and relationship (Keeler *et al.* 2015). In addition, incorporating the child's name into the lyrics (e.g., "Good morning to Peter") intensifies the sense of connectedness.

Check-up

The purpose of check-up is to connect with the child and show them that we are aware of how special they are. Listening is a powerful way to bond as well as to help a child build self-esteem.

The practitioner can watch a child sing a song or play an instrument. On a superficial level, the practitioner can simply name the song or instrument chosen by the child—for example, "You chose this big drum." On a deeper level, the practitioner might make comments on the process of what the child is doing—for example, "I noticed that you played a very loud sound followed by a softer section." In addition, the practitioner can pay attention to the tone of voice while commenting (e.g., the practitioner speaking relatively softly while reflecting on the softer section of the child's music), aiming to attune to the child's musical expression as closely as possible.

Activities addressing the session goal(s)

Structure: the adult takes the lead in the session and defines all rules and boundaries in order to promote feelings of emotional safety and predictability. It fosters the development of self-regulation in the child. Activities are alternated between active and quiet ones, thus providing opportunities for modulation of movement and energy.

The practitioner and child are watching, learning, and taking cues from each other. They are learning ways to have fun together while respecting the needs of all.

Table 14.1: Music in structure

Traditional Theraplay structure activities	Theraplay in a musical way
Hand clapping	• Use of musical instruments (such as small drums, rhythm sticks, wood blocks, or ocean drums) to imitate sounds
Hand stacking	• Sleigh bells around the arm, while doing the hand stack
Bean bag drop	• Adult holds the (buffalo) drum and child uses the mallet to play the drum
Move and freeze	• Children listen to the drum and move through the place when the drum tells them to move and freeze. Rhythmic patterns can be created for the children to model through actions: walk—run—hop—skip
Imitate sounds/match sounds	• Use instruments to match expressions of sounds— dynamics (loud and soft); drumming—allow children to use "big and strong" arm motions to release their anger, and eventually use quieter ways such as using palms to soothe the drum skin, returning their bodies to a calmer pace
Peanut butter and jelly	• Create a sound (possibly with the themes on animals, transportation, feelings, etc.) and respond in a musical way with voice
Matching sound/ matching pacing	• Use ocean drum, bongo drum, buffalo drum, sound tubes, wind gong

Engagement: the adult focuses on the child in a personal manner so the child knows they are seen and heard in the moment. There is shared joy, responsive companionship, and strong emotional connection between the adult and child. Music encourages emotional connections between those engaged in a musical activity.

Table 14.2: Music in engagement

Traditional Theraplay engagement activities	Theraplay in a musical way
Familiar action songs or rhymes	• Sing a song together a song—pause just before the last line of the song and wait for the child to fill in
Beep honk	• Playing xylophone on hand: touch fingers—using mallet on xylophone (doing on hand)—child plays, adult sings
Partner songs	• Hand clapping and partner dance encourage children to make eye contact, work cooperatively
Blow me over	• Child plays a recorder (no song is required, just a single note), creating a "sound wave" blowing the adult over
Creating a special handshake	• This is for an older child. Create a cool and special musical pattern together (e.g., bossa nova) on a drum, and play it together

Nurture: parent and child take part in soothing, calming activities that are believed to foster feelings of warmth, safety, and comfort. Soothing touch is a fundamental part of this dimension, and it can help a child develop an inner knowledge of being loveable, valued and special.

Lullabies are great examples of assisting children in modulating to a slower, more relaxed rhythm. Deep breathe to a slow, steady beat. Use your own sound as the metronome to maintain slow pace. Deep breathing provides a physiological benefit in helping you to feel calm (Russo, Santarelli, & O'Rourke 2017). Breathe in, breathe out, sing slowly. Examples of songs include: *Twinkle Twinkle Little Star*, *Frère Jacques*, and *Hush Little Baby*. In addition, you can consider making use of instruments that can create soothing sounds such as ocean drums and rain sticks to accompany the songs. We connect with the child through rhythms, melodies, volume, and tempo. We are showing that we hear them and that they are not alone. Making music together is an incredibly intimate experience. Modification includes gradually modulating to a different tempo, volume, etc.

Challenge: the child is helped to complete a fun but challenging task, or take a mild, age-appropriate risk in order to enhance feelings of self-confidence and competence. Activities are performed in an environment that is positive, fun, optimistic, and non-achievement-oriented.

In music, there is a saying: "Play what you know and practice what you don't know." Practitioners can encourage children to try out new things (instruments) and make music together.

The experience of playing instruments together motivates them to remain focused on a current activity. Successful experiences in using musical instruments help children acquire a sense of accomplishment. Easy, simple instruments include: hand drum, tambourine, jingle bells, egg shakers, wood block, and rhythm sticks. Harder ones include: finger cymbals, claves, and triangles. Non-pitched percussion instruments enable children to tap the beat in response to songs and singing. This leads to active participation in making music. It is especially good for children with ASD, as they may not be able to sing or may have limited verbal abilities.

Another musical activity in the challenge domain to consider is "being a conductor." The child can be a conductor and direct the adult to play various instruments such as hand drum, shakers, and triangles in the sequence the child prefers. Another version is to exchange roles and let the child be the musician instead, following the adult's conducting. Both can help the child to build up a higher sense of competence.

Feeding: cradle the child in your arms while gently rocking and humming a lullaby song.

Closing: ending can be "musical" through tailor-made rhymes or song or melody that signal the closing of a session. Example: goodbye songs, action songs, rapping to finish.

 ## CASE ILLUSTRATION
BACKGROUND
This illustrates how music and its elements can be incorporated into Theraplay to facilitate a child's social-emotional development as well as the interaction with family members. William, a three-year-old boy, was described as almost totally non-communicative and diagnosed with ASD. He demonstrated deficits in social behavior, and needed skills to connect with others, especially with increasing imitation skills and creating meaningful relationships. William's parents had been supportive and patient in providing a nurturing environment for William to develop structure for his daily routine and to relate to others. They sought therapeutic assistance hoping to enhance development associated with William's socializing with others.

William was extremely withdrawn and tense. He had no speech and was very anxious about staying in unfamiliar environments. He was, however, able to calm down with the presence of his mother. William had great difficulty in engaging with others. He was the elder child with one younger sibling, which left his parents feeling overwhelmed with his care, and consequently lead to much stress. The practitioner began sessions by sitting quietly on the floor with William in his mother's arms. The practitioner sang a lullaby softly, trying to connect with the child.

PROCESS

Early stage

William initially presented as a very distant and fearful child. Despite that, he was willing to go into the area for Theraplay. The physical setting was quiet and filled with different sizes of cushions, a few soft balls, and a small drum. For the first few sessions, William explored the balls and the drum. Sometimes the practitioner blew bubbles to get William's attention and to make him aware of the practitioner's presence. William kept his distance from the practitioner and simply ignored her. The practitioner called his name, but William didn't respond or make any eye contact. Slowly, over time, William began to raise his head in response to the practitioner calling his name, as he tried to make a connection. Gradually, William accepted the practitioner's presence and the sound of her voice. There was occasional eye contact. It was during this moment that the practitioner initiated further connection by calling William's name and rolling a ball towards him. Initially, he did not roll the ball back, but after several trials in different sessions, William began to pick up the ball and roll it back, though not in the practitioner's direction. That was the start of a connection between William and the practitioner. Later on, the practitioner called William's name and rolled the ball towards him. The rolling of the ball was later accompanied by singing out William's name. He responded back by "singing" his name with some sounds.

Middle stage

As the Theraplay sessions moved on, William increasingly spent time in close connection with the practitioner, initiating both eye and physical contact. William's social interaction increased. He reacted specifically with rhythm and other activities that included musical elements. For example, in singing songs together, William could sing along with some clapping (with the practitioner holding his hands to start with). He could also play the beat by clapping or tapping to accompany songs. He was also engaged in "Sound body part," as if singing a song. He could also use his voice (as an instrument) to match expressions of sounds (e.g., loud and soft).

Knowing that William was unable to make appropriate contact, the practitioner would model for William socially acceptable forms of making physical connection by singing action songs like *Row the Boat*, holding hands and moving to the rhythm. The following are a number of the musical activities incorporated into the Theraplay sessions during the middle phase of therapy:

Row the Boat: singing with different sounds by matching the mood (holding hands). William and the practitioner would jump or sit down when they heard a certain sound in the song. They would jump up and down on the cushions, walking tiptoe together, crawling when the practitioner used a low voice.

Weather report: the practitioner would use different sounds to call out 'blue sky', 'cloudy sky', 'rain', singing the song in a high/low voice, or fast/slow. Body parts could be used as a xylophone, to play out songs.

Body percussion: tapping the drum according to William's tempo...then the practitioner's tempo doubling William's tempo. William began to speed up his beat almost immediately, and though he did not match the beat, it showed that William responded with imitation. When we listen to a child playing their xylophone, we are showing we care, we are showing them that they are important and that their expressions matter.

Musical mat: William and the practitioner played out a melody together.

When it came to music time, the practitioner would ask William to sit in a relaxed manner, and to pick a song that he liked that the practitioner would then sing to him.

Towards the end
Echo songs: the practitioner would sing the first line of the song and then point to themself; they would then point to William and ask him to sing, encouraging him to echo the practitioner.

Freeze dance: William responded enthusiastically to a child when he hit a drum.

The practitioner made music together with William, integrating his sounds as well as calling his name, helping him build a sense of who he is as a unique individual and as a member of a family. Body percussion worked smoothly. Music helped William "engage" and improves his "focus," citing his undistracted attention to the drum during the musical Theraplay.

William responded to the steady beat. He loved moving a scarf according to a song (rhythm) with the practitioner's help. For William, music fulfilled a need for connection via expressions he could not yet achieve verbally. He realized that he would have others' attention as long as he continued to play the drum...he utilized the opportunity to show the practitioner what he could do. William had more interaction with his mother. His mother sang songs with him and used (finger) bells. They shared eye contact and that they were willing to share instruments...

On joining his peers for activities in the training center, William found it overwhelming, but he could sit down and observe what others were doing. Such a move initiated new relationships with his teachers and peers. As William's treatment continued, he began to take part, first as an observer and then as a participant in his class. He played games with his peers and participated in singing. He was less reluctant to relate to others and showed confidence in relating to this environment.

GENERAL SESSION OUTLINE AND SAMPLE ACTIVITIES
Welcome
Hello song: leader begins singing the hello song, encouraging the child(ren) to join, just singing, or with actions.

Check-up
Leader sings the song—call out names, child(ren) clap to respond or play the beat on the drum.

Activities
If You're Happy and You Know It (structure)

Freeze and go (with sounds, singing, drums, tambourine) (engagement)

Dance with a scarf (nurture), listen to a lullaby (e.g., *Hush Little Baby*)

Listen to an ocean drum (nurture)

Hold a drum for the child to play—tap to rhythm (challenge)

Be a conductor (challenge)

Feeding
Including soft music, a lullaby, while feeding the child

Closing/goodbye
Goodbye song; rap.

PRINCIPLES TO CONSIDER WHEN USING MUSIC IN THERAPLAY

Having fun instead of playing the "correct" notes; adhering to the four dimensions of structure, engagement, nurture, and challenge (SENC); if pure play doesn't work, try adding some music. If music doesn't work, drop the music—movement and songs are good partners too!

Conclusion

Both Theraplay and musical activities address the socio-emotional needs of children with ASD, such as their joint attention, initiation, and social interaction. In clinical practice, Theraplay provides a clear understanding of structure, engagement, nurture, and challenge to comprehend attachment relationship, while musical strategies of moving, singing, listening, and instrument playing can be incorporated perfectly into the framework. As readers can see from William's case, the use of the practitioner's voice, songs, rhythms, melodies, and various musical activities in Theraplay have helped the child to develop his socio-emotional competency, gradually transforming him from an observer in social interaction to an active participant. Indeed, music and play have always been indispensable elements in the history and culture of humans, suggesting that we may be born with an innate tendency to make music and play. After all, we might simply be helping our children to get in touch with their own human nature.

References

APA (American Psychiatric Association). (2013). *Diagnostic and Statistical Manual of Mental Disorders* (5th edn). https://doi.org/10.1176/appi.books.9780890425596

Booth, P. B., & Jernberg, A. M. (2010). *Theraplay: Helping Parents and Children Build Better Relationships Through Attachment-Based Play* (3rd edn). Jossey-Bass.

Corbeil, M., Trehub, S. E., & Peretz, I. (2016). Singing delays the onset of infant distress. *Infancy* 21(3), 373–391. https://doi.org/10.1111/infa.12114

Corke, M. (2002). *Approaches to Communication Through Music.* David Fulton Publishers.

Dimian, A. F., Symons, F. J., & Wolff, J. J. (2021). Delay to early intensive behavioral intervention and educational outcomes for a Medicaid-enrolled cohort of children with autism. *Journal of Autism and Developmental Disorders 51*, 1054–1066. https://doi.org/10.1007/s10803-020-04586-1

Elder, J. H., Kreider, C. M., Brasher, S. N., & Ansell, M. (2017). Clinical impact of early diagnosis of autism on the prognosis and parent–child relationships. *Psychology Research and Behavior Management 10*, 283–292. https://doi.org/10.2147/PRBM.S117499

Gaser, C., & Schlaug, G. (2003). Brain structures differ between musicians and non-musicians. *Journal of Neuroscience 23*(27), 9240–9245. doi: 10.1523/JNEUROSCI.23-27-09240.2003

Geretsegger, M., Elefant, C., Mössler, K. A., & Gold, C. (2014). Music therapy for people with autism spectrum disorder. *Cochrane Database of Systematic Reviews 6*, CD004381. doi: 10.100214651858.CD004381.pub3

Habibi, A., Damasio, A., Ilari, B., Veiga, R., Joshi, A. A., Leahy, R. M., Haldar, J. P., Varadarajan, D., Bhushan, C., & Damasio, H. (2018). Childhood music training induces change in micro and macroscopic brain structure: Results from a longitudinal study. *Cerebral Cortex 28*(12), 4336–4347. https://doi.org/10.1093/cercor/bhx286

Haslbeck, F. B., Jakab, A., Held, U., Bassler, D., Bucher, H. U., & Hagmann, C. (2020). Creative music therapy to promote brain function and brain structure in preterm infants: A randomized controlled pilot study. *NeuroImage: Clinical 25*, 102171. doi:10.1016/j.nicl.2020.102171

Hiles Howard, A. R., Lindaman, S., Copeland, R., & Cross, D. R. (2018). Theraplay impact on parents and children with autism spectrum disorder: Improvements in affect, joint attention, and social cooperation. *International Journal of Play Therapy 27*(1), 56–68. https://doi.org/10.1037/pla0000056

Hudson, M., Dallos, R., & McKenzie, R. (2017). Systemic-attachment formulation for families of children with autism. *Advances in Autism 3*(3), 142–153. https://doi.org/10.1108/AIA-02-2017-0005

Jones, E. A., & Carr, E. G. (2004). Joint attention in children with autism: Theory and intervention. *Focus on Autism and Other Developmental Disabilities 19*(1), 13–26. https://doi.org/10.1177/10883576040190010301

Keeler, J. R., Both, E. A., Neuser, B. L., Spitsbergen, J. M., Waters, D. J. M., & Vianney, J. M. (2015). The neurochemistry and social flow of singing: Bonding and oxytocin. *Frontiers in Human Neuroscience 9*, 518, 1–10. https://doi.org/10.3389/fnhum.2015.00518

Kern, P., Graham, F. P., & Alridge, D. (2006). Using embedded music therapy interaction to support outdoor play for young children with autism in an inclusive community-based child care program. *Journal of Music Therapy 43*, 270–294. doi:10.1093/jmt/43.4.270

Kim, J., Wigram, T., & Gold, C. (2009). Emotional, motivational and interpersonal responsiveness of children with autism in improvisational music therapy. *Autism 13*(4), 389–409. https://doi.org/10.1177/1362361309105660

Kreutz, G. (2014). Singing and social bonding introduction. *Music and Medicine 6*(2), 51–60.

Lense, M. D., & Camarata, S. (2020). PRESS-play: Musical engagement as a motivating platform for social interaction and social play in young children with ASD. *Music & Science 3*, 1–13. https://doi.org/10.1177/2059204320933080

Maenner, M. J., Shaw, K. A., Baio, J.,...Dietz, P. M. (2020). Prevalence of Autism Spectrum Disorder among children aged 8 years—Autism and Developmental Disabilities Monitoring Network, 11 Sites, United States, 2016. *Morbidity and Mortality Weekly Report. Surveillance Summaries 69*(4), 1–12. doi:10.15585/mmwr.ss6904a1

Mäkelä, J., & Hart, S. (2011). Theraplay: An Intensive, Engaging, Interactive Play that Promotes Psychological Development. In S. Hart (Ed.), *Neuroaffectiv psykoterapi med born* [*Neuroaffective Psychotherapy for Children*] (Chapter 7). Forlag Hans Reitzel.

Mössler, K., Schmid, W., Aßmus, J., Fusar-Poli, L., & Gold, C. (2020). Attunement in music therapy for young children with autism: Revisiting qualities of relationship as mechanisms of change. *Journal of Autism and Developmental Disorders 50*, 1–14. doi: 10.1007/s10803-020-04448-w

Ockelford, A. (2000). Music in education of children with severe or profound learning difficulties: Issues in current UK provision, a new conceptual framework, and proposals for research. *Psychology of Music 28*, 197–217. https://doi.org/10.1177/0305735600282009

Ofner, M., Coles, A., Decou, M. L., Do, M. T., Bienek, A., Snider, J., & Ugnat, A. (2018). *Autism*

Spectrum Disorder among Children and Youth in Canada 2018. Public Health Agency of Canada.

Raglio, A., Traficante, D., & Oasi, O. (2011). Autism and music therapy. Intersubjective approach and music therapy assessment. *Nordic Journal of Music Therapy 20*(2), 123–141. doi:10.1080/08098130903377399

Russo, M. A., Santarelli, D. M., & O'Rourke, D. (2017). The physiological effects of slow breathing in the healthy human. *Breathe 13*(4), 298–309. doi:10.1183/20734735.009817

Siu, A. F. Y. (2021). Does age make a difference when incorporating music as a rhythmic-mediated component in a Theraplay-based program to facilitate attunement of preschool children with social impairment? *International Journal of Play Therapy 30*(2), 136–145. https://doi.org/10.1037/pla0000131

Small, C. (1998). *Musicking: The Meaning of Performing and Listening.* Wesleyan University Press.

Stern, D. N. ([1985] 2018). *The Interpersonal World of the Infant: A View from Psychoanalysis and Developmental Psychology.* Routledge. http://dx.doi.org/10.4324/9780429482137

Wan, C. Y., Demaine, K., Zipse, L., Norton, A., & Schlang, G. (2010). From music making to speaking: Engaging the mirror neuron system in autism. *Brain Research Bulletin 82*, 161–168. doi:10.1016/j.brainresbull.2010.04.010

Williams, K. (2018). Moving to the beat: Using music, rhythm, and movement to enhance self-regulation in early childhood classrooms. *International Journal of Early Childhood 50*, 85–100. https://doi.org/10.1007/s13158-018-0215-y

Yau, K., & Fachner, J. (2019). Effects of motifs in music therapy on the attention of children with externalizing behavior problems. *Psychology of Music 49*(3). https://doi.org/10.1177/0305735619880292

Chapter 15

Theraplay with Gifted Children

Danielle H. Maxonight

Introduction

This chapter explores the benefits of Theraplay for gifted and twice-exceptional children. There are many definitions of "gifted." Sometimes this term is used to describe a child who has passed certain tests, whether measuring intelligence, aptitude, or achievement. In this chapter, the term will cover a broader group, indicating "asynchronous development in which advanced cognitive abilities and heightened intensity combine to create inner experiences and awareness that are qualitatively different from the norm" (Columbus Group 1991). For gifted children, uneven growth across areas of development can produce, for example, a ten-year-old who reads at a college level but functions emotionally and socially as a seven-year-old.

"Twice-exceptional" references gifted children who also present with a learning disability or mental health diagnosis. Gifted children in therapy are typically, therefore, twice-exceptional, and the terms will be used interchangeably in this chapter.

The therapeutic needs of this population will be examined within the existing literature, and various adaptations will be explored. Common presenting concerns and therapeutic approaches will later be contextualized with a case study.

Theoretical underpinnings

While the majority of treatment-seeking gifted children will experience some level of anxiety and will often benefit from Theraplay adaptations for anxiety (Glibota, Lindaman, & Coleman 2018; Maxonight 2021), these children also have unique, additional needs. Many gifted children struggle with some combination of heightened emotional intensity, sensory sensitivity, and adjustment concerns.

Overexcitabilities

In 1964, the Polish psychologist Kazimierz Dąbrowski began publishing works related to his theory of positive disintegration, a watershed framework conceptualizing the psychological development of gifted individuals. He surmised that several features of the nervous system differentiate these individuals from the neurotypical population, and he coined the term "overexcitabilities" to describe these distinctive features (Daniels & Piechowski 2009). Dąbrowski identified five overexcitabilities (OEs): psychomotor, sensual, intellectual, imaginational, and emotional (Falk & Miller 2009):

- Psychomotor OE involves heightened physical energy, movement, and communication. Children with psychomotor OE are known to be unusually alert, talking aloud rapidly, pacing while thinking. Sleep issues are common.

- Sensual OE refers to an intensified response to sensory input—for example, some children are distressed by fluorescent lighting and fussy about seams in their clothing, yet can be moved to tears of joy by a symphony or a sunset.

- Intellectual OE identifies individuals with an unquenchable thirst for knowledge and learning. These children sneak off to bed with books and flashlights under the covers, and can exhaust adults with their relentless curiosity. They fall in love with learning for learning's sake and often pursue special interest areas with great fervor.

- Children with imaginational OE have an extraordinary ability to imagine: daydreaming, worrying, and inventing in a profound and vibrant way.

- Lastly, the emotional OE, perhaps most central to the work of a Theraplay practitioner, conveys sensitivity and depth of feeling. A child with emotional OE might be inconsolable after accidentally stepping on a ladybug or have nightmares for weeks after watching an emotionally charged, though not classically "scary," scene in a G-rated movie. When well supported, children with emotional OE enjoy the gifts of advanced empathy, contentiousness, and kindness.

Across many dimensions of development, gifted children present with more sensitivity and intensity. Contributors to gifted literature often refer to OEs as "original equipment," as these differences appear quite early in infancy. OEs seem to be a matter of temperament or wiring of the nervous system rather than a response to lived experience, trauma, or parenting (Daniels & Piechowski 2009). Theraplay, with its focus on sensory integration and co-regulation of affect and arousal, is a powerful intervention for children with OEs.

Hyper brain/hyper body

The existence of OEs as a phenomenon is supported by a 2018 study by Karpinski et al. (2018) comparing self-report questionnaires from the American Mensa, a group of 3715 testing at or above the 98th percentile of intelligence, with national average statistics. The Mensa group reported significantly higher levels of both psychological disorders and certain inflammatory and autoimmune conditions. For example, the gifted group had 3.42 times the risk for anxiety disorders relative to the national average, and 4.33 times the risk for environmental allergies. The authors theorize that these correlations are the result of a "hyper brain/hyper body" association, and that the gifted neurology, particularly OEs and resultant rumination, creates a higher risk for certain health problems (Karpinski et al. 2018). A natural conclusion to draw here is that therapeutic intervention can mediate this process, serving as a protective factor for lifelong health.

Asynchronous development

Another hallmark of gifted children lies in their asynchronous development, in which some areas of development outpace others significantly. Consider, for example, a kindergartener who multiplies double-digit numbers in their head, yet struggles to zip their jacket or sit quietly during their classroom's "circle time." While they need much more advanced academic material to stay engaged with math, many essential motor and social skills are still emerging for this little one. Most mainstream educational contexts will fail to be a true fit across the board for a twice-exceptional child. This creates a dilemma when considering how to meet divergent needs: the majority of environments will adequately meet needs in some areas of development while severely neglecting others.

Theraplay practitioners become accustomed to differences between children's social-emotional and chronological ages. We design play sessions to create a welcoming environment for the "younger child" to emerge, be known, and grow. We carefully support children's sensory, emotional, and regulatory needs, and respond to each child as a multifaceted and complex individual. Fostering global adaptability, Theraplay builds increased synchrony, developmental integration, and felt safety for twice-exceptional children.

Social belonging, intersectionality, and systemic oppression

Gifted children often prefer gifted age mates or older children as friends, and as such they can struggle to make friends (Gross 2002). An Australian study found that children's conceptions of friendship grow in a hierarchy of age-related stages, from simple play partners to emotionally intimate, unconditionally accepting friends. The children's ideas on friendship seemed to mature alongside their IQ rather than their chronological age. So, in stages of development when neurotypical children were seeking simple play partners, many gifted children were seeking a "sure shelter," trusting their best friend. This discrepancy grew steeper for children alongside IQ, such that children with an IQ over 160 sought the "sure shelter" friendship four to five years earlier than neurotypical age mates (Gross 2001). Different friendship ideals can leave gifted children feeling socially dissatisfied or rejected by their peers.

An arduous quest for social belonging can also be complicated by neuro-discrimination, ableism, racism, classism, and intersectional identity. Gifted children can be viewed as a vulnerable and oppressed population (Chu & Myers 2015). Mainstream settings often thwart their needs for social belonging, intellectual stimulation and challenge, and expression of OEs. Gifted children can feel socially othered, and alienated. Many work diligently to blend in and camouflage their differences.

Children living in poverty, from working-class families, and of color, particularly Black and Latinx students, are vastly under-represented in gifted and talented school programs (Ford 2011; Grissom & Redding 2018; Grissom, Redding, & Bleiburg 2019). Classism and racism play a huge role in gifted gatekeeping. A 2019 study of 21,000 elementary-aged students, divided into five socio-economic status groups, found that placement in gifted programs correlated to the family's level of affluence. Students in the wealthiest group were placed in gifted programs at a rate of 12 percent, while students in the least wealthy group were placed at a rate of just 2 percent (Grissom & Redding 2018). This disparity leaves gifted children from working-class families with many social, emotional, and intellectual needs unmet.

Racial disparities also abound. In a 2018 sample of 10,000 elementary-aged children, Black students were less likely to be placed in gifted programming by 66 percent, and Hispanic students were less likely by 47 percent when compared to white students (Grissom & Redding 2018). Some would argue the racist biases of IQ testing as the primary issue (Kendi, 2018); however, in this study, white children were still twice as likely as Black children to be chosen for gifted programming even with identical test scores. Participating in a gifted program can increase interest in school, improve student–teacher relationships (Vogl & Preckel 2013), and meet emotional needs for self-understanding and social belonging. Not being identified as gifted in childhood is emotionally consequential, as it decontextualizes normative aspects of gifted development for children, caregivers, and teachers.

Some twice-exceptional children have a learning disability or mental health condition that precludes placement into gifted programs; for example, a gifted child with attention deficit hyperactivity disorder (ADHD) may not be permitted into a special program due to impulsive, non-compliant, or distracting behaviors. A gifted child who suffers from depression may not be identified due to underachievement or low motivation. A twice-exceptional child with paralyzing test anxiety may produce assessment scores that don't capture their ability or aptitude.

The glaring lack of diversity in gifted programs can leave young people feeling that "gifted" actually means white, wealthy, compliant, high-achieving, and socially privileged. Unsurprisingly, Black gifted children who are placed in special programs can struggle to find their place socially, noting that peers denigrate their intelligence or achievement as "acting white" (Ford 2011; Ford *et al.* 2008). Gifted children of color can feel social pressure to identify with one intersection, forsaking the other. This creates a double bind for a young person to escape social difficulties—one aspect of the self must be masked, yet, in hiding either their neurotype or culture, a child will never feel fully seen, known, or accepted. Gifted children can suffer social alienation and oppression within our society, undoubtedly. For some, twice-exceptionality, asynchronous development, and/or intersecting social identities will mean that there is no peer, teacher, or school environment that can celebrate all the idiosyncrasies of the child's self in an integrated, full way. For many, an entire part of their development, identity, and gifted neurotype will simply not be identified.

Theraplay helps caregivers to become a safe haven and secure base for their children. Through intense parental warmth and radical acceptance, Theraplay offers children increased resiliency against corrosive social environments. As caregivers come to deeply know their children's unique needs, vulnerabilities, and talents, they become more empowered and effective advocates with school counselors, teachers, coaches, and others. This is an identity-integrating process in which a child's whole self is seen and celebrated, and a caregiver feels empowered to support their child in new ways.

Additionally, because Theraplay targets issues of affect regulation, social-relatedness, sensory integration, and emotional resilience, a successful course of Theraplay can open up new academic options for children. For example, a second-grader performing academically as a fifth-grader but with significant social skills deficits is a poor candidate for grade skipping. However, if this same child developed enhanced social-emotional competencies through Theraplay intervention, skipping third grade could become a viable option. This would allow for less intellectual frustration and could protect against related concerns, underachievement, and perfectionism.

Underachievement and perfectionism

Teachers, caregivers, and therapists know that twice-exceptional children placed in traditional classrooms can stagnate in their learning for a number of reasons, including boredom or downplaying their intelligence in order to be socially accepted. Children often develop secondary problems with frustration tolerance, self-confidence, and perfectionism as a result of academically coasting. The many normal, everyday failures associated with learning a new skill can remain foreign to gifted children in the early grades; this sensitizes them to challenges and can lead to risk-avoidant behavior later on. Theraplay supports children in shifting their response to challenge, away from fear and perfectionism and toward increased playfulness, flexibility, and confidence.

Theraplay practitioners encourage children to take age-appropriate risks, using the caregiver as a secure base. This ultimately promotes a more stable and happy sense of self.

Could neuro-discrimination and other systems of oppression contribute to the gifted population's heightened risk for internalizing disorders and autoimmune conditions? Perhaps OEs on their own are not to blame. If our culture was created with the gifted neurotype in mind, children would have many positive outlets for OEs, adequate exposure to academic challenge, failure, intellectual stimulation, and deeper feelings of belonging and social acceptance.

Gifted children of all backgrounds would be readily identified and supported. Although we use the word "gifted," being part of this minority neurotype represents not only a gift but also many environmental and social obstacles. Therefore, any respectful therapeutic intervention with a gifted child needs to focus on ameliorating the child's symptoms, as well as on advocacy work within their greater social-emotional ecosystem. A child's neurotype is not something to be "fixed" but embraced, celebrated, and accommodated for by parents, teachers, and the world at large.

Theraplay with gifted children: therapeutic adaptations
Effective assessment and psychoeducation

In assessing gifted children, we should develop ways to inquire about OEs, intellectual interests, perceived stigma regarding the "gifted" label and/or intersectional identities, and autoimmune conditions. Given that feeding, laughter, heightened activity, and use of lotion are all prominent in Theraplay, it is essential to assess for food allergies, asthma, eczema, and other skin conditions prior to beginning the Marschak Interaction Method (MIM). Some children have sensitivity to common ingredients in lotion, such as fragrance, so in these cases, it is preferable to purchase the type used at their home prior to the MIM.

Clinicians can provide caregivers with great relief via the use of effective psychoeducation on the social and emotional aspects of giftedness. For most, it will be the very first time that they have encountered this information after experiencing many years of confusing difficulties with their child. Comparing their child's intense reactions, social differences, or educational problems to their neurotypical peers, they often wonder, "What am I doing wrong?" They also face judgment from other adults, about the child's perceived problems and about the child's intelligence. Some face accusations of under-disciplining their child (somehow creating their OEs) or "hot housing" their child (somehow creating their gifts through intrusive, accelerated teaching at home). In most cases, these assumptions are blatantly false. Despite this, many caregivers feel immense responsibility for their child's differences.

Therapists should not only normalize social-emotional issues within the context of the child's giftedness, but also support caregivers' understanding of how a second exceptionality fits into the full picture of their child's functioning. It is beyond the scope of this chapter to fully elaborate on the diagnosis, misdiagnosis, and missed diagnosis of gifted children, but these children often present very differently. Normative elements of giftedness in childhood, such as OEs, can both mistakenly appear to be ADHD, autism spectrum disorder (ASD), etc., and high intelligence can also easily mask these conditions, delaying diagnosis (Webb 2005). Many of our standardized instruments were normed using neurotypical children, not gifted children. So it is best to rely on a psychologist with significant experience testing gifted children in order to provide a clear and accurate diagnostic picture for families.

Complexity and pacing

Neurotypical children need six to eight repetitions of teaching for mastery; conversely, gifted children integrate new information after one to three repetitions (Kingore 2003). Much of life becomes about waiting and under-stimulation. For some, doing complex work at a faster speed will feel less frustrating and anxiety-provoking than doing simple, repetitive tasks slowly. In these cases, it will be effective to scaffold session activities from complex and fast-paced to simple and slow-paced as the child learns to manage OEs. For instance, early sessions might include a complicated hand-clapping game (boom snap clap) and build up to a much simpler one ("Miss Mary Mack"). The challenge lies in the ever-increasing level of repetition and under-stimulation, which can promote anxiety. This is an important adaptation to explore on a case-by-case basis, as some gifted children struggle with perfectionism, better served by a slow, rhythmic pace and low level of challenge to start, building later on to more speed, spontaneity, and risk of "failure." Complexity and pacing should be used intuitively, understanding that, paradoxically, complex is soothing for some gifted children, and simple is agitating. Every child is unique.

Helping a gifted child learn to emotionally regulate within some level of boredom or anxiety can be a helpful goal, but therapists, caregivers, and teachers will also need to make accommodations in the child's environment to meet their intellectual and emotional needs.

Without environmental changes, we are essentially helping a child learn to accept neuro-discrimination. Academic acceleration, differentiation, grade skipping, homeschooling, and extracurricular enrichment are all possible interventions beyond the scope of this chapter.

Cognitive interweaves

In Theraplay, we celebrate the uncelebrated aspects of a child. It will be helpful to consider which parts of the self are unidentified, ignored, devalued, or masked. Depending on the culture of the family, community, and school environments, this unsupported part could be the child's high intelligence, "strange" interest areas, OEs, learning disability, or social quirks. Throughout our typically non-speaking activities, we can interweave affirmations about the child's delightfulness through short, declarative statements that require no response from the child. We might use crepe paper to measure around the child's head, remarking, "This head is the home to a witty, funny, always-curious brain!" For a child with a deep but hidden-from-peers interest in *Star Wars*, we might adapt the words to the theme song, adding personalizing elements, in lieu of a standard lullaby. The office becomes a place to help the child and family accept and integrate the camouflaged or alienated parts of self.

Working with caregivers of gifted children

Ongoing research repeatedly proves that general intelligence is substantially genetic (Trzaskowski *et al.* 2013). For many reasons, caregivers will not typically identify as "gifted." However, as we provide caregivers with psychoeducation and explore their child's struggles to adapt to the neurotypical world, they will often draw parallels to their own experiences growing up. These resurfaced themes require careful attention, a nuanced approach, and some caregivers will benefit from their own individual therapy in addition to Theraplay. Here several adaptations within caregiver-only sessions are explored.

Invite skepticism

Theraplay is uniquely suited to support gifted caregivers because it follows a "caregiver-as-collaborator" approach, welcoming and celebrating their learning, skepticism, and curiosity. We should lean into this collaborative style and encourage deep questioning and exploration during caregiver sessions. For some, more detailed information will actually quiet the mind, rather than overwhelming. Adding additional caregiver sessions, suggesting books, and providing research articles written for a professional audience all go a long way toward maintaining solid rapport. Match a caregiver's intensity with intensity. Match their pace of learning and integrating. This is not about presenting oneself as an "expert" but about cheering on curiosity and accepting a caregiver's unique learning style.

Address over-responsibility

Anxiety is a common concern for gifted individuals. A few elements of anxiety, such as perfectionism and over-responsibility, create intense shame for gifted caregivers around being unable to help their child. These caregivers often present their child for treatment only after having scoured parenting blogs, books, and research, attempting multiple approaches on their own, and contending with feelings of great failure and self-reproach. Gifted individuals are often used to "getting it right," using logic and brainpower to solve problems rapidly. We need to help caregivers see that their family's concerns make sense only when appropriately contextualized, that sheer intelligence can't solve the family's problems, and that caregivers on their own are not to blame.

In order to help caregivers find the logic within their family's challenges, we must understand what drives caregivers' behavior. This means utilizing the Adult Attachment Interview (AAI) or a similar assessment tool as a standard part of the intake. This offers us invaluable information to reframe a caregiver's "imperfect" parenting as coherent and even expected, given their upbringing. Combined with psychoeducation on giftedness, gently processing key features of the AAI with the caregiver will aid their shift away from over-responsibility and into empowered self-compassion. The assessment phase of Theraplay offers families a great deal, building a clear and reasoned narrative around the problem's etiology, and thereby reducing confusion, over-functioning, blame, and shame.

CASE ILLUSTRATION: THERAPLAY WITH A TWICE-EXCEPTIONAL GIRL

BACKGROUND

Esme was a white seven-year-old girl who presented with symptoms of underachievement, poor attention, hyperactivity, and oppositional behavior at home. She had already navigated one change in school due to adjustment problems.

SESSION 1: COMPREHENSIVE CLINICAL ASSESSMENT

Esme's mother, Emily, described her as an infant "in need of constant stimulation." Esme slept little and poorly, and suffered from digestive concerns and eczema. While she struggled socially, by 14 months her preschool teacher deemed her a "master of sign language," and by age two, she had learned conversational French. The family consented to testing in preparation for kindergarten at the preschool's urging. Esme's achievement tests showed her performing at second-grade level by age four. In reviewing the testing, the local public school asked for a double-grade skip, but the parents declined, choosing kindergarten at a charter school for her social development. Here, she lacked friends, often taking charge of her peers' play. Due to a mismatch in the school's and family's culture and values, the parents moved her in first grade to a new school. Now in second grade, her achievement and interest in learning dwindled, and she often complained of hating school. In the past few weeks, this dread had escalated into multiple phone calls home each day with various somatic complaints. I offered preliminary psychoeducation on the social and emotional aspects of giftedness, and sent Emily home with several articles and books on the topic. I also shared scholarly articles on Theraplay's successful application with anxious children for review between sessions. Emily appeared relieved and curious.

SESSIONS 2–3: AAI AND MIM

In Emily's AAI, she shared about loving relationships with both parents. Absorbed in gymnastics, she had progressed to pre-Olympic levels by middle childhood. Emily recounted an incident at age six in which she had broken her arm at an invitational gymnastics workshop in Europe while her parents were off sightseeing. By the time her parents returned, she had been to a hospital, her arm set and cast, and she was back to training. Through examining this incident further, Emily acknowledged that her parents strongly emphasized achievement throughout her childhood.

During the MIM, Esme and Emily engaged in a fast-paced, highly verbal way. Esme appeared mildly anxious during the LEGO® task, copying her mother's quite elaborate sculpture perfectly, talking aloud to herself, and sustaining focused attention for more than 10 minutes. The imaginative play task with squeaky animals seemed taxing for both parties; this quickly turned into a typical conversation holding the animals. Throughout the feeding task, Esme sat at a distance and closed her eyes, guessing the flavor of the fruit snack and receiving Emily's praise.

SESSIONS 3–4: MIM FEEDBACK AND PARENT DEMONSTRATION

In watching the video clips together, we determined that nurture and engagement should be primary dimensions for focus. Our treatment objectives were to support Esme in accepting unconditional nurturing rather than praise for accomplishments; in tolerating silly, imaginative, and spontaneous engagement; and in finding a regulated state, even within slower-paced activities.

Outside of our Theraplay work, we would assess Esme's learning environment and advocate for adjustments to meet her needs. These objectives supported our overarching goals of reduced anxiety, improved adjustment, and increased self-esteem and social connectedness.

The parent demonstration session provided a space for dialogue about Theraplay and social-emotional aspects of giftedness. Emily began to spontaneously share elements of her own childhood that suddenly made sense, and her descriptions of Esme's difficulties became more compassionate. I focused with Emily on demonstrating nurture activities so that she could experience this firsthand. She noted her own nervousness around the intimate, slower-paced, non-speaking nature of Theraplay.

SESSIONS 5–7

In her first session, Esme moved at a breakneck pace through the activities, seeking out challenges at every turn. During "Simon says," she exclaimed, "Can you make this more difficult? This is easy!" I matched her intensity and speed, making a mental note to slow down and simplify over time. She appeared uncomfortable as Emily fed her and sang a lullaby, looking at her mother incredulously, as if to say, "Are you kidding me with this baby stuff?"

The following two sessions, Esme appeared more anxious, and her eczema flared a bright red; Emily reported that she had experienced headaches and stomach aches each day at school.

Within the comfort of her third Theraplay session, she spontaneously began to share about school, including previously undisclosed teasing and rejection by peers, feelings of social alienation, and longing for friends. Emily held her close in a soothing way.

SESSION 8: PARENT REVIEW

We watched clips in which Esme expressed discomfort with nurture by hiding beneath a blanket, speeding through activities, and talking rapidly to avoid resting in her mother's love and acceptance. Emily noted that as a result of Theraplay, she had realized how frequently she praised Esme for achievements, and she was working to curb this habit. Emily wanted her daughter to know that her delight in her was unconditional, not predicated on her accomplishments or good behavior. As a result of our advocacy work at school, Esme was trying out math lessons with an older grade to reignite and stimulate her intellectual interest in school; she enjoyed this a great deal.

SESSIONS 9–11

I used moments of heightened sensitivity to celebrate Esme's OEs as a positive force, her way of sensing things in a deep, unique way. While engaged in a texture-guessing activity, I exclaimed with a big smile, "Wow, your hand could tell the difference between these two paint brushes, even though they are so similar, and even with your eyes closed! You are so sensitive!" Esme beamed and nodded.

During this period, her resistance to nurture seemed to evaporate. Whereas Esme would scoff at having Band-Aids placed on little cuts in early sessions, she now eagerly presented injuries to her parents for care. Her parents intuitively began a routine of swinging her in a blanket and singing lullabies each night before bed. They carried a fanny-pack of Band-Aids everywhere, and Esme's somatic complaints declined. Her eczema healed noticeably.

SESSIONS 12–25

In parent review, Emily tearfully described Esme's reports of exclusion by peers and worries about her learning. While Esme had entered kindergarten testing significantly above grade level, her second-grade teacher was now recommending remediation because she had fallen so far behind. Her behavior in her main classroom continued to be overactive, disruptive, and unfocused. In contrast, during the pull-out math sessions, Esme was high achieving and compliant. Emily exclaimed, "In trying to help her socially by not grade skipping, I fear that we've failed her. Now she's bored, hates school, and is failing at everything, with academics and with friends!"

Emily shared that as a result of Theraplay, she was responding to Esme in a much more nurturing way, even when it felt awkward for her. Since Esme's behavior concerns softened via this new approach, it reinforced Emily, and she found it easier and easier over time. Esme's play with neighborhood children had also become more flexible, less controlling.

By the time Emily was confidently leading Theraplay sessions, the family decided on a transfer to a new school. The administration promised to allow Esme to continue on with accelerated math through an online curriculum while retaining her with same-age peers to meet her social needs. Due to the small size of the school, there were also opportunities for academic differentiation and cross-age friendships to develop during project-based learning.

At the end of Theraplay treatment, Esme smiled more. She seemed less stressed, sharing her thoughts and feelings more freely. She rarely complained of headaches or stomach aches; her skin was clear and bright. Emily, understanding her child's emotional and intellectual needs more deeply, felt comfortable advocating for her with school professionals. While still sensitive, spirited, and intense, Esme's defiant behavior at home softened. Her trouble with executive functioning continued to wax and wane, depending on her interests and the level of structure and challenge in her environment. As we concluded our process together, unsure whether the new school environment might resolve some of the focus issues, I referred Esme for further evaluation to rule out a second exceptionality or need for medication.

At a six-month follow-up, Esme was happily adjusted in her new school, excelling academically, and still quite ahead in math. Her hyperactive and inattentive symptoms were well controlled via a combination of academic differentiation, extracurricular enrichment, exercise, and stimulant medication. She enjoyed several meaningful friendships with same-age peers and with older children at her school.

Conclusion

In this chapter, the social-emotional vulnerabilities and therapeutic needs of gifted children have been investigated. While individuals with anxiety flourish in conditions of high predictability with clearly defined roles, gifted individuals often feel soothed by accelerated learning, complexity, intensity, and collaboration. In balancing the needs of twice-exceptional families with anxiety, Theraplay therapists must ascertain which parts of the work must be simple, slow, and direct, and which parts must be deep, multifaceted, and fast-paced. We must be keenly intuitive and flexible in approach. Given the vulnerable position of twice-exceptional children within society, Theraplay should not be a stand-alone intervention but part of a larger treatment plan that incorporates environmental accommodations and advocacy.

Key takeaways

- Gifted children have unique social-emotional vulnerabilities, including OEs and a heightened risk for internalizing disorders.

- The hyper brain/hyper body theory suggests that effective therapeutic intervention, such as Theraplay, can mediate health risks within the gifted population, including autoimmune conditions in adulthood.

- Asynchronous development, neuro-discrimination, and other forms of systemic oppression can create social and educational adjustment issues for gifted children.

- Theraplay supports caregivers in becoming an emotional refuge for their children; this increases the child's resiliency within ill-suited environments, and emboldens the caregiver's advocacy efforts.

- Theraplay adaptations for gifted families include adjustments in complexity and pacing, using nurturing cognitive interweaves, inviting caregiver skepticism, and matching intensity with intensity.

Questions for reflection and continued learning

1. Apply the core concepts of this chapter in treatment planning for the following case: Devon was a 10-year-old Black child presenting with poor impulse control, depressive symptoms, food allergies, and asthma. After behavioral difficulties in school at age five, he was diagnosed with oppositional defiant disorder and attention deficit hyperactivity disorder. During assessment, Devon paces back and forth, speaking rapidly, using eloquent metaphors and sweeping hand gestures. He identifies studying physics as his favorite hobby and laments his lack of "real" friends. While his grades have always been fair, his parents complain

about procrastination and underachievement. Devon has never been identified as "gifted" at school.

2. Describe three ways in which the development of gifted and twice-exceptional individuals differs from that of neurotypical individuals. Illustrate each difference with an example of how this may present within a Theraplay session with either a caregiver or child.

References

Chu, Y. H., & Myers, B. (2015). A social work perspective on the treatment of gifted and talented students in American public schools. *School Social Work Journal 40*(1), 42–57.

Columbus Group. (1991). The transcript of meeting of the Columbus Group. Unpublished document, July.

Daniels, S., & Piechowski, M. M. (Eds) (2009). *Living with Intensity: Understanding the Sensitivity, Excitability, and Emotional Development of Gifted Children, Adolescents, and Adults*. Great Potential Press.

Falk, R. F., & Miller, N. B. (2009). Building Firm Foundations: Research and Assessments. In S. Daniels & M. M. Piechowski (Eds), *Living with Intensity: Understanding the Sensitivity, Excitability, and Emotional Development of Gifted Children, Adolescents, and Adults* (pp.239–260). Great Potential Press.

Ford, D. Y. (2011). *Reversing Underachievement in Gifted Black Students* (2nd edn). Prufrock Press.

Ford, D. Y., Grantham, T. C., & Whiting, G. W. (2008). Another look at the achievement gap: Learning from the experiences of gifted black students. *Urban Education 43*(2), 216–239. https://doi.org/10.1177/0042085907312344

Glibota, L.C., Lindaman, S., & Coleman, A. R. (2018). Theraplay as a Treatment for Children with Selective Mutism: Integrating the Polyvagal Theory, Attachment Theory, and Social Communication. In A. A. Drewes & C. Schaefer (Eds), *Play-Based Interventions for Childhood Anxieties, Fears and Phobias* (pp.124–143). Guilford Press.

Grissom, J., & Redding, C. (2018). Discretion and disproportionality: Explaining the underrepresentation of achieving students of color in gifted programs. *American Educational Research Association 2*(1). https://doi.org/10.1177/2332858415622175

Grissom, J., Redding, C., & Bleiburg, J. (2019). Money over merit? Socioeconomic gaps in receipt of gifted services. *Harvard Educational Review 89*(3), 337–369. https://doi:10.17763/1943-5045-89.3.337

Gross, M. U. M. (2001). From "play partner" to "sure shelter": What do gifted children seek from friendship? *GERRIC News*, 4–5.

Gross, M. U. M. (2002). Social and Emotional Issues for Exceptionally Intellectually Gifted Students. In M. Neihart, S. M. Reis, N. M. Robinson, & S. M. Moon (Eds), *The Social and Emotional Development of Gifted Children: What Do We Know?* (pp.19–27). Sourcebooks.

Karpinski, R. I., Kolb, A. M. K., Tetreault, N. A., & Borowski, T. B. (2018). High intelligence: A risk factor for psychological and physiological overexcitabilities. *Intelligence 66*, 8–23. http://dx.doi.org/10.1016/j.intell.2017.09.001

Kendi, I. X. (2019). *How to Be an Antiracist*. One World.

Kingore, B. (2003). High achiever, gifted learner, creative thinker. *Understanding Our Gifted*.

www.westminsterpublicschools.org/cms/lib03/CO01001133/Centricity/Domain/21/Bertie%20Kingore.%20High%20Achiever.Gifted%20.Creative.pdf

Maxonight, D. (2021). Theraplay Adaptations for Anxiety Disorders. In S. Lindaman & R. Hong (Eds), *Theraplay: Theory, Applications and Implementation* (pp.157–173). Jessica Kingsley Publishers.

Trzaskowski, M., Yang, J., Visscher, P. M., & Plomin, R. (2014). DNA evidence for strong genetic stability and increasing heritability of intelligence from age 7 to 12. *Molecular Psychiatry 19*, 380–384. www.nature.com/articles/mp2012191

Vogl, K., & Preckel, F. (2013). Full-time ability grouping of gifted students: Impacts on social self-concept and school-related attitudes. *Gifted Child Quarterly 58*(1), 51–68. doi: 10.1177/0016986213513795

Webb, J. T. (2005). *Misdiagnosis and Dual Diagnoses of Gifted Children and Adults: ADHD, Bipolar, Asperger's, Depression, and Other Disorders.* Great Potential Press.

Chapter 16

Group Theraplay with Adolescents with Neurological Impairment

Daniel J. Cane

Introduction

Neurological disorders are common among school-aged youth and present challenges to the school system for both education and social integration. Neurological injury may present in obvious ways, such as with spastic cerebral palsy that affects easily observable motor skills, and in covert ways, such as with strokes or tumors that can affect social awareness, language comprehension, and impulse control. Medical advances in both emergency care and long-term care have ensured higher rates of survival, but many of these children live with chronic cognitive, motor, or sensory deficits that impact their learning, socialization, and community integration. Youth with a neurological injury can benefit from the Theraplay approach because it addresses neurodevelopmental needs at multiple levels. Activities based on Theraplay's four dimensions—structure, engagement, nurture, and challenge—are often useful in meeting the specific needs of young teens. This chapter outlines the principles of Group Theraplay as applied in a school setting. Neurological issues are specifically addressed as a specialized situation for therapeutic intervention. Key concepts are attunement, adaptation to physical limitations, and adapting to the developmental level of teen students with different cognitive abilities based on their injuries. Four case illustrations demonstrate how this innovative model can attain positive outcomes, facilitating social-emotional development in youth with neurological challenges.

Neurologically focused special education program

A Theraplay-trained school psychologist and a classroom teacher planned the group therapy activities in accordance with the Theraplay dimensions of structure, engagement, nurture, and challenge.

Any school district can expect that 2 percent of their students will have a neurological impairment that impedes functioning and learning, including tumors, aneurysms, brain infections, teratogens, and impact trauma (NCES 2022). Traumatic brain injury (TBI) is the leading cause of disability in young children and teens, and while the incidence of severe TBI is relatively small, at less than 691 per 100,000, the life impact can be enormous (ASHA n.d.). Seizure disorder is the most common neurological reason for pediatric hospital admission (Moreau *et al.* 2013). Other pediatric neurological illnesses include hydrocephalus, meningitis, stroke, cardiac arrest, and tumors (Fink *et al.* 2017). While a well-constructed Individualized Education Plan (IEP) can address the unique learning needs of this group, many of the youth feel isolated, embarrassed, or disconnected from the social milieu. Some may even be unaware of the social milieu or may spend considerable time in a small group or 1:1 learning situations that reduce their opportunity for social inclusion. The need for developing social skills is critical for this group of students to experience long-term, successful integration with society. They have the same desires for friendships, dating, and careers as other students their age, but their ability to achieve these basic human experiences is often attenuated.

Teens with neurological disorders face special challenges regarding social inclusion, as their cognitive and physical impairments can cause them to stand out or to be ostracized. Self-consciousness may arise in the face of motor problems or social awkwardness, causing an escalation of anxiety or depression. They benefit from sharing their experiences with others who can empathize. They also require very direct and clear corrective feedback regarding behavior. Providing the context of support from non-judgmental and accepting peers and adults leads to the development of a positive self-image. Caring and helping are vital for overall growth and development. The protective benefit of social support for physically impaired children and their families can offer improved functioning in school. For instance, children with impairments may avoid games with peers, play with younger peers, play overly aggressively, or appear depressed. Internalizing symptoms, such as depression, can ensue once a child with neurological impairment becomes aware of how different they are compared to typical peers. Developmental limitations can be more apparent as students age, which can resurface upon major transitions, such as puberty. Group programming has been acknowledged as an effective way to provide these youth with affirming and supportive social experiences, paving the way for confidence in relationships with all students in an educational school setting (Miyahara & Cratty 2004).

The students in this study were part of a centralized special education program within an Intermediate Unit, a program that draws special needs students from multiple districts. All students met the government classification criteria of "Other Health Impairment," meaning they had a neurological-medical disorder beyond the standard learning disability classifications. As a Nationally Certified School Psychologist who was also trained in Theraplay, I joined as the primary therapist in this program. A classroom teacher for a special education classroom dedicated to neurologically impaired youth assisted with the group therapy. The group therapy was once weekly, one-hour sessions, and ran continuously for a four-year period.

The neurologically focused special education program was designed for school-aged students identified through a neuropsychology or neurology clinic. A multidisciplinary team, including school psychologists with specialized neuropsychology training, along with speech and language clinicians and occupational therapists, would complete a neuropsychological evaluation. Generally, the evaluation process was used to determine acquired or traumatic brain injury, neurodevelopmental disorders, and orthopedic and speech and language impairments. Access to physical therapy or audiology evaluation was available depending on the student's need. The classes for this program would be housed in local public schools to provide specially designed instruction and related services, including speech and language therapy, occupational therapy, physical, and psychological services. Psychological services included weekly psychotherapy and support from multidisciplinary team members. The requirement was identified for an experiential or an authentic group program that could meet multiple needs, such as limited language skills, youth with orthopedic physical supports, and those needing wheelchair assistance.

Group Theraplay as the therapeutic modality

Group Theraplay was chosen as the primary psychotherapeutic intervention. Theraplay was identified as relevant because of the emphasis on non-verbal and experiential interactions rather than verbal discussion. Students with a range of neurologically involved medical conditions are able to participate in the Theraplay activities. Furthermore, Theraplay's emphasis on structure, engagement, nurture, and challenge meet the social-emotional needs of the students within the context of in-vivo, real-time, playful socialization. The lessons of a Theraplay group could be easily transferred into everyday classroom situations. The activities were determined to be easily adaptable to a variety of youth differences in emotional regulation, sensory–motor integration, communication, and social-emotional learning. This unique group of students benefits greatly from a nurturing community, structured playfulness, and gradual challenges in keeping with stages of recovery or development. Whether developing new skills, recovering old skills, or accommodating permanent skill loss, promoting acceptance of oneself in an atmosphere of joy and compassionate caring improves the chance for healthy outcomes (Miyahara & Cratty 2004). Active play in the context of structured group experiences and expert adult coaching is helpful to youth with neurological conditions and motor impairment (Larkin & Summers 2004), and reduces physical stress (Martikainen et al. 2013). These were additional reasons for choosing Group Theraplay as the therapeutic modality.

The neurobiological deficits that underpin behavioral inhibition and impulsivity are prominent in this group of at-risk students suffering from brain injury or strokes. Theraplay provides an evidence-based treatment that addresses deficient inhibitory processes that place the suffering person and others at risk for serious consequences that impact everyday life (Bari & Robbins 2013). Furthermore, neurodevelopmental problems, such as attention deficit hyperactivity disorder (ADHD) and Tourette syndrome, have adverse impacts on social wellbeing (Eapen, Cavanna, & Robertson 2016; Scott et al. 2015). Loss of skills and a long recovery from neurological injury or illness can delay the developmental experiences that typical students are able to draw on for healthy maturation. Recovery from childhood or adolescent aneurysm rupture can be quite long after discharge from hospital, and treatment with rehabilitative procedures can be protracted. Children with severe epilepsy may experience developmental regression at the time of onset of seizures (Schubert 2009). Understanding the irregular development, neurological symptoms, stages of recovery, and expected plateaus and regressions along the way were necessary when designing Theraplay experiences in a group setting. A reason for choosing Theraplay as the model was its flexibility in application across ages and developmental levels. Furthermore, the four key dimensions (structure, engagement, nurture, and challenge) can serve as a framework for addressing the developmental-emotional needs of individual children.

Group Theraplay for teens with a neurological disorder

Students in the neurological-impaired high school program included those with lobectomy, seizures, aneurysm, Tourette syndrome, brain injury, and severe developmental learning problems. A psychotherapeutic group format was chosen to best accommodate a wide range of neurological impairments and allow new students to enter throughout a nine-month school year.

This particular group presented with a unique shared experience of brain-related problems, including neurodevelopmental disabilities, acquired brain injuries, and TBI, laying the foundation for social connection and empathy. Group Theraplay illustrations are presented here, highlighting unique group dynamics, neurological medical-learning needs, and the expansive benefits of Theraplay with this critical population.

 ## CASE ILLUSTRATION 1: ENGAGEMENT AND NURTURE

The group developed special handshakes to bring a collective engagement and connection that is useful in bringing fun, arousal, and check-in with each other. The use of music to orient the group is a helpful transition into the session and to set the stage for whole group engagement.

Rodney was apprehensive and angry about returning to a public school even though he had already "graduated" from public high school. At the same time, he felt curious and encouraged about his last phase of recovery with peers who were close to his age in the neurologically impaired classroom. He was looking forward to leaving the nursing home where most of the residents were elderly. Rodney toggled with his now functional, non-dominant fingers to motor his wheelchair into the "neuro"-focused Theraplay group of high school students with a range of neurological impairments, ranging in age from 15 to 20. Rodney was able to enter this therapeutic program (addressing educational, medical, and psychological needs) with an IEP since special education can continue to 21 years of age.

Three students demonstrated the group's three-step signature handshake while Rodney followed the movements with his eyes. A nurturing high school senior, Richie, reached out toward Rodney's outstretched thumb, index, and middle fingers as his arm hovered over the toggle switch. As Richie locked finger grip with Rodney, he leaned down toward Rodney for a shoulder bump and a pat on the shoulder, and then slid his hand back to once again grip fingers. Rodney reacted with nervous laughter and called out an expletive conveying surprise and disbelief. Sensing Rodney's embarrassment, Richie backed away and expressed compassion, drawing on his own initial feelings of vulnerability as a new group member two years prior.

As music from Jack Johnson gradually filled the room, the student group members formed a circle around Rodney. A garbage bag of air-filled balloons was tossed into the air for members to hit back and forth to each other. If you attend a rock music concert event, you will find people hitting giant balloons in the air from one side of the venue to the other. The benefit of the very large balloon is that two people can safely hit it with greater strength, or one person has a large area to hit. Using the ideal technique for ascending the balloon can be noticed and replicated for increased accuracy and fun, especially for those with motor limitations.

As the therapist tossed a medium-sized garbage bag filled with balloons into the air, several group members excitedly yelled, "All right!" The teacher (assisting with the session) took a step and used two hands under the bag to loft it back to the therapist. Jeremy's name was then called out just before the bag went to him. He then hit the bag with his open hands so that it went straight to Rodney who used his fist in an uppercut movement that brought the bag up in the air for Terry to hit. A sense of awe or surprise was observed on the faces of members when Rodney engaged his strong punch. The game was paused as the therapist complimented Rodney's strong fist uppercut punch that made the air balloon ascend to the farthest member. To provide a nurturing touch and build his self-confidence, the therapist wrapped Rodney's fist and arm position in aluminum foil as a model for all to study. Rodney's foil was passed around for examination, students noticing the prominent middle finger knuckle and elbow position that reflected his unique punch that promised to deliver the bag to a member of the circle.

Theraplay and neuropsychological rationale 1

Although motor functions can be impaired in individuals with neurological disorders, Theraplay techniques can support improved functioning in daily living and in joyful movement activities. Hand movement strength and structured motor activities paired with fun and engaging social connection can offer support for improved functioning. For example, the use of a large bag of air-filled balloons enables paired group members to synchronize hitting the bag with their respective hands. Becoming more independent and controlled in his movement, one group member would hit the bag with his fist supporting relatively controlled arm and hand movement following practice rounds. McGowan et al. (2004) observed that frequent use of hand fist or grip activities embedded within various exercises is associated with the regulation of blood pressure and healthy blood vessel function. In 2021, a significant decrease in systolic blood pressure—that is, the heart pumping blood to the rest of the body—was found with isometric exercise, 12–20 minutes per day, three times per week (Rickson at al. 2021). As such, coordinated collaboration among the school-based physical therapist, occupational therapist, and school psychologist developed group activities with these observations in mind for maximum therapeutic benefit. This increased confidence in the therapists, while increasing the chance of success for group members with varying physiological, daily living, and social-personal needs.

It was observed that adolescents with neurological impairments experienced chronic feelings of insecurity stemming from a history of their parents' own anxiety around their child's developing autonomy and confidence due to neurological symptoms. Through Group Theraplay, adolescents developed personal security and assurance to the point of asserting leadership, making suggestions for Theraplay sessions. Upon accepting vulnerabilities and humanness through a shared therapeutic experience of Theraplay, group members develop a profound shift to a healthy sense of self and purpose in a social community. A sense of safety in a group allows an insecure member to embrace vulnerability that paradoxically brings about courageousness for improved social security and leadership. As a result, the group members grow to appreciate and accept their own shared feelings of security. They subsequently become more willing to risk vulnerability with challenge while also embracing nurturing members and therapists. Particular group members can develop attunement and responsiveness in caring for others. Members begin to observe a renewed sense of wholeness in their masculinity to one that includes emotional connection. The group process also helps members appreciate and resolve the question of "Who am I in this social world?"

CASE ILLUSTRATION 2: ENGAGEMENT AND CHALLENGE

From the start, face-to-face, bilateral, rhythmic hand clapping engaged group members getting the group into a cohesive sync. Members of the group paired off and used exercise grip chalk on one another's palms for the creation of various shapes. Samuel's partner attempted to draw a shape in a student's palm while Samuel's eyes were closed. Samuel leaned away while offering his hand to his partner. Samuel's shoulders dropped and his hand became supple with a very slow pace of writing on his palm. The designated shape "written" in chalk was "passed" from one person to the other within the circled group until all participants received and wrote the design in the palm of their hand. At the close to the sensory touch connection, Justin and Benjamin spontaneously created puffs of powder to arise from the hand contact in a "high-five" partner hand clap. Other members impulsively created multiple puffs without consideration of others' proximity. Responding to spontaneity, the therapist and assistant appealed to the interest of the group with the addition of safe structure. After providing safe distance of participants, the timing of members' puffs was calibrated to create a sequenced "'firework' cloud of chalk dust." Supporting the group's shared fun experience within a space-maintaining structure increased group cohesion and engagement. The circle transitioned from an energetic activity with low strength challenge to a seated line formation in preparation for a strength challenge event.

Following a transition to the seated position, a soft-grip athletic rope with bright strips of tape indicating hand placement was placed alongside group members' bodies as they sat on the floor in a line formation for "team"-based "pull-up." Participants sat on the carpeted floor, except for Rodney and Richie sitting on chairs on the ends of the line. To establish attention, self-control, synchronization, and safe participation, participants were not to reach for the rope until the key two-word phrase was called out. To capitalize on Richie's improved inhibition or impulsiveness, he was selected to call out a similar-sounding "distractor" or "false alarm" two-word command "Get it," so members could hold back from responding to distraction. The support of another member's unique voice and physical distance from Richie, Rodney, called out the actual command for correct responding. Immediately after hearing Rodney call out the pre-identified key phrase "Grab it," members successfully reached for the taped markers on the rope.

The tape ensured predetermined spacing for members based on distance. Pillows were placed between participants to maintain safety should a person fall backward during the activity. Subsequently, the therapist and/or teacher would "safety check" hand-to-rope grip, placing hands over each member's handgrip attached to the rope, offering nurturing touch for calm security and encouragement. Participant handgrips were also wrapped in foil to examine for handgrip form, including finger identification and placement for safe and ease of "team" pull-up.

After hearing the count down, "3, 2, 1, Go," from either chair-seated participant, a pair on one side of the rope—that is, half of the rope's length—would "pull up" the opposing pair holding on to the other half of the rope, lifting from lying back to full-seated position. For safety, the therapist and the teacher sat behind the chair-seated participants to ensure an adequate amount of tension and grip support needed for one side to lift the lying pair into a seated position. Assessment of the participants' handgrip strength and fatigue would trigger an end to the activity. Despite successful pair pull-up, members were surprised with the success of the "team" pull-up given the initial reluctance, increasing the group's mental and physical strength.

Theraplay and neuropsychological rationale 2

Brain injury from trauma, such as a cerebrovascular accident, anoxia, or a brain tumor, can occur in different areas of the brain that control functions such as sensory perception, motor control, cognition, emotions, personality, awareness, communication, and language. The grip chalk, a touch of fists and fingers, palm writing, and arm–hand motor activation all served to activate the sensory and/or motor systems of the brain and met the need to promote care for one another. The primary and secondary association areas of the parietal lobe and motor areas of the brain can become a focus of treatment. The identification of shapes on the palm directly activates the parietal lobe, related to graphesthesia. The use of safe, nurturing touch and attention to physical connection helped activate the essential sensory motor skills and increase the value of peer and adult support to meet challenges. Relatedly, the parietal lobe and the frontal lobe (the front part of the head) work together for execution of behavior. Executive functions in the front part of the brain are engaged in the format of selecting and executing a response and suppressing an impulse to move or speak (NIMH n.d.). Underlying brain circuitry involves the posterior parietal lobe, the dorsolateral prefrontal cortex, and the ventrofronto-striatal circuits of the brain. These higher-order or executive function areas are key behaviors for intervention in individuals with brain injury and many neurological conditions.

 ## CASE ILLUSTRATION 3: CHALLENGE AND STRUCTURE

BOBSLEDDING

The Theraplay approach to "Bobsledding" (Encyclopaedia Britannica n.d.) adapts a stationary, floor-based "pretend" bobsled that participants learn to run with and jump on in sequence for a simulated group sled ride. Alternating or random left and right movement of the "sled" through stimulated "curved turns" occur with the therapist or other adult leader guiding riders with athletic, soft ropes.

ISOMETRIC HOLDS

Isometric "holds" in-group involve solo, dyad, triad, or whole-group body position "holds" that use stabilization rather than moving for improved strength. According to Edward Laskowski, Co-Director of Mayo Clinic Sports Medicine Clinic, isometrics rehabilitates muscles, improves joint flexibility, and lowers blood pressure (Laskowski n.d.).

The use of structure helps to organize, regulate, and adapt to new situations that build essential confidence, growth, and safety. Beyond the fun favorite and challenging event, the bobsled is highly dependent on structured or scaffolded support activating individuals' personal sensory and motor capacities. This challenge is structured to create optimal success in a synchronized team fashion. Imagine group members working in unison using coordinated movement to create the real feel of a bobsledder. This appeals to athletic competency for students who may feel inadequate due to neurological injuries. Indeed, previously athletic students could feign illness to avoid "athletic" demands (Miyahara & Cratty 2004).

The winter season typically brought relevance to the bobsled event within the Group Theraplay session. The classroom winter theme of sledding events, including dog sled and bobsled, takes place within this high school class. Connecting with this theme, this Theraplay group becomes a bobsled team, learning the underlying bobsled techniques or foundational physical skills that will enable the team to perform a simulated bobsled run. After this activity the therapist and teacher observed group members demonstrating behaviors of safety and care for others. This demanding experience appeared to facilitate an increased degree of trust and emotional engagement with each other.

Preliminary isometric exercises were completed by participants at their desks rather than in small groups, providing practice for the movements involved in the bobsled activity. Students gripped the sides of the chair seat firmly and straightened their arms for reduced weight of the buttocks on the seat. They remained in the lift position for a count of five, and then returned to the original position while breathing out for a count of five. Members then transitioned to partner isometrics—paired members stood facing their partners and linked hands together with one palm facing upwards and the other down towards the floor. Samuel struggled with the additional challenge to maintain eye contact with his partner, increasing frustration and complaint of both parties.

Several practice rounds of maintaining eye contact with low-demand activities facilitated "readiness" for Samuel to meet the attention and the position awareness necessary for a return to the target goal. Using a cue word to trigger the start, partners leaned back until a strong pull was achieved and held for five counts. During this short time, they maintained eye contact for partner connection and signal support to begin, adjust, or end the isometric exercise.

For the bobsled event, able-body members would run or lightly jog in place next to the bobsled, and then serially hop into the imaginary bobsled in a sequenced, alternated (left and right sides of the sled) fashion, with close-seated positions behind one another "in" the sled. Except for the first member in the bobsled, all other members leaned on the person in front of them for added appropriate touch that occurs in a real bobsled to reduce wind drag and maintain speed.

For effect, I generated wind with a large pillow wave to create the effect of movement and sensory experience. In addition, soft athletic ropes on both sides of the bobsled (i.e., alongside the bobsled participants' bodies) were pulled by the co-leader in alternating left and right directional positions for a sensation of turning movement, simulating "slide curves" down the winding track. Surprisingly, Samuel could tolerate the multiple sensory experiences while sitting between two members and leaning onto one another while holding on to the ropes. All members supporting one another while managing movement and sensory demands helped the group gain cooperation, connection, and confidence. Members responded with enthusiasm and excitement, collaborating in the experience together, feeling relational connection and appropriate challenge.

Theraplay and neuropsychological rationale 3

Isolated and controlled stimulation with alternating degrees of intensity and rhythms are foundational for behavioral regulation. The alerting system and sensory motor control feedback (i.e., reticular activating system) assist the neurological system to adapt to simple and complex movements, including sitting or standing while performing occupational tasks in a workstation area.

Demands for balance and postural control training are critical areas for brain injury rehabilitation and for establishing a degree of challenge for stability and sensory support. Establishing appropriate challenges, with safety as a priority, builds self-esteem and confidence. Considering the physical limitations, modifications for Theraplay bobsled included one individual lying down on a thick yoga mat while members rock the "skeleton" racer down the track in unison based on rope movement under the mat for the sensory cue to move through "curves" down the simulated track.

CASE ILLUSTRATION 4: ENGAGEMENT AND STRUCTURE
STATUE

One or more people maintain a body position that is associated with a particular pose or cultural figure, such as a sports figure or superhero. Eyes are kept open, although they can be closed for increased challenge. The isolated body positional features of the particular or unique pose can be highlighted using aluminum foil.

IN AND OUT

This is a drill activity that skiers and soccer players learn. All it takes is some pylons or cone or bucket obstacles that are arranged into a pattern with a few feet of space between each of them. Participants weave in and out of the buckets as they walk or run. The closer the cones are to one another, the greater the degree of challenge. Placement of a book or an object on the head of the participant moving can be used to slow down the person with an additional challenge to balance while navigating the pylons or cones.

SALT AND PEPPER

Salt and pepper is a call-and-response activity. The identified "caller" speaks aloud (or holds up word cards) either "salt" or "pepper" and the group remains or moves to the designated season side, using lined tape or rope to separate the sides. Identifying salt as a mineral and pepper as a spice can be used for these seasonings. Additional demands can make this task more engaging and fun.

In the middle of the group, Justin stood and positioned himself in a baseball batter position or statue while members looked on. Benjamin called out, "Go Bucs!" Richie named the held position as the group therapist asked him to approach Justin as he held the statue position. Richie gave feedback to Justin, offering to reposition the right elbow and shoulders. I repositioned Justin for a more power-hitting statue pose that was held while the members noticed each position for the power stance. The use of a small stuffed or bean-filled animal placed on his elbow allowed Justin to "sense" the position to hold. Spontaneously, Justin tilted his chin up slightly once the pose was held without the supports, expressing a sense of pride on his face as the group looked at his held "hitting" pose. Justin held his position as if a statue on a baseball trophy for a one-minute hold. Richie then took a turn to hold the "superman" pose, placing one arm up in the air with the other arm bent, placing a fist on his hip. Security allowed him to accept feedback to grab a tossed bean bag in his direction while still holding a non-dominant hand fist in the air. The statue activity slows the body to a standstill for a holding of the position while not responding to distractions that would "break" the held pose. Shifting between slow or no movement to active movement can facilitate the growth of self-regulation (Bundy-Myrow 2010). Therefore, this in-and-out activity involves a transition to a faster pace alternating with being still.

The shift from structured slow-and-still pattern to stop-and-go movement (walking) substantially increased engagement and supported self-regulation. Group members and leaders followed each other walking in a line while weaving "in and out" of evenly distributed buckets placed in a pattern around the room. As Rodney lifted a traffic stop sign, the group could stop and hold the "freeze" position—that is, the skill related to in the above statue activity. Inconsistent with the goal or rule, Richie, Jeremy, and Justin spontaneously knocked down three buckets in the first two rounds. To support their success, I placed small paperback workbook(s) on their head to slow the pace and increase structure for improved self-control and confidence. Instead of knocking the buckets down, the participating members moved while either holding the workbook on their head or attempting to balance the book. This offered improved attention and sensory feedback for structured support to follow the "No hurts" safety rule—that is, knocking down buckets in the walking path.

Once Rodney raised the "go" traffic sign to a return to walking, all members—without books—successfully and efficiently weaved in and out of all "standing" buckets with safety structure intact. More importantly, members responded to the teacher and myself with physical structure to maintain cooperation and fun experience for similar subsequent group challenges. Moving from literal to relatable substituted words provided a concrete basis for Justin who struggles to respond with abstract words. In addition, the bucket placement offered spatial memory for the subsequent salt and pepper activity.

The alternating bucket–student placement pattern provided a safe distance for the next sequenced "go, no-go" experience of a safe salt and pepper activity. To provide further support, the teacher strategically placed bright duct tape on the floor, parallel to the lined buckets, while members were in the "ready" position. A line of tape was also placed on the floor parallel to the main dividing line. The words designated for each side were written on the tape for a supportive view. For several rounds, the salt and pepper game began with the group therapist calling out, "salt" and then "pepper." Members benefited from a slow-paced "call-out" for all members to successfully stay or move into the ruling "season." Benjamin impulsively began calling out the current season, confusing the group and the adults.

Responding to the need for greater structure and safety, I reiterated the rule of adult-only call-outs and looked for structured boundaries, minimizing the potential for "hurts." My leadership or the teacher's leadership to release students' expectation of taking on the call-outs allowed for the participants to focus their mental resources for learning and using the new skills. In addition, buckets were placed on both sides of the tape to increase the space among members and to further define the goal target area. Random call-outs for the mineral and the spice then ensued, engaging the "go, no-go" system of the executive brain. Several members committed several movement errors or false moves, mistakenly moving toward the designated spice side of the mineral. The words "salt" or "pepper" were written on carpet tape and then placed on the carpet target areas. Although a literacy or reading demand, this support significantly increased the likelihood of all students experiencing degrees of success. Next, the teacher alternated between raising separate signs with the words "salt" or "pepper," activating visual attention and concentration. Group members either jumped over or rolled over (i.e., the wheelchair) the duct tape based on the ruling "seasoning" poster card.

Rodney became frustrated as the poster cards were raised with increasing pace, as moving his wheelchair became more challenging. Kerry became discouraged from making more errors with the introduction of the cards-only situation. As a result, Richie offered a signal to direct Rodney, using cards in proximity. Accepting the accommodation, Rodney laughed aloud while Richie took over assisting Rodney's movement. Kerry began lifting cards in the air, watching classmates look to him for direction. He began to laugh in unison with all members. The teacher and I shared in the humor of the escalating fun to remain in this activity while not taking ourselves too seriously, allowing ourselves to connect to vulnerability and humanness.

In subsequent weeks, members became quite adept at the card-only condition, allowing the words on the card to reflect the opposite color of the seasoning. The box font letters were filled with the color black and the box font letters in "pepper" were left white to match the poster card color. This changed the rule to do the opposite of what the seasoning reads. For example, if the original poster card, "salt," was side A, then the filled black font letters of "salt" become side B. In other words, doing the opposite of what is stated becomes the demand. Developmentally, some adolescents enjoy doing the opposite of social, imposed rules, which adds to the attraction of this activity. The teacher and I modeled vulnerability, sending the message that it can be safe being confused and frustrated when having to adjust on the fly. Having student participants challenge us adults with the highest demand of activity sequence helped them to value persistence in the face of failure.

Theraplay and neuropsychological rationale 4

The statue activity engages the interests of participant members, including superheroes and sports figures (Cuddy 2015), and incorporates body awareness, attention, and motor persistence (Mahone *et al.* 2006). Motor persistence is holding or maintaining eyes closed on verbal command, associated with diffuse brain damage or right hemisphere impairment (Joynt, Benton, & Fogel 1962). Carney, Cuddy, and Yap (2010) conducted research on the benefits of holding "power" poses for one minute. The benefits of improved psychological, physiological, and behavioral systems of the participants were affirmed. The statue activity also incorporates a pose hold with distractors while eyes are occluded or closed. The therapist initially conceptualized the statue activity within Theraplay as a treatment for adolescents who struggle with concentration and motor control, such as impulsivity, and/or adolescents who feel insecure and powerless. Children with high-functioning autism have greater problems with motor persistence than impulsivity. However, children who have an ADHD are found to have greater problems with motor persistence and conflicting motor response. This was certainly the case for students from the neurologically impaired classroom.

The ability to start a new action—that is, moving or speaking, in a way that competes or conflicts with an old way of acting or speaking—is impaired for those with TBI or prefrontal brain-related problems, such as ADHD. Difficulty in adjusting to rule changes or ways of doing something can generate frustration and withdrawal. Increasing structure support within an atmosphere of fun and targeted challenge appeals to adolescents to optimize the feeling of success. It builds personal and social acceptance. Kerry benefited from structures to become the "leader," after modeling, rehearsal, and practice created predictability and reduced the chance for error. This effect was observed during the salt and pepper activity, a classic "go, no-go" format that engages the motor and behavior controls associated with the prefrontal lobe. Despite the engaging and appealing format, Kerry struggled with the visual rather than the auditory demands on attention. Auditory stimuli can be easier for some students to hold attention as there is no need to maintain continuous eye contact for visual cues (Sandford & Anton 2020). As a result, the group leader challenged Kerry to take the "lead" and release the additional burden on the group participants.

As success improves and confidence ensues, the last modification of the salt and pepper activity is safely challenged once again. Participants and leaders are engaged in challenging the impulse to move and the need for mental flexibility. The "Stroop effect" (1935) paradigm challenges these behaviors as they are important for quick and accurate decision making when faced with opposing rules ("If you hear salt, go to pepper side"). Related to prior brain anatomy around inhibition, this skill of inhibiting a response involves a critical mesial frontal circuit, important for emotional regulation, impulse control, and decision making (Chevée *et al.* 2022; de la Vega *et al.* 2016; Waugh, Lemus, & Gotlib 2014). These types of games exercise these executive abilities. A significant amount of practice for the therapist and co-leader to model the task with vulnerability (i.e., making mistakes and corrections) sends the message that it can be "okay" to feel uncertain or frustrated due to mistakes, but that these feelings should not deter participation and persistence. Accepting challenging feelings while flexibly accessing therapeutic support and structure from others, either adult group facilitators or peer members, can lead to primary feelings of pride, confidence, and joy.

Conclusion

Theraplay provides a naturally engaging and nurturing psychotherapeutic approach to provide fun and targeted challenges relevant to adolescents with neurological impairments. The social format provides experiences in cooperation, emotional connection, and compassion for group members' unique yet shared neurological impairment experiences. The format provides opportunities for fun and nurturing relationships while maintaining the dignity of learners as they adapt and relate to each other's experience. These adolescents had a fresh awakening to the melding of neuropsychological techniques from a rehabilitation framework into Theraplay's theory and neurodevelopmental considerations. This is a stark contrast to the traditional rehabilitation treatment to meet neurological needs that often focuses on medical improvement or cognitive skills in the absence of social-peer context. Integrating techniques from psychotherapy, neuropsychological rehabilitation, group therapy, and Theraplay proved an ideal method of promoting social rapport, therapeutic motivation, and school integration. This is consistent with literature discussing the integration of psychotherapy and neuropsychological rehabilitation in the context of a structured play format in school for improved adaptive functioning (Ylvisaker 2003; Ylvisaker *et al.* 2005).

The positive impact on the students was accentuated following an announcement near the program end that the group psychotherapist was being reassigned based on organization needs. As the final group preparation began, the students approached the psychotherapist to declare that the Theraplay materials were staying in a hidden part of the classroom so the Theraplay group could remain part of their class. The grief of ending our Theraplay time became an unexpected focus that motivated the group to continue planning events that could replicate what was learned and apply it with the support of the teacher. Working toward acceptance and using gradual release helped the group value what they learned and incorporate it into a shared value for future students.

References

ASHA (American Speech-Language-Hearing Association). (n.d.). Pediatric traumatic brain injury. Clinical Topics. www.asha.org/practice-portal/clinical-topics/pediatric-traumatic-brain-injury/#collapse_1

Bari, A., & Robbins, T. W. (2013). Inhibition, and impulsivity: Behavioral and neural basis of response control. *Progress in Neurobiology 108*, 44–79. doi:10.1016/j.pneurobio.2013.06.005

Bundy-Myrow, S. (2010). Theraplay for Children with Self-Regulation Problems. In C. Schaefer, J. McCormick, & A. Ohnogi (Eds), *International Handbook of Play Therapy: Advancements in Assessment, Theory, Research and Practice* (pp.35–64). Jason Aronson.

Carney, D. R., Cuddy, A. J., & Yap, A. J. (2010). Power posing: Brief nonverbal displays affect neuroendocrine levels and risk tolerance. *Psychology Science 21*(10): 1363–1368. doi: 10.1177/0956797610383437

Chevée, M., Finkel, E. A., Kim, S., O'Connor, D. H., & Brown, S. P. (2022). Neural activity in the mouse claustrum in a cross-modal sensory selection task. *Neuron 110*(3), 486–501. doi:10.1016/j.neuron.2021.11.013

Cuddy, A. (2015). *Presence: Bringing Your Boldest Self to Your Biggest Challenges.* Little, Brown Spark.

de la Vega, A., Chang, L. J., Banich, M. T., Wager, T. D., & Yarkoni, T. (2016). Large-scale meta-analysis of human medial frontal cortex reveals tripartite functional organization. *Journal of Neuroscience 36*(24), 6553–6562. doi:10.1523/JNEUROSCI.4402-15.2016

Eapen, V., Cavanna, A. E., & Robertson, M. M. (2016). Comorbidities, social impact, and quality of life in Tourette syndrome. *Frontiers in Psychiatry 7*, 97. doi:10.3389/fpsyt.2016.00097.

Encyclopaedia Britannica. (n.d.). Bobsledding. www.britannica.com/sports/bobsledding

Fink, E. L., Kochanek, P. M., Tasker, R. C., Beca, J., Bell, M. J., Clark, R. S., Hutchison, J., Vavilala, M., Fabio, A., Angus, D. C., & Watson, R. S. (2017). International survey of critically ill children with acute neurologic insults: The prevalence of acute critical neurological disease in children: A global epidemiological assessment study. *Pediatric Critical Care Medicine 18*(4), 330–342. https://doi.org/10.1097/PCC.0000000000001093

Joynt, R. J., Benton, A. L., & Fogel, M. L. (1962). Behavioral and pathological correlates of motor impersistence. *Neurology 12*(12), 876. https://doi:10.1212/WNL.12.12.876

Larkin, D., & Summers, J. (2004). Implications of Movement Difficulties for Social Interaction, Physical Activity, Play, and Sports. In D. Dewey and D. Tupper (Eds), *Developmental Motor Disorders: A Neuropsychological Perspective* (pp.443–457). Guilford Press.

Laskowski, E. R. (n.d.). Are isometric exercises a good way to build strength? Healthy Lifestyle, Fitness. Mayo Clinic. www.mayoclinic.org/healthy-lifestyle/fitness/expert-answers/isometric-exercises/faq-20058186

Mahone, E., Powell, S., Loftis, C., Goldberg, M., Denckla, M., & Mostofsky, S. (2006). Motor persistence and inhibition in autism and ADHD. *Journal of the International Neuropsychological Society 12*(5), 622–631. doi:10.1017/S1355617706060814

Martikainen, S., Pesonen, A.-K., Lahti, J., Heinonen, K., Feldt, K., Pyhälä, R., Tammelin, T.,

Kajantie, E., Eriksson, J. G., Standberg, T. E., & Räikkönen, K. (2013). Higher levels of physical activity are associated with lower hypothalamic-pituitary-adrenocortical axis reactivity to psychosocial stress in children. *The Journal of Clinical Endocrinology & Metabolism 98*(4), E619–E627. https://doi.org/10.1210/jc.2012-3745

McGowan, C. L., Visocchi, A., Faulkner, M., Rakobowchuk, M., McCartney, N., & MacDonald, M. J. (2004). Isometric handgrip training improves blood pressure and endothelial function in persons medicated for hypertension. *Physiologist 47*, 285. doi:10.1007/s00421-006-0337-z.

Miyahara, M., & Cratty, J. B. (2004). Psychosocial Functions of Children and Adolescents with Movement Disorders. In D. Dewey and D. Tupper (Eds), *Developmental Motor Disorders: A Neuropsychological Perspective* (pp.427–442). Guilford Press.

Moreau, J. F., Fink, E. L., Hartman, M. E., Angus, D. C., Bell, M. J., Linde-Zwirble, W. T., & Watson, R. S. (2013). Hospitalizations of children with neurologic disorders in the United States. *Pediatric Critical Care Medicine 14*(8), 801–810. https://doi.org/10.1097/PCC.0b013e31828aa71f

NCES (National Center for Education Statistics). (2022). Students with disabilities. Condition of Education. US Department of Education, Institute of Education Science. https://nces.ed.gov/fastfacts/display.asp?id=64

NIMH (National Institute of Mental Health). (n.d.). Motor persistence paradigms. Research Domain Criteria Initiative. www.nimh.nih.gov/research/research-funded-by-nimh/rdoc/constructs/suppression

Rickson, J. J., Maris, S. A., & Headley, S. A. E. (2021). Isometric exercise training: a review of hypothesized mechanisms and protocol application in persons with hypertension. *International Journal of Exercise Science 14*(2), 1261–1276. www.ncbi.nlm.nih.gov/pmc/articles/PMC8758172/

Sandford, J. A., & Anton, S. E. (2020). *Brain Train IVA-2 Integrated Visual and Auditory Continuous Performance Test Manual*. Brain Train.

Schubert, R. (2009). Cognitive Dysfunction and Other Comorbidities: Attention Deficit Disorder and Epilepsy in Children. In P. A. Schwartzkroin (Ed.), *Encyclopedia of Basic Epilepsy Research* (pp.141–146). Academic Press.

Scott, J. G., Mihalopoulos, C., Erskine, H. E., Roberts, J., & Rahma, A. (2016). Childhood Mental and Developmental Disorders. In V. Patel, D. Chisholm, T. Dua, R. Laxminarayan, & M. E. Medina-Mora (Eds), *Mental, Neurological, and Substance Use Disorders: Disease Control Priorities* (Third Edition, Volume 4) (Chapter 8). The International Bank for Reconstruction and Development/The World Bank. www.ncbi.nlm.nih.gov/books/NBK361938

Stroop, J. R. (1935). Studies of interference in serial verbal reactions. *Journal of Experimental Psychology 18*(6), 643–662. https://doi.org/10.1037/h0054651

Waugh, C. E., Lemus, M. G., & Gotlib, I. H. (2014). The role of the medial frontal cortex in the maintenance of emotional states. *Social Cognitive and Affective Neuroscience 9*(12), 2001–2009. https://doi.org/10.1093/scan/nsu011

Ylvisaker, M. (2003). Context-sensitive cognitive rehabilitation: Theory and practice. *Brain Impairment 4*(1), 1–16. https://doi.org/10.1375/brim.4.1.1.27031

Ylvisker, M., Andelson, D., Braga, L. W., Burnett, S. M., Glang, A., Feeney, T., Moore, W., Rumney, P., & Todis, B. (2005). Rehabilitation and ongoing support after pediatric TBI: Twenty years of progress. *Journal of Head Trauma Rehabilitation 20*(1), 95–109. doi: 10.1097/00001199-200501000-00009

Chapter 17

The Case for Theraplay within Homeless and Transient Housing Services

Joanna Fortune

Introduction

With the rising numbers of families and children experiencing homelessness and for longer periods of time, the need for trauma-informed and evidence-based therapeutic models has become more pronounced. Theraplay's status as an evidence-based model (SAMHSA 2017[1]) that is embedded in attachment and trauma theory made it the ideal framework for our project. If "home is feeling connected and safe," and we know that play fuels connection, we wanted to bring trauma-informed play to the forefront of this sector. Furthermore, parenting is about connection, and we know that the parent–child relationship is the most powerful and influential element for change in outcomes for children's lives. As an evidence-based, attachment- and trauma-informed, relational, play-based therapeutic model, Theraplay is the perfect fit. This chapter presents a specific program using a modified Group Theraplay Training format that I applied with a broad range of staff who work within homeless services in a specific geographical area. I present how this program was funded, supported, and facilitated as well as the modifications involved and lessons learned as a template for others to apply within their countries and work settings.

---

1   Substance Abuse and Mental Health Services Administration, USA has rated Theraplay "effective" (highest rating) on the National Registry for Evidence-Based Programs and Practices.

Why Group Theraplay, and why the +?

Janet Healy and I[2] have been working collaboratively with Nuala Nic Giobúin, the coordinator of CYPSC (Children and Young People's Services Committee, a state organization) in Dublin City South on a program to deliver a modified three-day Group Theraplay training that includes a trauma-focused third day to organizations working within the homeless sector in Ireland.[3] This program began in 2019 and is ongoing at the time of publication (2023). It is our assertion that this modification of the Group Theraplay model is a format that is easily adaptable in other countries and in other social environments.

Using Theraplay's three types of Theraplay intervention, pyramid tier two was identified as the most appropriate for this project. Tier two is the application of the Theraplay model most suited to focused Theraplay intervention—family or group work. This is because most of the staff we were training hold a variety of therapeutic roles but are not therapists or mental health clinicians. The service users' present needs are more complex than tier one's Group Theraplay or Sunshine Circles for general populations. This is a focused intervention for a specific population, and we were starting from a place of acknowledging and accepting that experiencing homelessness is a trauma in and of itself, regardless of other traumatic experiences that led up to or contributed to the family experiencing homelessness. Moreover, homelessness is a complex trauma, and as such, the solution is more complex than a bricks and mortar house (FEANTSA 2017).

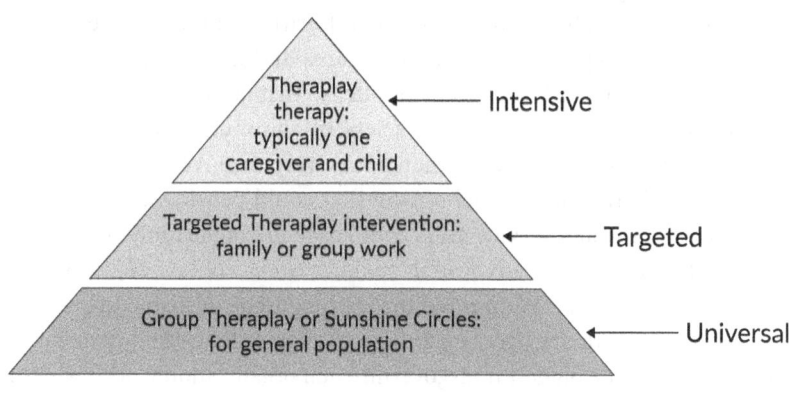

Theraplay intervention pyramid
SOURCE: THE THERAPLAY INSTITUTE

---

2   Janet Healy, Psychoanalytic Psychotherapist at Reflecting Minds Psychotherapy, collaborated on the development and delivery of this program from the outset.

3   This program was supported with funding from the Healthy Ireland Fund supported by the Department of Health and the Department of Children and Youth Affairs Ireland.

Based on the above, we decided that our specialized Theraplay program would be a Group Theraplay+ three-day training model. This meant that we would deliver the classic two-day Group Theraplay training program but add a bespoke third day that would speak directly to the experience of homelessness as a trauma.

Our goal was to create a critical mass of Group Theraplay-trained professionals within the homeless sector resulting in "Theraplay-informed care" across the community. It should be noted that with minor changes this format could be used within other community sectors too, such as domestic violence, addiction, youth justice, etc.

Why homelessness?

The number of families experiencing homelessness in Ireland increased from 429 in February 2015 to 1707 in February 2019, an increase of 298 percent. This figure lowered slightly to 1488 families (that is, 3355 children) in April 2020, a slight reduction in figures, but still representing far too many families (Siersbaek & Loftus 2020). The number of children living in emergency accommodation has quadrupled, from 938 children in February 2015 to 3784 in February 2019. By April 2020, 3355 children comprised one-third of the entire population of people experiencing homelessness (Siersbaek & Loftus 2020).

Over three-quarters of families in emergency accommodation are living in one of the four Dublin region local authorities. Therefore, we decided to spotlight one regional local authority area and grow a critical mass of professionals all trained in the same model so that families who experience homelessness and engage with a variety of community services in this area would receive a consistent therapeutic response. We were motivated to roll out a therapeutic model of care that could provide a safe, holding environment in which service users could have the opportunity to heal and work. In this regard, we advocated "making every contact count because every contact matters." We wanted the training to be available to everyone who worked within services, regardless of their role in the organization. Focus Ireland is the biggest non-governmental organization working within the homeless sector in Ireland. In 2017, they commissioned specific research to better understand families' pathways in and out of homelessness (Walsh & Harvey 2017). A key finding was that the experience of homelessness affects families in multiple ways. Significantly, parents identified many different ways in which homelessness affected their children, themselves, and their relationships with each other, and they identified how homelessness impacted their broader social networks. A range of practical issues arose, as well as impacts on emotional functioning and mental health. Common themes running through these observations were that, for some, many of these issues became more manageable once the family had made the transition to secure housing, and that staff attitudes—whether positive or negative—had the "biggest impact" on parents.

Two factors were highly significant in the parental statements. One was the impact parents reported that homelessness had on their relationship with their children, and the second was the impact that staff attitudes had on the families' experiences. Theraplay, be it dyadic or group format, is focused on strengthening and enhancing relationships. Further, we are a "right here, right now" therapeutic model promoting opportunities for shared joy within moments of meeting and connection. We work on the understanding that communication can be expressed in actions and without words or having to talk about what is going on or what has happened. This principle enables a parent and child who may struggle to engage in cognitive or talk therapy to process difficult experiences using a bottom-up approach in the brain, entering through the brainstem with sensory input over words. In 2016, I ran a 14-week parent–child Theraplay group for parents who were parenting beyond addiction, and this aspect of the intervention, the practical play, the opportunity to connect and laugh with their children, and "do" rather than "speak," was cited as the most beneficial aspect and the reason that seven-eighths of the parent–child dyads completed all 14 weeks of the program. When everything around you is chaotic, unstable, and uncontained, the transformative power of a "right here, right now," joyful opportunity to connect is extremely powerful. This is an invitation to come out of your head and take a reprieve from the worries and stresses of your physical situation. To play.

The second point about the importance of staff attitudes is another reason to advocate for Theraplay being the ideal therapeutic model in such settings. Theraplay offers something to staff as well. When working in frontline trauma-based services, the exposure to vicarious trauma and risk of compassion fatigue is high.

> The problem for the worker is that such un-housedness, insecurity, and nihilism cannot be split off and got rid of precisely because there are parts of all our minds that remain insecure, un-housed and intensely fearful. As a consequence, individual workers, teams and organisations working with these dynamics inevitably find themselves caught up in related states of un-housedness or incohesion. (Scanlon & Adlam 2019, p.11)

Hughes and Baylin (2012) explained that continually offering a relationship or continually offering care that is not reciprocated can push the carer into a place of "blocked care," whereby the carers protect themselves from further rejection by emotionally stepping back and providing the basics of care without the over-and-above care that is necessary for a relationship to grow and flourish. This is functional care without a bid to connect. Stephen Porges stated at the Theraplay Conference in 2017 that trauma is a chronic disruption to connectedness, so we cannot expect recovery from trauma to take place in the absence of (re)establishing connection.

Group Theraplay offers the opportunity to experience connection within the cohesion of the group. Furthermore, Theraplay offers staff a way to stay emotionally grounded and self-regulated and work through the brainstem upward to process what they are holding themselves. It is fair to assert that by training staff to practice Group Theraplay and some dyadic activities with service users, they will feel better equipped and empowered to respond to the needs of those accessing their services.

Training paraprofessionals

Most of the staff working in the homeless sector are not trained or qualified psychotherapists or psychologists. The services working in this sector are frontline, trauma-based providers responding to the basic needs of those experiencing homelessness. They are not positioned to provide access to long-term or ongoing psychotherapy to service users. This is another reason that the Group Theraplay+ model can be so effective within the homeless sector. The model we proposed aimed to build an attachment environment within the services and equip staff with skills and a practical toolkit that would be therapeutic without crossing into therapy. I suggested that there could be two ways of rolling out the Theraplay groups:

- Open groups: the Theraplay group would run weekly indefinitely on the same day at the same time, and anyone who was present in the service at that time would be welcome to participate.

- Targeted groups: a selected group of participants would be invited to participate in a time-focused group, i.e., once or twice weekly for a set number of weeks ranging from 12 to 20 weeks or longer, if wished.

Suggesting two different applications or group structures reflected those services operating more of a drop-in type of service and those running specialized family hubs or medium- to long-term residencies. While the desire is that families avoid spending prolonged periods of time in a state of homelessness, the statistics show that the majority spend in excess of six months in so-called emergency accommodation, with 30–40 percent spending longer than a year in emergency accommodation (Long *et al.* 2019).

By training all staff in trauma-informed Group Theraplay skills, each of the service users would benefit from accessing services that are embedded in an attachment - and trauma-informed framework, again, advocating that every contact matters.

Parenting without a home

While modifying the Group Theraplay model, I was introduced to a startling statistic (Long *et al.* 2019)—11 percent (of respondents) were classified as new family formations. This means that their entry into homelessness was on the arrival of a new baby. In such an instance, what does this baby come to represent to their parents? How does this impact the parent–child relationship and early attachment formation? We can broaden this question beyond parenting newborns and look at the parent–child relationship through the lens of homelessness in general.

Research by Walsh and Harvey (2017) showed that parents identified that their family's experience of homelessness had impacted their parent–child relationship. Other research from the USA (Faed, Murphy, & Nolledo 2017) found that without access to trauma-informed responses to homelessness, children suffer serious deleterious consequences that can persist into adulthood and can damage their mental, physical, cognitive, and social functioning. This same research also found that mental health challenges were commonplace in children who experienced homelessness, and that such mental health issues increase the older the child is while experiencing homelessness. They highlighted that one-fifth of children aged three to six and two-thirds of adolescents would need mental health treatment.

These findings are consistent with the work of Stephen Porges and Deb Dana (2018) in the field of polyvagal theory. Dana (2018) refers to our ventral vagus as our place of safety and regulation, as our "home," and refers to each of us having a "home away from home" in either sympathetic or dorsal vagus arousal. Of course, the idea is that we can anchor ourselves in our ventral "home," or at least develop a pathway to bring us back to our ventral home after stress. But what of the parent who is parenting in a state of homelessness? A parent who cannot be anchored in their ventral "home" and is in a physical and emotional state of homelessness can find a ventral home, a ventral experience perhaps, within the cohesion and containment of the group dynamic. The space of the Theraplay group can provide a badly needed ventral experience for an un-housed parent and child.

Parenting in an unhoused state of mind

"When a homeless Mother gazes at her child, her own pain and sadness are mirrored back" (Smolen 2015, p.xii). This quote reminds me of the phrase "an un-housed state of mind" (Brown 2019). An unhoused state of mind highlights the psychological underpinnings of current societal problems, and the experience of being homeless can make it hard for the parent to hold a child's needs within their mind.

A state of mind can be defined as your emotional state. I understand an unhoused state of mind to mean a mind that is uncontained and therefore, in the context of the parent–child relationship, it cannot contain a mind in mind—that is, the parent cannot mentalize the experience of the child in order to reflect that back to the child with meaning.

Including parents in Theraplay groups, even if the group structure is child-only rather than a group of parent–child dyads, is vital. If running a child-only Theraplay group, consider starting with one to two group sessions for the parents of those children, to introduce them to the model and orient them to the type of play experiences their children will have. As they play, invite them to pay attention to how the act of playing feels for them now, what it was like as a child for them, and what it might be like for their child. Allow time to share these thoughts at the end of your parent sessions. Consider building in another parent session halfway through and at the end of your Theraplay group. At the end, you could present the parents with a small, basic take-home kit of Theraplay props (a feather, two straws, a toilet roll, small bubbles, balloon, and some lotion) along with some of the activities they have experienced that they can continue to do with their children. With groups such as those experiencing homelessness, I always emphasize activities that require no props. Activities to play with your body or face or hands are very useful in this regard, so build such activities into your groups too.

An unhoused state of mind is something I have seen in the homeless sector but also the domestic violence sector, and within a Group Theraplay program I ran in 2016 with parents who were all parenting beyond addiction.[4] The program we ran, and continue to run at the time of this writing, with staff in the homeless sector is focused on training and supporting them in developing Theraplay groups. This application of Group Theraplay also worked well for the parents recovering from addiction. In the addiction program the goals were the following:

- to improve the parent–child relationship through fun, interactive play

---

4   This was a 14-week Group Theraplay program I delivered in collaboration with two community organizations in 2016. I presented a poster on this work at the Theraplay conference in Chicago 2016.

- to empower the parents to assume their parental role

- to maintain existing levels of access between the parents and children by the end of the group and at least three to six months beyond.

Our results were very positive:

- Seven out of the eight parent–child dyads completed the group work.

- All participants reported a marked improvement in their relationship with each other.

- All maintained existing levels of contact or access throughout the group, and were continuing to maintain it six months later.

At the end of the 14-week program, I concluded that Group Theraplay was a highly effective therapeutic program with families living in complex conditions. Working in a group was experienced as less intense than individual work for all participants. They reported that they didn't feel "monitored," which was important for many of them who had had access with their children supervised at some point. All participants identified the practical play skills Theraplay gave them as the "highlight of the program" and "the aspect they got most benefit from." The debriefing sessions highlighted how participating in a group like this was a learning experience that enhanced their relationships with their children and their first experience of playing and being played with. In addition to the addiction we knew about, we learned that each participating parent had some unresolved childhood trauma. Appropriate follow-up measures were put in place around this fact, and a follow-up mentalization group work for parents was developed. The outcome is best summarized in the words of one participating parent, who said, "This group has shown me that I can be a good parent and that I can enjoy being a parent. I never believed that before," and the eight-year-old child, who said, "Thank you for showing my dad and I how to have fun together. I never saw him laugh before this and he has a great laugh."

The role and function of the "Group"

It is our belief and assertion that the Theraplay Group can accommodate the unhoused state of mind. Take the structure of Group Theraplay:

- *Play groups adapted from Theraplay:* we take the practices and principles of the dyadic model and apply it to the group format.

- *Play groups are 99 percent interactive, 1 percent talking:* we remove the expectation or demand that participants "tell" their story or attend to the administration of the situation, and instead participants get the opportunity to emotionally exhale and be in the moment.

- *Adult-directed and structured:* the group facilitator(s) are there to structure, contain, and guide the group activities, giving participants a break from holding responsibility.

- *Support positive mental health through boosting self-esteem, trust, positive sense of self, self-regulation:* participants are welcomed and accepted as they are, without demands or expectations that they "earn" the opportunity to participate in the group. Nor is participation in the group dependent on any behavioral transgression that may occur outside the group. The group is an autonomous, safe, therapeutic space, free of judgment.

- *Teach pro-social skills for successful social interactions—attention, cooperation, turn-taking, waiting, sharing, etc.:* participation in Group Theraplay will have a positive impact on all aspects of participants' lives outside the group.

- *Build positive relationships and communities:* the experience of homelessness, and in particular prolonged homelessness that can result in that unhoused state of mind, can result in a terrifying internal sense of there not being an inside that can contain "me"/"my child"/"my family." Participation in a group like this can build a sense of community, togetherness, and connections that bring a sense of belonging and feeling claimed, part of something, on the inside of something again, rather than feeling on the outside looking in.

- *Improve group functioning and individual learning:* participants (re)learn the value of being part of a system bigger than themselves. Participants learn about themselves through shared learning and engagement with each other. Theraplay groups are about fun and shared joy. In order to enjoy life and others and ultimately themselves, participants have to experience being enjoyed by others. Group Theraplay makes this possible.

Homelessness is a trauma. And in recovery from trauma, it is important to focus on the person who has been traumatized rather than on the memories of the trauma itself. Following trauma, the body's warning system often gets stuck on high alert, so we need effective ways for "speaking" directly to a trauma survivor's nervous system. Hence, we "do" communication starting with sensory input from the brainstem upwards rather than expecting participants to "speak" communication relying on a neocortex area of the brain that is often offline in such situations. Things like tone of voice, certain gestures, and even the use of music can help someone re-establish a sense of safety after trauma. Group Theraplay uses rhythm/synchrony in the activities that are patterned and congruent with the sub-systems of our brains that trigger emotional regulation. Our groups are heavily structured to ensure predictability, bringing a sense of inner-state safety and containment. Our groups are fun and pleasurable, to promote a sense of enjoyment through being enjoyed. Our groups are respectful of participants' cultural and religious beliefs, to promote a sense of acceptance, belonging, and community.

Marc Bekoff (Bekoff, Newberry, & Spinka 2001), an evolutionary biologist at the University of Colorado, described play as "training for the unexpected." Living in a state of homelessness is a constantly rolling state of the unexpected. Bekoff (in the *New York Times*, 2008) spoke of play resulting in mental suppleness and a broader behavioral vocabulary. A broad behavioral vocabulary is akin to a deeper level of emotional fluency, but we find the means to say it in actions rather than words.

Group Theraplay and trauma recovery

Trauma affects all aspects of a person's life and can underpin a myriad of overt behavioral issues that serve as layers of defense against a shame base. These experiences can result in a negative internal working model (IWM), a belief that "I am the bad thing," that other people are unsafe, untrustworthy and will "hurt/disappoint me," and that the world is a scary, threatening place to either retreat from or fight against. To affect a shift from a negative to a positive IWM takes time and exposure to repeated positive experiences that consistently *model* a different way of relating and reflecting to the individual a more positive view of themselves that is authentic and meaningful.

Group Theraplay creates an atmosphere that makes the above possible. The group facilitator is positive and upbeat without being hyperarousing. This means that the group facilitator models positive and engaging behavior to connect and co-regulate the group dynamic. The group facilitator is trained to work with any resistance the group members present and, as best they can, to understand resistance as communication of discomfort or struggle, and to prescribe that resistance into an activity rather than issuing consequences or behavioral corrections. When redirecting a group member from distracting and sabotaging behavior, the group facilitator is trained to do so with positively reframed language—for example, "I see you have very strong hands. We have a 'No hurts' rule in our group, but I wonder if you can use your strong hands to punch this balloon/punch through this paper?" Our "rules" in Group Theraplay are not the rigid and inflexible type of rules many people are used to, but are flexible and adaptable to the needs of group members while holding the group boundary gently, yet firmly, in place.

Group rules: "No hurts," "Stick together," "Have fun"

These playful, gentle, yet firm rules help provide the boundaries and limits we all need to feel safe and contained. When (not if) the group cohesion slips and tensions bubble over, they give us a solid baseline to refer back to. The group will need to repeatedly return to the rules and start afresh from that baseline. Boundaries and limits remind us that we are part of a system bigger than ourselves. It helps to know that there is someone bigger, stronger, and kinder who will ensure that neither the situation nor our behavior will get out of control. This is the role of the group facilitator(s).

The case for a trauma-informed model that affects meaningful and sustained change in the parent–child relationship for those who experience homelessness is pronounced. It is imperative that the model in question avoids replicating patterns of exclusion and the "othering" that have been used by societal systems to maintain the status quo. Play is a language, and it is an accessible and universal language that enables participation and fuels connection and cohesion. All are welcome; there is a place for everyone in play. This is why a Group Theraplay+ model is vital in such settings and will effect sustained and meaningful change.

An overview of Group Theraplay delivery in Ireland

We had/have clear goals in rolling out Group Theraplay+ training for as many staff as possible in this sector. Rolling this out as a global pandemic started could not have been anticipated and has slowed progress, but our goals remained the same. Here are the steps in our process:

Step 1: Stakeholder meeting

This was an initial meeting with those in decision-making roles within all organizations working within the homeless sector within our geographical area. My colleague Janet Healy and I outlined the case for this model within homeless services as well as detailing the Group Theraplay model itself, and being Theraplay trained, we included a balloon relay as part of this initial presentation!

Step 2: Funding confirmation

Taking time to ensure adequate funding is made available to facilitate the execution of the program is critical. This includes delivery of the training and a follow-up day approximately six weeks after the training to provide a reflective space to process initial learning and the challenge of getting groups started. Our experience was that it could be easy to underestimate the administrative time in liaising with multiple organizations, so be aware of this. Our ongoing relationship with Nuala Nic Giobúin, the coordinator of the umbrella service (CYPSC Dublin South City), of which all attendees were members, was invaluable in this regard, as was having the ongoing program support of Janet Healy. It was important to calculate time and funding to review organizational policies that ensure the model can be fully integrated within the organization's ethos. If possible, we would suggest also considering the costs of including supervision for those running groups and providing access to certification.

Step 3: Clinical vs. community application

Spend time on your program design. For us, this was the two-day classic Group Theraplay training plus a third day focused on trauma. This is an area of complex trauma, and, as such, we anticipated that a standard two-day Group Theraplay training would be inadequate to fully meet the needs of this sector. This assumption was confirmed during our experience. The additional third day was trauma-focused material. The training material was taken from Theraplay literature and from literature specific to the trauma of homelessness.

Step 4: Deliver the training program

Ensure that all dates are booked and confirmed and then reconfirmed well in advance. Ensure that the venue being provided is adequate for the delivery of the Group Theraplay program. Ensure adequate breaks are provided for the group with access to water and that bowls of sweets/candy of varied texture are available. This helped with co-regulation of the group, particularly on trauma day, resulting in people needing to leave the room for the bathroom a lot less.

Step 5: Follow-up consultation day

We felt strongly from the outset that it would be invaluable to check in with participants approximately six weeks post training to provide a reflective space to share early learning and challenges and allow group participants to learn from each other's experiences. The feedback from those who have participated in this aspect (the majority of those trained) was been very positive and seemed to have served as a motivational space for some.

Step 6: Organizational policy review

In order for the Group Theraplay model to be fully integrated into the organization, and for those staff rolling out the Group Theraplay program to feel fully supported, we believed that this would be helpful. It would allow us to identify any incongruencies between the model and the organizational policies. It provided a forum to suggest Theraplay concepts and touch-affirming statements that could be added to organizational policy manuals.

Conclusion

Most participants felt they could run a targeted parent–child group (single parents/first-time parents/first-time homeless/long-term homeless, etc.) or a targeted child group (set number of sessions with a specific age range and presenting symptom such as anxiety/school refusal/parentified children, etc.). We also explored and planned for the provision of an open-ended group format. This would be a general Theraplay group that would run on a set day or time each week, and whatever families were in the hub or center could attend and participate. This would be open-ended and run indefinitely, offering a positive play experience on the premise that play itself is transformative.

Our conclusion, thus far, is that community-based Group Theraplay can be done very successfully within complex populations.

References

Bekoff, M., Newberry, R. C., & Spinka, M. (2001). Mammalian play: Training for the unexpected. *Quarterly Review Biology 76*(2), 41–68. doi:10.1086/393866

Brown, G. (Ed.) (2019). *Psychoanalytic Thinking on the Unhoused Mind*. Routledge.

Dana, D. (2018). *The Polyvagal Theory in Therapy*. W.W. Norton & Co.

Faed, P., Murphy, S., & Nolledo, R. (2017). *Child Homelessness and Trauma: The Connections and a Call to Action*. www.first5la.org/files/ChildHomelessnessTrauma.pdf

FEANTSA (European Federation of National Organisations Working with the Homeless). (2017). FEANTSA Position: Recognising the link between trauma and homelessness. www.feantsa.org/en/feantsa-position/2017/02/28/recognising-the-link-between-trauma-and-homelessness?bcParent=27

Henig, R. M. (2008). Taking play seriously. *The New York Times*, February 17. www.nytimes.com/2008/02/17/magazine/17play.html

Hughes, D., & Baylin, J. (2012). *Brain-Based Parenting: The Neuroscience of Caregiving for Healthy Attachment*. Norton.

Long, A. E., Sheridan, S., Gambi, L., & Hoey, D. (2019). *Family Homelessness in Dublin: Causes, Housing Histories, and Finding a Home*. Focus Ireland. www.focusireland.ie/wp-content/uploads/2021/09/Research-Briefing-No-1-Interactive.pdf

Porges, S. W., & Dana, D. (2018). *Clinical Applications of the Polyvagal Theory: The Emergence of Polyvagal-Informed Therapies*. W.W. Norton & Co.

Scanlon, C., & Adlam, J. (2019). Housing Unhoused Minds. In G. Brown (Ed.), *Psychoanalytic Thinking on the Unhoused Mind* (Chapter 1). Routledge.

Siersbaek, R., & Loftus, C. (2020). *Supporting the Mental Health of Children in Families that Are Homeless—A Trauma Informed Approach*. A discussion paper. Focus Ireland. www.focusireland.ie/wp-content/uploads/2021/09/Supporting-the-mental-health-of-children_FINAL.pdf

Smolen, A. G. (2015). *Mothering Without a Home: Attachment Representations and Behaviours of Homeless Mothers and Children*. Rowman & Littlefield.

Walsh, K., & Harvey, B. (2017). *Finding a Home: Families' Journeys out of Homelessness*. Focus Ireland. www.focusireland.ie/knowledge-hub/research

Chapter 18

Theraplay with Older Adults

Philip F. Daniels

Introduction

Theraplay with older adults encompasses working with individuals over the age of 65, and across the spectrum of emotional, mental, and physical disabilities, and illnesses. Additionally, Theraplay can be provided in a variety of locations, from the home to the hospital and all spaces in between. Specifically of interest is training Theraplay practitioners in working with formal (e.g., paid care providers) and informal (e.g., unpaid care providers) caregivers of older adults. This chapter provides an overview of aging theories and how play can be integrated into daily life with older adults, specifically with individuals with neurocognitive disorders and their caregivers. Readers will gain insight into attachment theory, physical and mental changes of aging, consideration of individual and cultural differences, emotional regulation, and Theraplay principles such as structure, engagement, nurture, and challenge. A case illustration is provided that describes how Theraplay can be incorporated into Activities of Daily Living (ADLs) for individuals with neurocognitive disorders and their informal caregivers.

Journey of using Theraplay with older adults

According to the 2010 US Census, by 2035, for the first time in American history, older adults will outnumber children under the age of 18. Specifically, in 2011, baby boomers had begun reaching the age of 65; by 2020, all boomers had reached the age of 65 and over. Consequently, by 2050, the number of Americans aged 65 and older is estimated to be 88.5 million (Vincent & Velkoff 2010). This projection results in almost one in four Americans being 65 and over by 2060 (Federal Interagency Forum on Aging-Related Statistics 2016). From an international perspective, in 2015, the worldwide population was 7.3 billion; of these individuals, 617.1 million were 65 and older (Roberts *et al.* 2018). By 2030, the worldwide older adult population is projected to be around 1 billion, and estimated to increase to 1.6 billion by 2050.

A 2012 report from the US Institute of Medicine indicates the rise of dementia, substance abuse, and mental illness such as depression among the older adult population. Of individuals over 85, roughly 69 percent experienced at least one type of disability. In comparison, only 9 percent of individuals under 65 experienced one type of disability (Roberts *et al.* 2018). Thus, a need arises for healthcare practitioners to discover ways to help individuals and families cope, manage, and heal a wide variety of mental health issues. Specifically, for dementia, best practices call for the first-line approach to be non-pharmacological interventions, whereas depression and other health issues such as anxiety can be treated with integrated care, including counseling and possible medication. No matter the mental health issue, Theraplay can be a first attempt to enhance the quality of life and to bridge a connection between older adults and their caregivers.

I found myself interested in Theraplay through my personal experience of caregiving for both my maternal and paternal grandmothers while they were suffering from progressive dementia. As a caregiver, I found ways to have fun in times that seemed so dark because I was losing the ability to communicate with two of the most important people in my life. After becoming a mental health professional and marriage and family therapist, I knew I wanted to earn my doctorate and focus my dissertation on people with dementia and their caregivers. Thus, after many years of research, I was referred to look into Theraplay. Once I was connected with Theraplay, I traveled to the Theraplay Institute for my Level 1 training. After completing my training, I practiced Theraplay-informed principles and practices in nursing homes while completing my dissertation research. I was also connected with Michele Robison, who invited me to conduct my dissertation study at her memory care community, the only one in the nation known to actively implement Theraplay-informed principles and practices with their older adults with progressive dementia.

Theoretical rationale for using Theraplay with older adults

Theraplay has been used in a wide variety of settings that serve older adults (Adamitis 1982, 1985, 1986; Kim 2011; Robison 2015; Savola 2015). Play is fundamental and universal. Thus, anyone at any age can find enjoyment and fun through playful activities. Attachment bonds are present across the lifespan, and although personalities may change as we grow older, relationships are vital. Social engagement is a primary source of sense of belonging and acceptance. Based on attachment theory, humans thrive on social connection. Without social connections, individuals can lose the will to live and thrive. Therefore, Theraplay is a way to maintain attachment bonds throughout the lifespan.

Aging is a result of biology, passage of time, existentialism, and society. Among the many theories of aging, there are biological, psychological, and sociological theories. The biological theories of aging are separated into major categories of programmed theories and damage or error theories (Jin 2010). Programmed theories of aging imply a biological timeline based on genetic predispositions that regulate systems responsible for maintenance, repair, and defense responses, whereas damage or error theories assume aging occurs based on external damage affecting living organisms and the cumulative damage of cells throughout our lifespan. Therefore, according to biological theories, exercise and movement could be viewed as having positive and beneficial outcomes; however, there are also limitations if there are physical disabilities. In the case of physical disabilities, therapeutic touch could be utilized to establish and maintain engagement and nurture (Bush 2001; Field 1998). Field's (1998) review of studies of children and infant populations concluded therapeutic touch was effective in reducing stress, focusing attention, and decreasing pain and cortisol. Bush's (2001) review of studies provides various methods of using touch to improve the wellbeing of older adults. Additionally, music, song, and reminiscing are all appropriate methods to connect with an older adult, with or without physical or cognitive limitations.

Other theories of aging include psychosocial theories, such as the classical theories of disengagement, activity, and continuity (Franklin & Tate 2009). Disengagement theory differentiates between middle and old age. As a person ages, disengagement is assumed to be a natural process for individuals to withdraw from society and relationships. Activity theory is known as successful aging in which the assumption is for the older adult to remain active and add new roles to their life, identity, relationships, and behaviors. According to the continuity theory, older individuals typically maintain and manage their activities and relationships within their environment. In each of these theories, there is room to grow and add new experiences as we age, in which Theraplay could be utilized to gain new ways to have fun and build social connections.

When considering individuality, culture, and positive aging, Lars Tornstam (1994, 2011) developed gerotranscendence theory. According to this, aging occurs within three dimensions: the cosmic level, the self, and social and individual relations. Within each dimension new feelings, thoughts, beliefs, and values develop based on current and past experiences. From the perspective of healthy and positive aging, there is a wide variety of applicable areas in which Theraplay can be incorporated into the daily lives of older adults.

Polyvagal theory can provide a conceptual understanding of emotional regulation through sensation known as neuroception when determining the safety of a social situation (Porges 2001, 2009, 2011; Porges & Dana 2018). Polyvagal theory, developed by Stephen Porges (2001, 2009, 2011), supports the use of Theraplay as a means to connect with individuals to help emotional regulation and establish and maintain attachment bonds. Mammals have a mind–body connection with feelings and emotions. We have a natural affinity to connect through playing, evident by playing since birth. Thus, play can be enjoyed at any age and can be utilized to nurture and engage older adults. Polyvagal theory has evolved, and clinical applications have become increasingly explored and applied. See Porges and Dana (2018) for a guide to effective polyvagal-informed therapies.

Effectiveness of Theraplay in working with older adults

Theraplay with older adults is a specialty that has been used in dyadic and group settings within nursing homes (Adamitis 1982, 1985, 1986; Kim 2011; Robison 2015; Savola 2015). Lindaman and Haldeman (1994) wrote the first, and, to date, only, textbook chapter on geriatric Theraplay. They provide five guidelines for using Theraplay when working with older adults: slow the pace; value spontaneous reminiscence; conduct activities in a manner allowing face saving; be alert to diminished sensitivity in sight, hearing, smell, taste, and touch; and give special consideration to feet and hands. Guidelines for geriatric Theraplay were developed from anecdotal evidence and case studies that indicated positive results such as increased social engagement, reduced behavioral and psychological symptoms of dementia, and improvements in the caregiving relationship (S. Lindaman, personal communication, November 6, 2017). Additionally, older adults appear to follow the same phases as children in the traditional Theraplay process, evidenced by some older adults questioning the activities when introduced to the playful activities (Adamitis 1982, 1985, 1986; Franke 1991; Jernberg 1988; Lindaman & Haldeman 1994).

Although research is scarce on the use of Theraplay with older adults, there are anecdotal positive results. Robison (2015) and Savola (2015) provide examples of their use of Theraplay with older adults in a *Theraplay Institute Newsletter*. Robison designed and implemented two groups daily (before lunch and dinner) for individuals with progressive dementia living in a residential memory care community (M. Robison, personal communication, November 13, 2017). Savola (2015) provided an overview of her work in

Finland with group Theraplay and nursing home residents as being powerful and touching as she was able to connect through words or simply through the eyes of those who could not speak.

In sum, an international community of researchers have reported promising efforts and results. These suggest older adults can benefit from an emotionally focused, attachment- and play-based intervention that can be implemented in both healthcare and home settings. Theraplay is an accessible and affordable intervention for informal and formal caregivers. Additionally, Theraplay can be adapted and supported by organizations because of the psychoeducation component that is included in the Theraplay training.

Special considerations or adaptations of Theraplay in working with older adults

Keep in mind culture and how this will impact the treatment of an older adult. This pertains to how younger individuals interact with older adults relating to respect and gender differences. Cultural appropriateness of interventions can predict successful outcomes and treatment compliance within non-minority caregivers. As such, introducing play-based interventions to caregivers and care receivers may be welcomed or resisted depending on cultural and generational differences. According to the literature, similarities exist among caregivers such as family involvement in care, filial piety, and religion or spirituality. However, Gallagher-Thompson *et al.* (2003) found differences between the top three minority populations in the US—Black Americans, Mexican-Americans, and Cuban-Americans—in terms of cultural perceptions, stereotypes, and asking for and receiving professional help. Therefore, practitioners need to be aware of, respect, and modify play-based interventions based on care receiver and caregivers' perception and understanding of aging, physical and mental illness, neurocognitive disorders, and the role of family systems and individuals regarding receiving care and caregiving (Brooke *et al.* 2017; Gallagher-Thompson *et al.* 2003; Rivera & Marlo, 1999). Practitioners may also address cultural differences by gaining awareness through talking to the client and their families with respect and curiosity to better understand the family's needs and desires and develop culturally appropriate interventions.

Additional considerations when using Theraplay with older adults include being aware of how past traumas may impact the interactions in relationships, such as veterans and survivors of trauma or torture (e.g., Holocaust survivors). For example, touching certain body parts can trigger traumatic memories. Furthermore, consider the family of origin, cultural values, and personal preferences of how fun or play is perceived and utilized.

Finally, take into account personal histories and childhood games that could bring back memories and reminiscence of enjoyable past times. There are traditional and folk games that can be utilized to individually tailor activities for the older adult or group of older adults. Knowing about different cultures and international games is helpful in the development and structure of activities. Families can help inform care providers of specific games to be used and incorporated into Theraplay activities.

CASE ILLUSTRATION

BACKGROUND

This account describes Theraplay with a family in which the 83-year-old mother has progressive dementia. Lucinda is a Hispanic female who has been married to Steven, a Caucasian male, for 65 years. Together they have four children, one daughter and three sons. The sons live out of state. The daughter, Brigida, who is the oldest sibling, still lives close and visits as often as she can. Lucinda and Steven still reside in their home even though Lucinda has progressive dementia that is severe and requires 24/7 care from a home health aide. As a therapist familiar with Theraplay principles, and since I know the family, I offered my assistance in using a Theraplay framework to deal with difficulties the family was experiencing.

THERAPLAY PROCESS AND PROGRESSION

In the beginning, I introduced the family to Theraplay principles and practices. I worked with the family to help them reframe their attitudes, beliefs, and perspectives of how play could be used in their family relationships. I used reframing to help the family view play not as infantilizing, but as a new way to connect and have fun together. For example, Brigida initially was not comfortable playing with her mother because they had not played together when she had been a young girl. Therefore, I worked with Brigida to teach her how play is essential and can be incorporated into everyday activities. I also had to work with Steven to gain acceptance of the value of play. Steven is considered a traditionalist and is in denial of the progression of dementia. However, he had noticed that Lucinda has memory loss and some personality changes. To begin with helping the family understand the value of play, I used psychoeducation and provided some examples and opportunities to observe playful activities among themselves or with Lucinda. Additionally, I took the time to learn about their cultural beliefs and traditional games that could be incorporated into the playful activities.

Throughout this time, I encouraged the family members to observe and embrace Lucinda's strengths to individually tailor playful activities. After introducing the family to the four dimensions of Theraplay, they could discover ways in which play can naturally be incorporated into their daily rituals and caregiving tasks. By the end of this introduction period, the family would be able to use Theraplay-informed principles and practices in ways that were comfortable, and as they continue to practice, they will be confident to use playful activities on a daily basis.

SESSION OUTLINE AND ACTIVITIES

On a daily basis, Lucinda needs assistance getting dressed in the morning and eating breakfast. Between breakfast and lunch, she has time to relax by watching TV and enjoys time outside walking around in her backyard garden. Later in the evening, she has dinner and then takes a shower to get ready for bed. At each of these times, she needs some assistance and reminding of what to do next. Brigida and Steven assist her as much as they can, but they also have a home health aide who helps with bathing and feeding. Brigida and Steven sing traditional songs to help great Lucinda in the morning and wake her up. They use these songs to incorporate music at the beginning of the day, and this helps Lucinda wake up in a positive mood. They play a game of tossing clothes back and forth, which originally Steven thought was childish, until he saw how Lucinda laughed when they played catch with the balled-up clothes. Lucinda was more willing to get dressed without a fight after she was laughing and having fun.

For breakfast, sometimes Lucinda will not eat with utensils, so Brigida has incorporated eating together with their fingers, as well as changing the food so that it is easy to grasp. For example, before, she would try to feed Lucinda oatmeal with a spoon. So she started breaking up pieces of soft granola bars that she would eat with her fingers, which essentially means both Lucinda and Brigida share a meal together as they eat with their fingers. Here, again, Steven thought it was childish to eat with his fingers, yet after a while he came to understand that it was more important to connect over a meal made of finger food rather than making Lucinda angry by trying to force her to eat with a utensil.

Later in the afternoon, Brigida and Lucinda spend time outside in the garden. A game that was incorporated was catching bubbles and popping them. Brigida blows bubbles and Lucinda catches them on her hands and pops them while laughing from the small tickles. Another game was developed using a towel and a small ball. Steven and Lucinda hold a towel while Brigida places a small bouncy ball on it. Steven and

Lucinda play together while trying to keep the ball on the towel. Another game was developed for them to stay outside and it consisted of sitting in chairs and kicking a ball back and forth. Brigida retrieves the ball if it goes too far away. During this time, Steven and Lucinda are able to continue connecting through play while still enjoying the outside. Once inside, Brigida uses a puzzle to entertain Lucinda. Although the puzzle is never completed, it calms Lucinda and brings her pleasure as she sorts the puzzle pieces. Lunch and dinner are also made of finger food to accommodate Lucinda. It has become a custom for Steven and Brigida to eat with their fingers to share meals together rather than forcing Lucinda to eat with utensils.

To get ready for bed, a song is used to connect and bring fun to shower time. Brigida has taught the home health aide the songs that Lucinda had sung as a young girl, which helps calm her during her shower. Finally, Steven gives Lucinda a lotion massage afterward, to nurture and engage Lucinda before bed. The lotion massage provides Steven and Lucinda with a moment of intimacy and connection as he engages and nurtures his wife before bed.

OUTCOME AND EVALUATION

After Steven and Brigida implemented Theraplay principles and practices, they noticed Lucinda was more joyous during the day and more amiable during getting dressed and eating. Steven has become more accepting of his wife's situation and has fun playing with Lucinda. Brigida found herself having fun with her mother that was different from when she was growing up as a little girl, and has embraced play. Lucinda has become familiar with the fun activities and has made comments about having fun, which indicates to Steven and Brigida that Theraplay has made a difference in their lives.

Conclusion

When considering a method of connection and care, Theraplay with older adults is an appropriate method to structure activities and engage, nurture, and challenge individuals of any age. Depending on the cognitive and physical abilities of older adults Theraplay can be tailored to enhance the strengths of individuals while improving the quality of life for older adults and their families. Additionally, Theraplay is a method to help individuals emotionally regulate through structuring activities that are upregulating and downregulating. Using this type of structure allows for the intentional tailoring of activities to best serve the needed purpose at the moment. Simple materials can be used to create games, such as balls, cloth, bubbles, and paper products. Theraplay is an intervention that is taught and translatable to use in a variety of settings. Having fun is an essential need, and play is a natural way to have fun. No matter the age of an individual, Theraplay is a way to facilitate a social connection to have fun through engagement and nurturing.

Five key takeaways of using Theraplay-informed principles and practices with older adults

- Attachment theory is relevant across the lifespan. However, a difference in working with older adults is that their personalities, attitudes, and attachment styles are based on a lifetime of experiences, and continue to change. Moving beyond theory into reality, older adults experience loneliness and the loss of attachment through changes in relationships. Theraplay can create moments of connection with structured activities that engage and nurture the older adult, and provide opportunities for meaningful challenges.

- Physical and mental changes are inevitable as we age. Thus, a key component of using Theraplay with older adults is helping family and friends learn how to structure activities that engage, nurture, and challenge the person they love, all while coping with the new reality that comes with age.

- Considering individual and cultural differences is of key importance in reducing the risk of infantizing older adults. Individually tailor and structure Theraplay sessions based on individual and cultural sensitivity and awareness, yet be flexible and remain attuned to the older individual to make the necessary changes. This can be accomplished by talking with the individual and, when appropriate, their family members, to gain insight and understanding of their likes and dislikes. This also allows individual tailoring depending on what the person enjoys.

- When using Theraplay with older adults with cognitive impairments, such as progressive dementia, the caregiver is the emotional regulator in the relationship. This means that sometimes an older adult is unable to emotionally self-regulate. In this case, the role of the caregiver is to balance their own emotions while engaging and nurturing the person receiving care. A sensation of danger will supersede any sense of safety, thus leading the individual to feel the cascade of physiological symptoms, which removes the individual from a desire to connect and into a protective state (Porges & Dana 2014). A Theraplay practitioner must find balance between what can be controlled, such as structured activities, and what must be accepted, such as progression of the disease.

- Theraplay's focus on warm, interpersonal engagement, nurturing language, and gentle, physical contact provides a new way to manage difficult behaviors rather than relying on commands and questions, medication, isolation, or restraints. Additionally, if possible, learn about past physical or sexual trauma and how this may impact the use of therapeutic touch. Utilize a strengths-based approach by adapting Theraplay activities to the older adults' abilities, such as sight, hearing, mobility, taste, and smell.

References

Adamitis, C. (1982). Theraplay with the elderly: A case study. *The Theraplay Institute Newsletter*, Spring, 2–3.

Adamitis, C. (1985). Theraplay with an older adult. *The Theraplay Institute Newsletter*, Winter, 2–4.

Adamitis, C. (1986). The use of Theraplay with older adult women in a group setting. Unpublished paper.

Brooke, J., Cronin, C., Stiell, M., & Ojo, O. (2017). The intersection of culture in the provision of dementia care: A systematic review. *Journal of Clinical Nursing 27*(17–18), 3241–3253. https://doi.org/10.1111/jocn.13999

Bush, E. (2001). The use of human touch to improve the well-being of older adults: A holistic nursing intervention. *Journal of Holistic Nursing 19*(3), 256–270. doi: 10.1177/089801010101900306

Federal Interagency Forum on Aging-Related Statistics (2016). *Older Americans 2016: Key Indicators of Well-Being.* https://agingstats.gov/docs/LatestReport/Older-Americans-2016-Key-Indicators-of-WellBeing.pdf

Field, T. M. (1998). Touch therapy effects on development. *International Journal of Behavioral Development 22*(4), 779–797. https://doi.org/10.1080/016502598384162

Franke, U. (1991). Theraplay mit Elisabeth Miaer, 79 Jahre alt [Theraplay with Elizabeth Maier, 79 years old]. *Theraplay Journal 4*, 9–11.

Franklin, N. C., & Tate, C. A. (2009). Lifestyle and successful aging: An overview. *American Journal of Lifestyle Medicine 3*(1), 6–11. https://doi.org/10.1177/1559827608326125

Gallagher-Thompson, D., Haley, W., Guy, D., Rupert, M., Argüelles, T., Zeiss, L. M., Long, C., Tennstedt, S., & Ory, M. (2003). Tailoring psychological interventions for ethnically diverse dementia caregivers. *Clinical Psychology: Science and Practice 10*(4), 423–438. https://doi.org/10.1093/clipsy.bpg042

Institute of Medicine of the National Academies. (2012). *The Mental Health and Substance Use Workforce for Older Adults: In Whose Hands?* The National Academies Press.

Jernberg, A. (1988). Theraplay for the elderly tyrant. *Clinical Gerontologist 8*, 76–79. https://psycnet.apa.org/record/1989-30250-001

Jin, K. (2010). Modern biological theories of aging. *Aging and Disease 1*(2), 72–74. www.ncbi.nlm.nih.gov/pmc/articles/PMC2995895/pdf/ad-1-2-72.pdf

Kim, K. Y. (2011). The effect of group Theraplay on self-esteem and depression of the elderly in a day care center. *Korean Journal of Counseling 12*(5), 1413–1430.

Lindaman, S. L., & Haldeman, D. (1994). Geriatric Theraplay. In K. O'Connor & C. E. Schaefer (Eds), *Handbook of Play Therapy: Advances and Innovations* (pp.207–228). John Wiley & Sons.

Porges, S. W. (2001). The polyvagal theory: Phylogenetic substrates of a social nervous system. *International Journal of Psychophysiology 42*(2), 123–146. doi: 10.1016/s0167-8760(01)00162-3

Porges, S. W. (2009). The polyvagal theory: New insights into adaptive reactions of the autonomic nervous system. *Cleveland Clinic Journal of Medicine 76*(Suppl 2), S86. doi: 10.3949/ccjm.76.s2.17

Porges, S. W. (2011). *The Polyvagal Theory: Neurophysiological Foundations of Emotions, Attachment, Communication, and Self-Regulation.* W.W. Norton & Co.

Porges, S. W., & Dana, D. (2018). *Clinical Applications of the Polyvagal Theory: The Emergence of Polyvagal-Informed Therapies.* W.W. Norton & Co.

Rivera, P. A., & Marlo, H. (1999). Cultural, interpersonal and psychodynamic factors in caregiving: Towards a greater understanding of treatment noncompliance. *Clinical Psychology & Psychotherapy 6*(1), 63–68. https://doi.org/10.1002/(SICI)1099-0879(199902)6:1<63::AID-CPP185>3.0.CO;2-I

Roberts, A. W., Ogunwole, S. U., Blakeslee, L., & Rabe, M. A. (2018). *The Population 65 Years and Older in the United States: 2016.* American Community Survey Reports, ACS-38, US Census Bureau. www.census.gov/content/dam/Census/library/publications/2018/acs/ACS-38.pdf

Robison, M. (2015). Group Theraplay with elderly. *The Theraplay Institute Newsletter*, Summer.

Savola, S. (2015). Group Theraplay with seniors. *The Theraplay Institute Newsletter*, Summer.

Tornstam, L. (1994). Gerotranscendence—A Theoretical and Empirical Exploration. In L. E. Thomas & S. A. Eisenhandler (Eds), *Aging and the Religious Dimension* (pp.203–225). Greenwood Publishing Group.

Tornstam, L. (2011). Maturing into gerotranscendence. *Journal of Transpersonal Psychology 43*(2), 166–180. www.atpweb.org/jtparchive/trps-43-11-02-166.pdf

Vincent, G. K., & Velkoff, V. A. (2010). *The Next Four Decades: The Older Population in the United States: 2010 to 2050* (No. 1138). US Department of Commerce, Economics and Statistics Administration, US Census Bureau. www.census.gov/content/dam/Census/library/publications/2010/demo/p25-1138.pdf

Chapter 19

Men in Theraplay

THE CASE FOR BIG MUSCLES

David L. Myrow

Introduction

Research has demonstrated that fathers typically have a different approach to play from mothers (Grossmann *et al.* 2002; Paquette & Dumont 2013). While early maternal interactions play a central role in children's development, healthy fathers engage children in experiences that also have enormously positive effects on children's development. Could there be an advantage in bringing Theraplay into the lives of children and teens in ways that mirror the ways of attuned, skillful fathers?

In three decades as a Theraplay therapist, my view has been influenced by the male tendency to like large muscle activities more than is typically taught in Theraplay training. Activities that resemble familiar games and sports are inviting and can pave the way for older children who may at first be uncomfortable with the intimacy of Theraplay. In support of this, child development research has shown that many fathers engage children in rough-and-tumble and gross motor play that can promote attachment, help with self-regulation, increase self-confidence, and reduce negative behavior.

How this works in the playroom

It is easy for many Theraplay therapists to have a shy seven-year-old stand as tall as a soldier and fall into our arms. But some therapists will take the next step and have the child fall into outstretched arms—and then fly him around the room. Another example—it is a familiar Theraplay strategy to help a depressed preschooler to gain confidence by jumping from some pillows into the therapist's arms. But some of us have a timid six-year-old practice jumping from a table into our arms, and we gradually move step by step, further from the table, until she starts to feel quite brave indeed. And some therapists are likely to heft a depressed first grader onto our shoulders for a motorcycle ride, giving a child the experience of an adult who inspires trust while having some hearty laughs together. Those with adequate physical strength may fly a second-grade bully on a pillow *up in the air, off the floor* when he makes eye contact. (The child sits on a large pillow that has handles at the corners. When he makes eye contact, the pillow moves. The longer the child looks, the faster the therapist pulls it until the therapist actually swings the child, on the pillow, up to a foot or more off of the floor. It's not as hard as it sounds.) Thus, this "tough" kid can experience the joy of letting go with an adult who can safely challenge him to discover real courage.

This tendency toward gross motor engagement seems to be a prevalent play style among fathers across cultures (Masaki Kawakami, personal communication, 2019). Based on an informal survey, this type of play is more commonly used among male than among female Theraplay therapists. Some children appreciate this show of physical prowess. It suggests strength— enough to help them when they get out of control. This kind of strength is itself well regulated, attuned, and in the context of laugh-out-loud fun. Furthermore, children often admire therapists who are strong enough to pick them up and move them around. It helps younger children be comfortable with the reality of their relative size. They appreciate it when an adult uses strength for structure, protection, and fun, not to bully and demean. The tendency of male therapists to like games has also been confirmed by my Theraplay colleague Masaki Kawakami: "Especially with boys and older children, I tend to include activities that resemble clients' familiar games or sports. Those activities seem to help children get less guarded and more comfortable with me" (personal communication, 2019).

Research on how fathers play with children

A considerable amount of research has shown that fathers who are engaged with their children usually offer play that is more physical (rough-and-tumble, running, jumping, challenging abilities, respectfully competitive) and promotes children's development in useful ways. Golding and Fitzgerald (2017, p.7) introduced a special issue of the *Infant Mental Health Journal* by noting that, according to the (US) Centers for Disease Control and Prevention, boys are more likely than girls to be diagnosed with attention deficit hyperactivity disorder (ADHD), to smoke cigarettes, and to die by suicide. They noted that fun, physical play enhances father–son attachment and promotes self-regulation. This special issue focused on profound issues for children, especially boys growing up without male role models, and made a case for finding ways to fill this void. There is great potential for male therapists to help children who have not had a constructive and positive relationship with a father or father-figure.

Based on Porges' (2017) polyvagal theory, the evidence indicates that when a parent and child engage in interactive play where the child feels safe, there are increased opportunities to practice self-regulation and to develop comfort in social engagement. These seem to be critical concerns, especially for boys' development. Safe play that has a more physical component addresses this need.

While mothers typically play a pivotal role in building initial trust and attachment, fathers can play a significant role in expanding those skills to peer and, later, adult interaction. Fathers who are engaged with children tend to be more physical, boisterous, creative and unpredictable, and more energizing (Brizendine 2010, p.88).

Paquette and Dumont (2013) studied what they call the activation relationship between children aged 12–18 months and fathers. They developed a procedure called the "Risky Situation." It was designed to look at the role of fathers in attachment as a companion to the "Strange Situation" (Ainsworth *et al.* 1978). The activation relationship theory claims that when parents encourage exploration of the environment, while protecting them by setting limits, children increase their self-confidence.

It seems likely that challenges arise in the ordinary give-and-take of physical play (e.g., someone accidentally gets hurt), which provides opportunities to repair misunderstandings. Also, it may be easier for some fathers to become invested in treatment when the therapist is a man. When the treatment is Theraplay, because it is directly playful and physical, many fathers find the work more ego-syntonic than verbal therapy. Therapists wrestle with the fact that many men struggle to accept addressing their feelings (Pappas 2019). Theraplay offers a different point of entry. In my experience, it is not unusual to find that just observing physical behavior in a Marschak Interaction Method (MIM) review helps engage fathers in the therapeutic work. The invitation to play in ways that many men find more familiar offers them an avenue to help both themselves and their children.

Many children have little experience with a father who is emotionally attuned and nurturing. Theraplay therapists can offer these children experiences that can broaden their internal working models of what men have to offer. For boys, this can expand their view of male behaviors.

Some of these ideas can be seen in a project Sherman (2009) described with a father–son Group Theraplay program conducted with two male colleagues at a Toronto-area clinic. The boys were aged six to nine, and presented with a wide range of problems, including low self-esteem, ADHD, depression, tantrums, and poor school performance. The fathers reported struggling in their relationships with their sons. Many of the fathers experienced personal struggles, including histories of neglect, abuse, substance issues, and trouble managing their tempers. Among the goals established for the group was to help them feel more comfortable in expressing affection as a way to promote father–son attachment (Sherman 2009, p.241). One of the co-therapists, Doug Lowen (personal communication, 2019), told me that the group content emphasized "gentle, persistent nurturing and engagement... We were very aware that we were dealing within a context of socially-reinforced male parenting norms." Lowen stated that when the leaders modeled nurturing and empathic behavior, they were profoundly impressed at how the fathers seemed to open themselves to more options in parenting. The group was evaluated with pre- and post-testing. Among the positive outcomes were the boys' decreased externalizing behavior and increased acceptance of their fathers' affection.

CASE ILLUSTRATION

BACKGROUND

Mom and Dad brought Frank, an eight-year-old boy, for a consultation after meltdowns in school left his teachers baffled. When tested, he was found to have high average intelligence, but would avoid doing a task, hide under his desk, or yell out when a task seemed frustrating. Sometimes he ran out of the classroom. Behavior reward systems were unsuccessful. His teacher had been reduced to tears as she struggled to find a way to engage and calm Frank. At home, his parents reported that Frank tended to quit games quickly when he didn't think he would win. The family was intact, with three older siblings, all of whom were doing well in school, enjoyed activities, and had friends. Dad had immigrated to the USA with his family from a South American country at age six. Mom was born in the US and worked as a paralegal. Dad worked in construction, so he was somewhat less available in the summer. Dad had been unsuccessful in engaging his son in sports, especially soccer, which Dad had learned from early childhood. At the first meeting, Dad expressed his disappointment that his son was hard to relate to.

MIM ANALYSES

MIM analyses revealed that Frank was mostly engaged, but his mood was subdued in that setting. Mom took some leadership, but it was inconsistent, and when she stumbled, Frank drew inward. With Dad, Frank smiled a few times, and there was some eye contact. Frank leaned in toward Dad physically. Dad seemed surprised, but smiled. Dad spontaneously tousled Frank's hair at one point. For the bean blow game, Dad gave Frank only a little room to compete, and Frank quit early. Dad stopped the game, looking disappointed. Notably, Dad sometimes struggled to read the instruction cards correctly, and Frank patiently, but somewhat persistently, helped Dad read the instructions and tried to explain to Dad what was meant. Dad seemed a little embarrassed about this.

After reviewing the MIM with Mom and Dad, I followed my usual practice in developing treatment goals with the parents. We agreed on the following: (1) Frank will show increased capacity to regulate frustration and to persevere on tasks; (2) Mom and Dad will provide better organization and more consistent structure at home; (3) Dad will work with Frank to find more ways that he and Frank can have fun together; and (4) Frank will show signs of increased self-esteem and will try new things.

When school-age children present with more typical (e.g., less trauma-driven) concerns, after the MIM review, I start treatment with some individual Theraplay sessions. After 25–30 minutes in an individual session, I show the parents the video of the session and explain what is going on. Individual time can give the child a chance to feel special outside of the family dynamics and help reframe the child's concerns with the parents. After there is some improvement, parents come into the sessions to finish bringing the work home.

FIRST THERAPLAY SESSION

Frank's first session began when I took Frank's hand and walked him down the short hallway to the large playroom. I explained that the carpeted floor had extra padding underneath to keep it safe. As I took off my shoes, I asked him to do the same. He seemed a little puzzled, balked, but then took off his shoes. We sat on stacks of pillows. I explained that we sit cross-legged and touch knees. "There are rules in the playroom," I said. "Number one, no one gets hurt, not you (as I gently touched his chest) or me (as I touched mine). Rule two: everyone has fun." As I paused, Frank seemed a bit vigilant, as if waiting for the rest of the rules. "That's it." He smiled broadly. "Okay with you?" I asked. He nodded "yes."

With school-age children, it is my custom at the first Theraplay session to review the treatment goals that have been established with the child's parents in words that would make sense to the child. Frank nodded "yes" to all the goals.

In classic Theraplay fashion, we started with a check-in. When I rolled up Frank's shirtsleeves and measured his biceps with my thumb and forefinger serving as a caliper, he smiled broadly. We quickly started work on the goals of increasing self-esteem and self-confidence.

The next activity in the first session was a cotton ball blow. Early on, Frank jumped the start. "Oops! We'll have to start over," I said. We played to the end, laughing often. With this experience, Frank discovered that he could succeed at a new game, even with a mistake or two. He practiced self-regulation and managing frustration.

Since Frank tended to pull inward, I chose to continue with another activation experience. I had him stand facing me for a game of "I say, you say." "I will say something and make some kind of movement. When I'm done, you do exactly the same thing." I loudly said, "Boo!" while raising my hands. Frank copied this but in a whisper. "Around," I said, as I spun around in an about-face. He copied this, but in a slightly louder voice. Then, facing him, I traced a square with my fingers: "A square." To my surprise, Frank got the joke and chuckled to himself. Then, "No!" I proclaimed, shaking my hands and arms a little in the air. He followed suit. Then, "Never!" I yelled, waving my arms harder. He smiled and copied this. Finally, "Ne-e-v-e-r!" I screamed while I jumped in the air and waved my arms, temper tantrum-style. Frank laughed, tried to do this, and fell to the carpet laughing. We followed the pattern in several more examples.

After all of this action, we returned to the pillow stacks to sit down and do something calmer, thumb wrestling. It would be less intimate than the last game, but would still give Frank a chance to be physically proximate and be able to win. The first session was closed with guess the goodies. This activity was designed to help Frank continue to build trust and accept some nurturing from an adult male. By adding the challenge of the guessing aspect, an older child can accept the nurturing part. After working with Frank, I met with his parents to discuss the session. The goal was for them to know what he was experiencing, and to connect the process in the session with the goals and with their experiences at home. Mom and Dad seemed relieved to understand their son as anxious rather than damaged, and to start seeing his needs as something they could address.

SECOND THERAPLAY SESSION

At the second individual session, during the check-in, Frank volunteered to show me how big his biceps were. I got a tape measure, and we measured each upper arm. After wrapping it around each one, I would hold out the tape to its length, showing it to Frank and comparing the two arms' biceps. (Since the circumference is much longer than the diameter, the length is quite impressive!) We then played football tag. In this scenario, a child is positioned across the room as far away from the therapist as the room allows. The therapist is the "quarterback" and the child is the "receiver." The child is told to clap twice when he is ready to receive the football. (This maneuver, learned from a child via a gym teacher, sets up the child perfectly to catch the ball.) The therapist throws the child a soft, Nerf-type ball (always a soft ball, to keep it safe). When the child catches the ball, he and the therapist race to the "goal," a third point in the room, to see who gets there first. If the child reaches the goal (usually a bean bag chair or something else soft), he gets a "touchdown." If the therapist tags the child before he gets to the goal, the child does not get a touchdown but does get a gentle tag...or a shoulder hug...or, for a smaller child, even a little swing in the air as the therapist gently puts him back down. Football tag was followed by a staring contest. Seated on pillows, knees touching (which gives just enough closeness), I explained that on "Three!" we would keep our eyes open. The last person to blink would win. To keep it interesting, I varied the starting rhyme. The first time it was, "One for the money, two for the show, four to get ready...three!" The next time: "I like you and you like me, here we go, it's one, two...three! I made sure that Frank won most of the rounds. At the end, I congratulated him with high-fives. At this point, as with other children this age, I gave him a chance to talk with me about his life since our last session. This is a departure from a typical Theraplay routine, but for many young people it is beneficial to have an opportunity to verbalize their experience with a trusted adult outside the family. The role of Theraplay is attending directly to the goals of self-confidence as well as taking the initiative and quickly building trust in the therapeutic relationship.

After this, a more active game, pillow balance, was used. I explained that it was like riding a skateboard or a snowboard. Frank stood on a large pillow with handles. When he made eye contact, I slowly pulled the pillow around the floor, varying the direction and speed. When he looked away, we stopped. Frank's job was to balance on the pillow.

We concluded this second session with eating M&Ms with a straw: "In this [business-size] envelope I have some M&Ms. Your job is to see if you can lift them out of the envelope with the straw by sucking on the straw like it is a vacuum cleaner and lifting it out of the envelope so that I can grab it. First, see if you can get the orange one..." After half of the eight M&Ms were achieved, I noted: "You're really good at this. You must have done it before." Frank said he hadn't. After he lifted out the rest, I said, "I'll have to get some harder ones for you." I brought over another envelope marked "Hard ones." "I think you will be able to get these, but we'll see." The second envelope contained a goldfish cracker, a miniature Oreo cookie, a Necco Wafer, a peanut M&M (larger than the regular ones), a grape (from my lunch box), a tiny pretzel, and a Hershey's Kiss, which I unwrapped. Frank worked to get them all, then smiled broadly as I said, "Wow! You got all of the hard ones!"

WORKING WITH PARENTS

There were three more individual Theraplay meetings. In the second half of each meeting, I met with Mom and Dad to connect what happened with their experiences with Frank at home. We worked on strategies for managing frustrating situations. I joined with Dad to help him develop approaches for engaging Frank in fun activities. I worked with Mom on how to structure. We role-played an activity introduced in the play with Frank so that Mom and Dad could use it at home.

At this point, when Frank's behavior had started to improve, his parents were brought into the playroom for part of each session. The format was changed so that I would meet initially with one or both parents to see how things were going at home and school, and then prepare them for the activities we would do jointly with Frank. Then I would see Frank for a shorter time, following which a parent would join us. At the end of the last individual session, I prepared Frank for his parents to be joining us. He was delighted.

PARENT-INVOLVED SESSIONS

At the first conjoint meeting, after preparing Mom for her role later in the session, I had a short time with Frank. After doing two activities together, we got ready for Mom. Frank and I made a box out of large pillows, in which Frank would hide, like a human version of the Jack in the Box toy. When I would say the secret code word, he would jump out and give Mom a big hug. Frank liked my suggestion of "bathroom" for the code word. After hiding the "Frankie in the Box," I brought Mom into the playroom, and we unsuccessfully hunted for her son. Soon I proclaimed, "Maybe he went to the BATHROOM." Frank jumped out and scurried over to give Mom a huge hug, which she returned. I led Mom through a check-in, and then coached the two through a cotton ball blow, crawling into arms, and guess the goodies. Mom needed a little help maintaining the structure of the cotton ball blow, and I reminded her to make eye contact on guess the goodies, but otherwise, the time together went smoothly. In the end, Frank jumped gleefully into the air a few times before leaving.

At the next session, Dad was the one to join in. It turned out to be enlightening. As I prepared him to come into the room, Dad revealed that he had been working on his relationship with Frank. Dad said that, as part of our discussions, he remembered how hard it was for him when, at age six, he had immigrated with his family to the USA. He had no English. He struggled in school and could not understand what was going on. Dad said that as he had come to remember his own experiences, he realized how he felt unsure of himself as a father and generally felt inferior. When he was critical of his son, he realized it often came out of his own hurt and sadness as a boy. At the same time that Dad became more mindful of his own past, he had also been working to be more engaged with Frank. He had taught Frank soccer basics. They had hiked in the woods nearby. Dad was starting to feel close with his youngest child. In theoretical terms, this session helped change Dad's mentalization of his child and his relationship with him.

I prepared Dad for what we would do together. Then I saw Frank. We set up a "Frankie in the Box." When Dad came into the room and after we pretended to be looking for Frank, I gave the code word. Frank sprang out of the pillow box to Dad's arms, and Dad hefted this big kid up in a big bear hug. Then Dad swung him around in a circle before setting him down. Such joy! When we did the check-in, I noted that the two guys had the same eye color. I made sure Dad used his fingers as calipers to admire Frank's big biceps. When Dad did this, Frank beamed. Dad told me that Frank had been admiring his growing muscles in the mirror at home for months. Next, we played football tag. With each catch-and-run cycle, there was a great deal of anticipation. As with Mom, we finished up with guess the goodies. Dad seemed surprised at how comfortable his eight-year-old son was in being fed by his big Dad.

FINAL SESSION

In a subsequent session with Frank and Dad, I was able to add a pillow ride for Dad to try. As with nearly every child I have worked with, this was Frank's favorite. And Dad could do it in our playroom. I suggested that Dad try a variation of it in the swimming pool, where the child lies on a kickboard, and when he looks at the parent, the parent pulls the child around the pool. Or on a snow disk in the winter, with similar rules.

Conclusion

Adding large muscle, sports-like activities to the Theraplay repertoire can have tremendous benefits. Especially for school-age children, these approaches can quickly build trust and confidence. Children who are already capable of real-world games and sports are immediately drawn to these activities. These Theraplay activities can help children who have not had positive experiences with popular games to develop self-confidence to be comfortable with them. Research has shown that children benefit when parents (typically fathers) engage in similar playful interactions. For children who have not had the benefit of this kind of parental play, Theraplay can fill a void and provide a simulation that is likely to enhance their self-confidence and coping skills down the road.

References

Ainsworth, M. D., Blehar, M., Waters, E., & Wall, S. (1978). *Patterns of Attachment: A Psychological Study of the Strange Situation.* Lawrence Erlbaum.

Brizendine, L. (2010). *The Male Brain.* Harmony Books.

Golding, P., & Fitzgerald, H. E. (2017). Psychology of boys at risk: Indicators from 0–5. *Infant Mental Health Journal 38*(1), 5–14. doi:10.1002/imhj.21621

Grossmann, K., Grossmann, K. E., Fremmer-Bombik, E., Kindler, H., Scheurer-Englisch, H., & Zimmerman, P. (2002). The uniqueness of the child–father attachment relationship: Fathers' sensitive and challenging play as a pivotal variable in a 16-year longitudinal study. *Social Development 3*(3), 307–331. https://doi.org/10.1111/1467-9507.00202

Pappas, S. (2019). APA issues first-ever guidelines for practice with men and boys. *Monitor on Psychology*, January, 34–39.

Paquette, D., & Dumont, C. (2013). The father–child activation relationship, sex differences, and attachment disorganization in toddlerhood. *Child Development Research*, 1–9. https://doi.org/10.1155/2013/102860

Porges, S. W. (2017). *The Pocket Guide to the Polyvagal Theory: The Transformative Power of Feeling Safe.* W.W. Norton & Co.

Sherman, J. (2009). Father–Son Group Theraplay. In E. Munns (Ed.), *Applications in Family and Group Theraplay* (pp.237–248). Jason Aronson.

Subject Index

Entries in *italics* indicate tables and figures.

Author Index